Endodontics

Commissioning Editor: Michael Parkinson
Project Development Manager: Barbara Simmons
Project Manager: Nancy Arnott
Design Direction: George Ajayi
Illustration Manager: Bruce Hogarth
Page layout: Kate Walshaw, Jim Hope
New illustrations: David Graham

Endodontics

THIRD EDITION

Christopher J R Stock BDS MSc DGDP (UK)

Specialist Endodontist
Heath Dental Suite, Fleet, Hampshire, UK

Kishor Gulabivala BDS MSc FDS RCS (Edin)

Consultant in Restorative Dentistry
Eastman Dental Institute for Oral Health Care Sciences
University College London, UK

Richard T Walker RD BDS PhD MSc FDS RCS (Eng) FDS RCPS (Glasg)

Formerly Centre Director, International Centre for Excellence in Dentistry
Eastman Dental Institute for Oral Health Care Sciences
University College London, UK

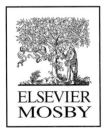

ELSEVIER
MOSBY

EDINBURGH   LONDON   NEW YORK   OXFORD   PHILADELPHIA   ST LOUIS   SYDNEY   TORONTO   2004

ELSEVIER
MOSBY

An imprint of Elsevier Limited

First edition 1988
Second edition 1995
Third edition 2004

ISBN 0723432031

British Library Cataloguing in Publication Data
A catalogue record for this book is available from the British Library

Library of Congress Cataloging in Publication Data
A catalog record for this book is available from the Library of Congress

Notice
Medical knowledge is constantly changing. Standard safety precautions must be followed, but as new research and clinical experience broaden our knowledge, changes in treatment and drug therapy may become necessary or appropriate. Readers are advised to check the most current product information provided by the manufacturer of each drug to be administered to verify the recommended dose, the method and duration of administration, and contraindications. It is the responsibility of the practitioner, relying on experience and knowledge of the patient, to determine dosages and the best treatment for each individual patient. Neither the Publisher nor the authors assumes any liability for any injury and/or damage to persons or property arising from this publication.

The Publisher

Printed in UK

Preface

Rational endodontic therapy must be founded upon a sound understanding of the biological concepts of disease, its natural history and the physical, chemical and therapeutic basis of treating infection. Much fundamental biological and clinical endodontic research still remains to be undertaken. The principles of endodontic therapy have not changed greatly since the beginning of the twentieth century. However, research findings and collective clinical experiences have prompted a re-evaluation of treatment concepts. Modern approaches to treatment, together with the large array of new equipment and materials, have resulted in a need to rewrite and update most of this third edition.

This book has been designed to lead both the undergraduate student and the general dental practitioner, in a logical fashion, through the subject of endodontics. Chapters 1 and 2 outline the biological basis of endodontics, as it is understood today. The remaining chapters provide practical details, describing the current techniques and materials used in the treatment of patients. The text is liberally illustrated with photographs and colour diagrams to convey an effective message.

The standard of endodontic teaching and practice has improved considerably over the past few years. This is due in part to a heightened patient awareness of the benefits of dental care and a rise in the demand for procedures that help to retain teeth longer. The restoration of aesthetics and function is now commonly practised. With the prevention of dental disease and the decline in dental caries, an increasing number of patients present with problems that relate to the 'natural wear and tear' of teeth due to attrition, abrasion, erosion and trauma. Patients of all ages now expect to receive treatment that is successful. The vast need for endodontic treatment globally is certainly matched by the demands of informed patient population bases for predictably reliable conservative treatment.

Endodontics, together with periodontics, forms an essential foundation for restorative management of patients. Apart from the root canal treatment that forms an integral part of a restorative plan, there is also the treatment of pulp and periapical disease consequent upon the restorative procedures. Students and practitioners of the subject must, therefore, be competent to carry out root canal treatment of both anterior and posterior teeth, in order to cope with the increasing number of difficult cases that present before, during and after complex restorative care.

The overall success rate of conventional root canal treatment has been shown to range from about 65% to 95%. Successful outcome of treatment is influenced by the preoperative state of infection, technical quality of root canal treatment, apical extent of the root filling and the design and technical quality of the subsequent restoration. Poorly adapted root fillings and those short by more than 2 mm from the root apex are correlated with higher failure rates, which increases the risk of tooth loss.

Book learning alone cannot convey clinical skills, however practical the information. Theory has to be assimilated into a working knowledge by vigilant practice. Some individuals have an innate ability to make this transition, whereas for others the process is facilitated by further hands-on instruction. The acquisition of practical skills requires a constant disciplined effort to achieve a preconceived end result. The scientific rationale behind the strategy required to attain the preconceived end result should be continuously reviewed in the light of new knowledge. There is nothing new in this general concept, which is embodied in the following age-old adage from Aristotle:

'Excellence is an art won by training and habituation. We do not act rightly because we have virtue or excellence, rather we have those because we acted rightly. We are what we repeatedly do. Excellence then is not an act but a habit'.

We hope that this book will be only the beginning for the reader's development in this fascinating field.

Christopher J R Stock
Kishor Gulabivala
Richard T Walker

Acknowledgements

We would like to thank the following for their help:

Miss Noushin Attari for assistance with clinical photographs (Carol Mason), Dr Margaret Byers, Dr Melody Chen, Angela Christie, Dr Michael R N Collins, Dr Peter Endo, Dr David Dickey, Dr Jane Goodman, Dr Ben Johnson, Dr Paul King, late Professor Ivor Kramer, Dr Lars Laurell, Dr Koos Marais, Dr Ramanchandran Nair (for contributing so many excellent illustrations of the relationship between bacteria and host tissue structures), Dr Joe Omar, Dr Paul O'Neilly, Professor Tom Pitt Ford, Dr Alastair Speirs, Dr Elisabeth Saunders, Professor Michael Tagger, Dr Peng Hui Tan, Dr J Woodson, Dr Callum Youngson, late Dr Jakob Valderhaug, and finally the Department of Oral Pathology, Eastman Dental Institute, for their permission to use much of the histological material in Chapters 1 and 2.

Contributors

Jackie E Brown BDS, MSc, FDS RCPS, DDR RCR
Consultant in Dental Radiology, GKT Dental Institute;
Senior Lecturer in Dental Radiology,
Eastman Dental Institute for Oral Health Care Sciences,
London, UK

Ian Cross BDS, MDent Sci, MRD RCS
Specialist Endodontist and Prosthodontist
Postgraduate Clinical Tutor, Leeds Dental Institute
The Bramhope Dental Clinic, Leeds, UK

Ulpee Darbar BDS, MSc, FDS RCS
Consultant, Department of Periodontology
Eastman Dental Institute for Oral Health Care Sciences
University College London, UK

Carol Mason BDS, FDS RCS
Consultant in Paediatric Dentistry
Great Ormond Street Hospital for Children
Eastman Dental Hospital
London, UK

Yuan-Ling Ng BDS, MSc, MRD RCS
Clinical Lecturer in Endodontology
Department of Endodontics
Eastman Dental Institute for Oral Health Care Sciences
University College London, UK

Shahrzad Rahbaran BDS, MSc, FDS RCS, MRD RCS
Specialist Endodontist
Honorary Clinical Lecturer in Endodontology
Department of Endodontics
Eastman Dental Institute for Oral Health Care Sciences
University College London, UK

John D Regan BA, BDentSc, MSc, MS, DGDP
Assistant Professor
Baylor College of Dentistry
Texas A&M University System
USA

Paul R Wesselink PhD
Professor and Chairman
Department of Cariology, Endodontology and Pedodontology
Academic Centre of Dentistry Amsterdam
The Netherlands

Contents

Introduction to endodontology and endodontics

DEFINITION OF ENDODONTOLOGY AND ENDODONTICS

The Consensus report of the European Society of Endodontology (1994) defines this discipline thus:

'**Endodontology** is that branch of dental science concerned with the study of form, function, health of, injuries to and diseases of the dental pulp and periradicular tissues, and their treatment. The aetiology and diagnosis of dental pain and disease are considered to be integral parts of **endodontic practice**. **Endodontic treatment** encompasses any procedure that is designed to maintain the health of all, or part of, the pulp. When the pulp is diseased or injured, treatment is aimed at maintaining or restoring the health of the periradicular tissues. When pulpal disease has spread to the periradicular tissues, treatment is aimed at restoring them to normal; this is usually achieved by root canal treatment or in combination with endodontic surgery.'

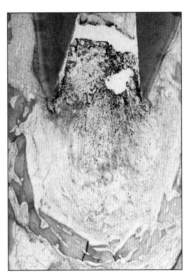

I.1 Periapical lesion

BRIEF INTRODUCTION TO PULPAL/PERIAPICAL DISEASE

Pulp disease consists of inflammation of connective tissue (the pulp), which in common with inflammatory responses in other parts of the body can be caused by any type of injury. Persistent and permanently damaging inflammation is, however, caused principally by unremitting stimulation of the pulp by oral bacteria. As yet ill-defined pathogens interact with the pulp, either directly or via the medium of dentine and lead to its demise. Death and necrosis of the pulp tissue leaves a moribund space in the central cavity of the tooth allowing bacteria to invade, colonize and infect the root canal space, eventually leading to periradicular inflammation which manifests clinically as a radiographic radiolucency, with or without symptoms.

In summary, therefore, a breach in the integrity of the tooth (first line of defence), exposes the dentine and allows the pulp to be stimulated. Death of the pulp tissue removes the second line of defence and leads to the final and third defensive barrier, the periradicular inflammatory lesion (**I.1**).

The dental pulp may also be killed by acute traumatic injury to the tooth, where infection may be delayed for six years or longer unless there is a breach in the tooth structure allowing bacteria to invade. A rational approach to the management of these inflammatory diseases requires an understanding of the normal structure and function of teeth and their supporting structures and the pathogenesis of the diseases. In principle, the treatment approaches consist of eradication of the bacterial infection using biomechanical debridement, in conjunction with chemical antibacterial agents, to help decontaminate the dentine and prevent its recontamination by using various obturation or filling materials that create an environment within which the body is able to effect healing. Treatment of pulp inflammation by preserving the pulp tissue is called *pulp therapy* and treatment of periapical inflammation by eradicating infected pulp tissue to allow periradicular tissues to heal is called *root canal treatment*.

Reference

European Society of Endodontology (1994) Consensus report of the ESE on quality guidelines for endodontic treatment. *Int Endod J* **27**, 115–24.

Chapter 1

Biological and clinical rationale for pulp therapy

K Gulabivala

The aim of this chapter is to outline the biological basis for prevention and management of pulp disease. A rational approach to the treatment of disease requires an understanding of the pathological process and this in turn demands knowledge of the normal anatomy and physiology of the involved tissues.

ANATOMY AND PHYSIOLOGY

The dental pulp

The dental pulp is a minute piece (approximately 25 mm³) of connective tissue akin to any other in the body and consists of cells, nerve fibres and blood vessels embedded in a gel-like ground substance. However, its unique characteristic is that it is encased in a rigid hard tissue called dentine (**1.1**). The pulp is normally considered together with the dentine, which it both secretes and is surrounded by. The dentine and pulp are therefore referred to as the pulp–dentine

complex (**1.2, 1.3**). The dental pulp is covered on its outer periphery by a layer of specialized cells called odontoblasts. These have the function of secreting the mineralized but resilient hard tissue called dentine, which forms the bulk of the tooth. The initial three-dimensional distribution of the odontoblasts, which is genetically determined, maps out the final shape of the tooth (**1.4**). Dentine is laid down by odontoblasts in such a way that they leave an extension of their cell body, called the odontoblastic process (**1.5**), at their origin. As dentine matrix is progressively laid down, the odontoblastic process simultaneously grows longer and the cell body recedes centrally. Mineralization of the dentine matrix causes a hard, calcified tissue to form but the advancing front of dentine matrix remains unmineralized and is called predentine (**1.3**). The net effect is that as each of the millions of odontoblasts lay down dentine

1.1 Ground section of crown of tooth: A = enamel; B = dentine; C = pulp

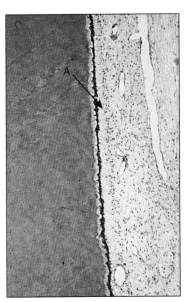

1.2 Low-power view of pulp–dentine complex:
A = cell-free zone

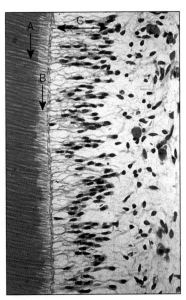

1.3 High-power view of pulp–dentine complex:
A = mineralized dentine;
B = predentine; C = odontoblasts

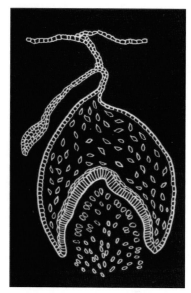

1.4 Developing tooth germ at the 'Bell Stage'

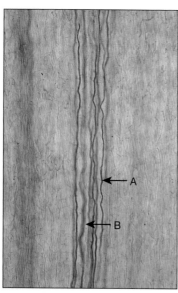

1.5 High-power view of odontoblast process (B) in dentinal tubule (A)

of the total surface area near the dentine–enamel junction. The dentinal tubules, which are interconnected by lateral tubules, (**1.7**) make up 20–30% of the volume of dentine. In the crown, the tubules follow a gentle 'S' shaped curve (**1.6**) and therefore trauma to one part of the crown affects the pulp at a more apical level (**1.8**). A deeper cavity would also traumatize more tubules and cause greater damage (**1.9**).

There is controversy about the persistence of the odontoblast processes through the full length of the dentinal tubules during the life of the tooth. Some believe they recede midway to the enamel–dentine junction and others that they extend the full distance. The remainder of the tubule is filled with a unique protein-rich, dentinal fluid that is normally under positive pressure. Fluid exchange may take place either from the pulp outwards or in the reverse direction.

The name peritubular dentine is given to the tissue laid down by the odontoblast process, which lines the tubules and is 40% more mineralized than intertubular dentine (mineralized tissue between tubules) (**1.10**). The formation of peritubular dentine is thought to be a normal age change and may be accelerated by stimuli such as caries, attrition and abrasion. Occlusion of the dentinal tubules by this process and by mineral crystals is called sclerosis and gives aged root apices their characteristic translucency (**1.11**).

Primary dentine formed during the development of the tooth is laid down at a rate of 4 µm per day. Secondary dentine is formed after the teeth are fully developed and is laid down at a rate of about 0.8 µm per day. It is formed evenly over the entire pulpal surface and is also known as physiological or regular secondary dentine. It may be distinguished from primary dentine by the slight and sudden change in the direction of the tubules (**1.12**). Irregular secondary dentine, as the name implies, is laid down unevenly at a rate of 3 µm per day, in response to noxious external stimuli such as dental caries, attrition, and abrasion (**1.13–1.15**).

matrix and withdraw towards the centre of the pulp tissue, a hard shell of dentine is created, permeated by millions of tubules (with an approximately radial distribution), each containing a cellular process.

Dentine is, therefore, a specialized connective tissue of mesenchymal origin that contains thousands of tubules radiating outwards from the dental pulp to the enamel in the crown and the cementum in the root (**1.6**). There may be up to 65 000 tubules per square millimetre at the pulpal end and 15 000 tubules per square millimetre at the dentine–enamel junction. The diameter of the tubules is about 3 µm near the pulp and less than 1 µm peripherally. The dentinal tubules account for 45% of the surface area near the pulp and 1%

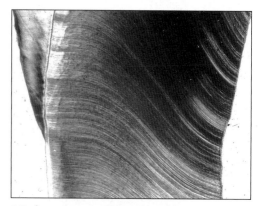

1.6 Ground section of tooth at the cemento–enamel junction

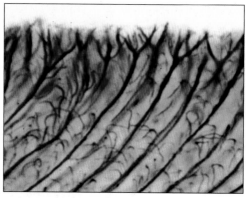

1.7 High-power view of lateral communication between dentinal tubules

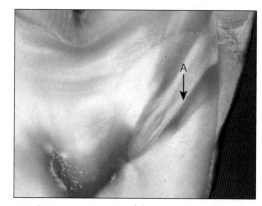

1.8 Sclerosis of dentine (A) caused by caries

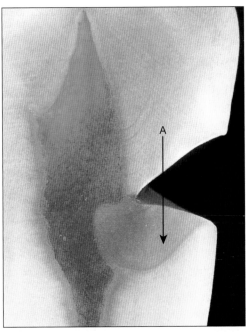

1.9 Sclerosis of dentine (A) and pulp calcification caused by cervical abfraction

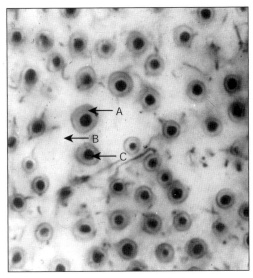

1.10 Cross-section of dentinal tubules:
A = peritubular dentine; B = intertubular dentine;
C = odontoblast process

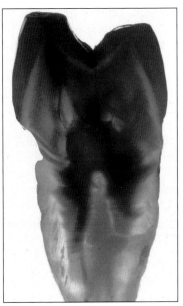

1.11 Translucency of root caused by sclerosis of dentine

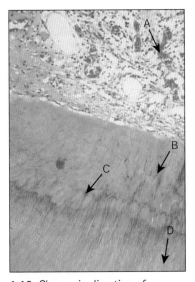

1.12 Change in direction of secondary dentinal tubules:
A = pulp; B = secondary dentine;
C = change in direction of tubules;
D = primary dentine

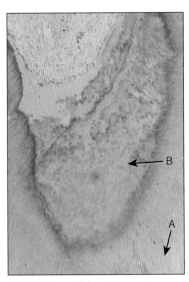

1.13 Primary (A) and irregular secondary (B) dentine

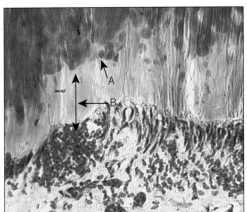

1.14 Active deposition of irregular secondary dentine: A = globular dentine at mineralizing front; B = widened predentine

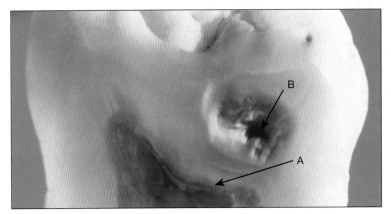

1.15 Irregular deposition of secondary dentine (A) due to caries (B)

The odontoblast bodies are separated from the mineralized dentine by a layer of unmineralized dentine, 15 μm wide, known as predentine (**1.16**). The odontoblasts form a single layer of cells but, because of the differences in the level of the nuclei, an illusion of a multilayered structure is created in histological section (**1.16**). Odontoblasts are incapable of further division once fully mature and if damaged may be replaced from undifferentiated mesenchymal cells.

Immediately adjacent to the odontoblastic layer is a zone of connective tissue, which is relatively free of cells, called the 'cell-free zone' (**1.2**). It tends to disappear during periods of cellular activity in a young pulp or in older pulps where reparative dentine is being formed (**1.13**).

The remainder of the pulp consists of ground substance in which are embedded cells that include fibroblasts and inflammatory cells, collagen fibres and a complex network of blood vessels and nerve fibres (**1.17**). The ground substance contains the fibroblasts responsible for producing the proteins and carbohydrates that form the viscous substance of the matrix. The ground substance accommodates humoral and immune cellular infiltrates produced during inflammatory responses. Lymphatic vessels help to clear away exuded fluid and macromolecules and return the tissue to status quo.

Biological or chronological aging may reduce the cellular and neurovascular elements and thereby reduce the ability of the aged pulp to respond to injury but it is possible that there is no direct correlation between such cellular content and ability of pulp to defend itself. The pulp tissue has a rich neurovascular supply that reaches it via arterioles and nerve bundles through the apical foramina and lesser accessory supplies via lateral canals in the root. These allow an exchange of tissue fluid between the periodontal and pulpal tissues, otherwise the cementum is impervious to macromolecules (a feature that makes root canal treatment feasible).

The vascular supply

The arrangement of the vascular system in the pulp is unique in order to help overcome the problems of its non-compliant encapsulation within the rigid dentine shell. The main vessels, which are branches of the dental arteries consisting of arterioles, enter through the apical foramina and pass centrally through the pulp giving off lateral branches which divide further into capillaries (**1.18–1.21**). Some minor vessels may enter through lateral canals but these cannot provide sufficient collateral circulation (**1.22**). The smaller terminal vessels reach the odontoblastic layer where they divide extensively to form a plexus below (**1.23**) and within (**1.24**) it. The venous return is collected by a network of capillaries that unite to form venules that primarily course down the central portion of the pulp (**1.25**).

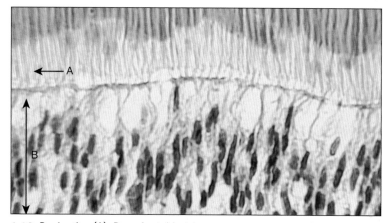

1.16 Predentine (A): B = odontoblast layer

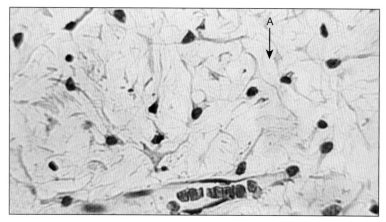

1.17 Pulp tissue elements: A = ground substance

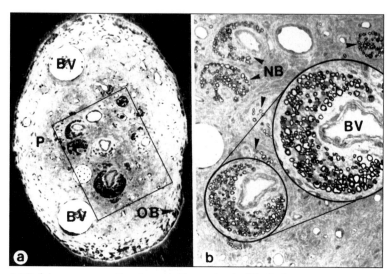

1.18 A transverse section through the root pulp (P) of a human mandibular premolar. The rectangular demarcated area in **a** is magnified in **b**. Note the numerous nerve-fibre bundles (NB), some of which are closely associated with blood vessels (BV) to form neurovascular bundles (inset in **b**). OB = Odontoblasts. Magnifications: **a** × 55, **b** × 130, *inset* × 225. (From Nair & Schroeder, 1995)

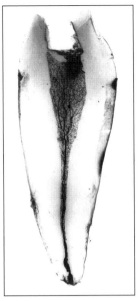

1.19 Network of blood vessels in the pulp (courtesy of Prof. I Kramer)

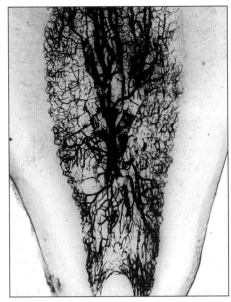

1.20 High-power view of network of blood vessels in the pulp (courtesy of Prof. I Kramer)

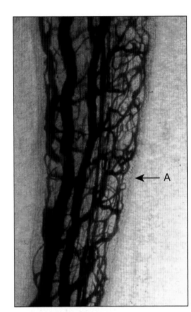

1.21 Relationship of arterioles and capillaries in the pulp to dentine (A) (courtesy of Prof. I Kramer)

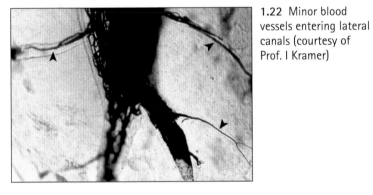

1.22 Minor blood vessels entering lateral canals (courtesy of Prof. I Kramer)

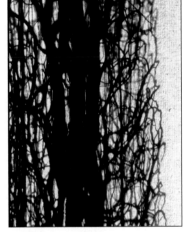

1.23 Capillary plexus adjacent to the dentine (courtesy of Prof. I Kramer)

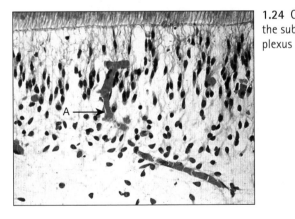

1.24 Capillary (A) from the subodontoblastic plexus

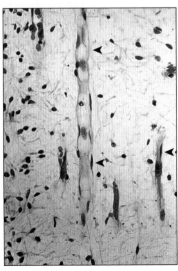

1.25 Venules (arrowed) coursing through centre of pulp

Functional aspects of the blood supply

A unique feature in this arrangement is that blood can be shunted directly from the arterioles to the venules via arteriovenous shunts. This design helps prevent a build-up of unsustainable pressure in the non-compliant environment. The pulp was originally thought to be a fragile tissue, susceptible to rapid death as a result of even minor inflammation, by virtue of its encasement in a rigid dentine shell. Elegant experiments demonstrated that apical strangulation of blood vessels was not inevitable because of the arteriovenous shunts. Recent evidence has shown the presence of lymphatic vessels that facilitate return of larger molecules and blood cells back to the circulation. Tissue pressure changes are localized not only by the shunting away of blood and fluid from the inflamed area but also by the barrier effect of the ground matrix. These mechanisms are so effective that localized inflammation (**1.26**) and even localized pulp abscesses may be surrounded by normal tissue. These insights have changed the perception of the pulp to that of a very resilient tissue.

The nerve supply

The dental pulp is richly innervated with both sensory (large diameter, myelinated A-fibres and small diameter, non-myelinated C-fibres) and autonomic nerve fibres (serving the vascular supply) (**1.27, 1.28**). The nerve fibres enter the pulp through the apical foramen together with the blood vessels (**1.18**). As the nerve bundles pass through the pulp coronally they divide into smaller branches until ultimately single axons form a dense network near the pulp–dentine border called the plexus of Raschkow (**1.29**). Furthermore, individual axons may branch into many terminal filaments, which in turn may enter the dentinal tubules (**1.30**). One axon may innervate up to a 100 dentinal tubules. These usually only penetrate the tubules up to 100 or 200 µm. Some of the tubules may contain several nerve fibres. The true contribution to the functions of the pulp by the nerve supply is probably more complicated then originally thought, considering the diversity of the neuropeptides they produce. Apart from their sensory function they play an important part in neurogenic inflammation (**1.31**).

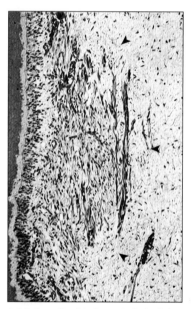

1.26 Localized inflammation of the pulp (arrowed)

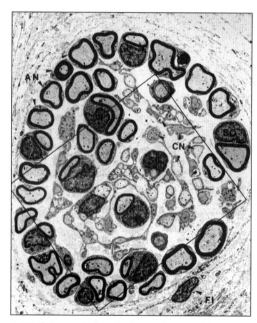

1.27 A transmission electron micrographic reconstruction of an axon-bundle containing both myelinated (AN) and non-myelinated (CN) axons. Note the absence of a perineureum around the nerve fibre bundle. The demarcated area is magnified in **1.28**. (FI = fibroblasts, SC = Schwann cells). Magnification: × 5360. (From Nair & Schroeder, 1995)

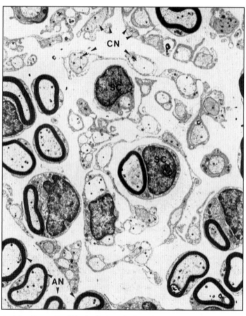

1.28 A magnified view of the demarcated area in **1.27** showing detail of non-myelinated axons (CN) in a nerve-fibre bundle. Note the wide variation in size of the non-myelinated axons. (AN = myelinated axons, SC = Schwan cells). Magnification: × 9110. (From Nair & Schroeder, 1995)

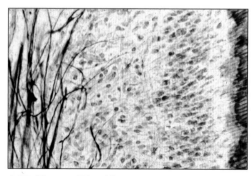

1.29 Plexus of Raschkow

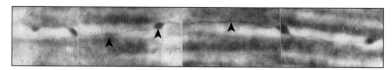

1.30 Nerve axon in dentinal tubule (arrowed)

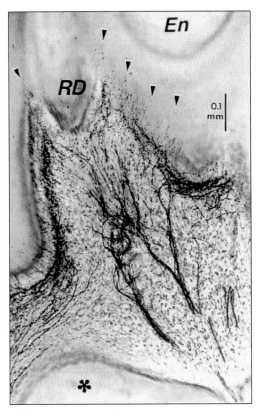

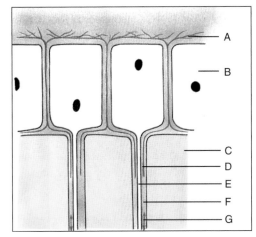

1.31 Immunocytochemical sections showing CGRP-IR nerve fibres branching extensively in the coronal pulp and entering into dentine for up to 0.1 mm but avoiding reparative dentine (RD). (From Byers *et al.*, 1990)

1.32 Hydrodynamic theory: A = nerve plexus; B = odontoblast; C = dentine; D = A-δ-nerve-fibre; E = odontoblast process; F = dentinal tubule; G = fluid movement stimulates A-δ-nerve-fibre

Functional aspects of the nerve supply

The autonomic nerve supply consists of sympathetic fibres that control the microcirculation. The sensory innervation consists of at least two, and possibly three different types of fibres. The faster conducting myelinated A-δ-fibres are thought to be responsible for the sharp, localized dentinal pain. The slower conducting, unmyelinated C-fibre is thought to give rise to the duller throbbing less localized pain. Drilling, probing, air-drying, heating and cooling dentine stimulate the A-δ-fibres. Application of hyper osmotic fluids to the exposed dentine surface may also stimulate the A-δ-fibres. This sensitivity of dentine is explained by the 'hydrodynamic theory' (**1.32**). The common feature of the above stimuli is that they all cause a rapid movement of fluid in the dentinal tubules. This causes a mechanical distortion of the tissue in the pulp–dentine border that results in the stimulation of the A-δ-fibres. Dentine sensitivity may therefore be increased by opening up the dentinal tubules by acid etching; conversely, blockage of the tubules by composite resin or potassium oxalate crystals prevents fluid flow and leads to desensitization of dentine. Blockage of the dentinal tubules by sclerosis would also lead to desensitization.

During electric pulp testing, the A-δ-fibres are stimulated first because they have a lower threshold. As the stimulus intensity is increased not only are more A-δ-fibres activated but some C-fibres may also be stimulated giving rise to a strong unpleasant sensation. The relative unreliability of electric pulp testing young teeth with immature roots may be explained by the scarcity of A-δ-fibres in their pulps at this stage of development.

The C-fibres may be activated by thermal, mechanical or chemical stimuli reaching the deeper parts of the pulp. Dentinal stimulation does not activate the C-fibres unless some element of damage occurs to the pulp tissue such as raising the pulp temperature to about 44°C. Similarly, extreme cold temperatures reaching the pulp may stimulate the C-fibres. The C-fibres are thought to play an important role in the development of the dull and poorly localized symptoms associated with pulp inflammation.

The third type of nerve called the A-β-fibre is myelinated and has the fastest conduction velocity. They are thought to respond to non-noxious mechanical stimulation of the intact crown and may be important in the regulation of mastication and loading of teeth. They do, however, also respond to stimulation, of dentine. In addition to the different nerve fibres and the types of their stimulation, their threshold of stimulation may also vary, as may that of the patients' perception and tolerance of pain. This results in a wide range of pain descriptors and makes diagnosis of conditions of the pulp on the basis of the symptoms unreliable.

The normal pulp contains few inflammatory cells, the exception being some dendritic antigen-presenting cells and T-lymphocytes which are probably recirculating rather than resident. At early stages of pulp infection there is a non-specific inflammatory response dominated by polymorphonuclear leucocytes and macrophages. A specific antibacterial immune response follows and consists of lymphocytes, macrophages and plasma cells.

FUNCTIONS OF THE PULP

The functions of the pulp are stated to be formative (dentine) and defensive (through the pulp–dentine complex). Once the tooth is fully formed, the pulp mainly serves a defensive function. It is unlikely that the pulp is a vestigial organ. The definite change in the rate at which dentine is deposited suggests that the pulp tissue has a lifetime role. Hypothetically, if secondary dentine deposition continued at the rate of primary dentine, the almost complete obliteration

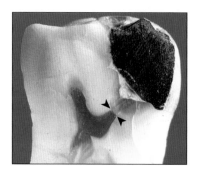

1.33 Secondary dentine deposition caused by caries and its treatment

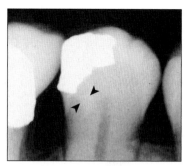

1.34 Sclerosed dentinal tubules (arrowed)

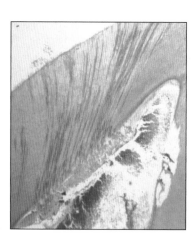

1.35 Bacteria in dentinal tubules (low–power view)

of the pulp would result in a tooth with very different mechanical properties. By inference, the *raison d'être* of the pulp and dentine must be to provide a tooth with the resilient characteristics necessary for withstanding masticatory load. The slight deformation of the tooth must be detectable by proprioceptors in the pulp. There is only indirect evidence of the existence of proprioceptive mechanisms in the pulp but it is an attractive explanation for the apparently greater susceptibility of pulpless teeth to fracture.

Defence reactions are essential for the survival of the pulp. The most obvious and widely described defence reactions include: the initial inflammatory response; blockage of the dentinal tubules by large molecular substances; the sclerosis of the dentinal tubules by the formation of peritubular dentine; and the formation of secondary and tertiary dentine (**1.13**).

The pulp has been thought of as a sensory organ that warns against disease (e.g. caries or the loss of tooth tissue) by eliciting pain. This is a relatively poor warning system considering the number of teeth whose pulps become irreversibly inflamed apparently without warning.

The pulp is therefore considered to be a sensory organ serving to forewarn the owner of damage or impending damage, although this is not always foolproof. The first line of sensory defence involves stimulation of the low-threshold A-δ-nerve-fibres, responsible for the sensation of the characteristic sharp dentinal pain elicited by stimulating dentine by probing, air blast, application of hyperosmotic fluids, extreme temperatures or occlusal loading in the cracked tooth syndrome. Inflammation of the pulp reduces their threshold and leads to hyperalgesia or hypersensitivity. In addition, it also allows stimulation of the higher threshold C-fibres that are responsible for the deep-seated, less localized, duller, throbbing pain of pulpitis. Stimulation of proprioceptive A-β-nerve-fibres may forewarn the owner of impending overloading of the tooth.

In addition to sensory defences, the inflammatory response of the pulp contributes to recruitment of the full array of non-specific and specific immunological responses. This system protects the pulpal soft tissue against external molecular or microbial stimuli. An extremely important function of the pulp–dentine complex, which works in concert with inflammation, is secondary (reactionary) and tertiary (reparative) dentine formation (**1.33**) together with dentinal tubule sclerosis (calcification) (**1.34**) to block off further ingress of noxious factors.

Reparative processes within the pulp–dentine complex mimic developmental processes. During tooth formation, molecular signals (growth factors) between epithelial and mesenchymal cells control the induction of odontoblast differentiation. The growth factors have a profound effect on various cellular activities and are found throughout the body. A sub-class of these molecules called transforming growth factor-beta (TGF-β) family are responsible for signalling odontoblast differentiation. The differentiated odontoblasts synthesize and secrete the TFG-βs together with other growth factors and sequester them into the dentine matrix, which is then calcified. The subsequent dissolution of the dentine matrix as a result of caries releases these molecules again to exert their influence on healing. TGF-β molecules released by mild dentine-pulp injury diffuse along a concentration gradient down the dentinal tubules, against the outward flow of dentinal fluid, and stimulate viable odontoblasts to lay down reactionary dentine. Injury that is severe enough to damage odontoblasts irreversibly requires their replacement from the mesenchymal cell pool. This is a lengthier and more complex process requiring the migration and differentiation of new cells followed by secretion of a new matrix. The resulting dentine is therefore less well organized and known as reparative dentine (**1.13**). An important factor that may interfere with the reparative process is a continuing microbial challenge as a result of coronal leakage (**1.35**).

CAUSES OF PULP INJURY

The pulp may be injured in a variety of direct and indirect ways. These are summarized in **Table 1.1** below (**1.36–1.38**). The relative importance of the different factors causing pulp injury has been debated at length and over time, the emphasis has changed from one set of factors to another. In the 1950s and 1960s, the effect of restorative procedures was considered to be of predominant importance with the toxic effect of restorative materials uppermost in the minds of practitioners. The observation of pulp necrosis

Table 1.1 Pulp injury

Relation to treatment	Damaging agent	Studies
Preoperative factors	Cervical exposed dentine (genetically determined)	Ten Cate 1994
	Tooth surface loss (acquired) erosion attrition abrasion abfraction	Tronstad & Langeland 1971 Meister *et al.* 1980 Rosenberg 1981 Stanley *et al.* 1983
	Caries	Brannstrom & Lind, 1965 Reeves & Stanley 1966 Massler 1967 Langeland 1987
	Trauma Tooth subluxation or avulsion Tooth fracture enamel dentine pulp exposure	Andreasen & Andreasen 1994
	Periodontal disease	Seltzer *et al.* 1963 Mazur *et al.* 1964 Rubach & Mitchell 1965 Bender & Seltzer 1972 Langeland *et al.* 1974 Czarnecki & Schilder 1979 Dongari & Lambrianidis 1988
Intraoperative factors	Tooth preparation Intracoronal Extracoronal Iatrogenic pulp exposure	Marsland & Shovelton 1957 Shovelton & Marsland 1958 Langeland 1959 Hartnett & Smith 1961 Morrant & Kramer 1963 Hamilton & Kramer 1967 Marsland & Shovelton 1970 Morrant 1977 Turner *et al.* 1989 Ohshima 1990
	Other restorative procedures Local anaesthesia Pin placement Cavity cleaning Impression taking Temporization Electrosurgery Orthodontics	Langeland & Langeland 1965 Suzuki *et al.* 1973 Cotton & Siegel 1978 Spangberg *et al.* 1982 Kim *et al.* 1984 Plamondon *et al.* 1990 Nixon *et al.* 1993 Odor *et al.* 1994
	Restorative materials Dentine liners Temporary materials Permanent materials	Cox 1987 Cox *et al.* 1987 Qvist 1993 Smith *et al.* 2002
Postoperative factors	Microbial microleakage Any preoperative factor	Brannstrom & Nyborg 1971 Vojinovic *et al.* 1973 Bergenholtz *et al.* 1982 Browne & Tobias 1986 Mejare *et al.* 1987

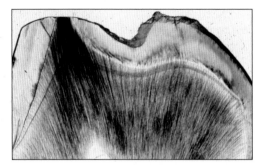

1.36 Effect of attrition on dentine

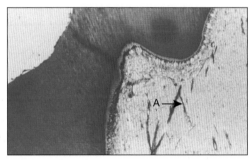

1.37 Effect of caries on the pulp: A = inflamed pulp tissue

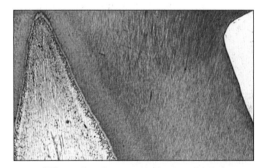

1.38 Effect of cavity preparation on the pulp

associated with silicate and zinc phosphate cement restorations reinforced these views. The notion that pulp damage was a matter of accumulative injury became established; often beginning with caries or trauma and then being superimposed by a series of restorative procedures. A point would then be reached when the inflammatory response of the pulp became chronic and spread through the tissue leading to chronic total pulpitis. If the pulp survived the restorative procedures, then slow recovery would occur leaving the pulp fibrosed, compromised and more susceptible to necrosis with further insults.

The above view changed as a result of studies at the end of 1960s and early 1970s. Controlled animal and human histological studies revealed that pulp injury caused by restorative procedures and toxic restorative materials was reversible provided that microbial leakage was eliminated. In 'worst-case-scenario' studies involving exposure of the pulp and capping with a range of restorative materials, it was shown that the restorative procedures and materials were not the most important factor, the controls consisted of similar tooth samples but with the outer part of the restorative material cut back and restored with zinc oxide/eugenol cement.

The relative importance of initial pulp inflammation, restorative procedures and postoperative factors is still not well understood. Current understanding is that there is a complex interplay between the size of cavity, remaining dentine thickness, restorative material, microbial leakage and presence of pulp inflammation.

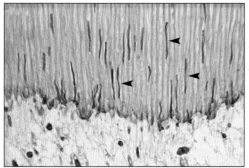

1.39 Aspirated odontoblasts in dentinal tubules as a result of injury

The degree of injury to the pulp and its ability to survive is dictated in large part by the amount of remaining dentine (**1.37, 1.38**). It is therefore important to preserve as much dentine as possible as it provides a natural buffer to further injury. Cutting deeper cavities or crown preparations increases the number of dentinal tubules involved, reduces the survival of odontoblasts (**1.39**) and increases the degree of pulp inflammation. This is probably due to a combination of direct injury by transsection of the odontoblasts, dehydration, heat generated during cavity preparation (**1.40**) as well as subsequent microbial and chemical stimuli that are now able to reach the pulp more easily (**1.41, 1.42**). Factors such as type of bur (diamond or tungsten, large or small), rotation speed (type of handpiece), duration and nature (intermittent or continuous, high or low interfacial pressure) of bur contact (e.g. stalling bur causes high temperatures and dentine burns), cutting technique (slot versus surface removal), amount of vibration and adequacy of coolant spray may all contribute to the amount of heat generated. Although it is difficult to quantify the threshold of dentine thickness that is critical to pulp survival, it is estimated that dentine thickness less than 0.25 mm results in severe inflammation. Teeth with cavities that are also contaminated by microbial leakage have even more severe pulp inflammation.

A functional pulp–dentine complex requires responsive and vital odontoblasts that are able to lay down protective secondary or tertiary dentine. Their conservation is enhanced by an absence of pulp inflammation and cavity restoration with a sublining of calcium hydroxide, zinc polycarboxylate or zinc oxide/eugenol cements (in decreasing order of influence). Use of composite resins, enamel-bonded resins and resin-modified glass ionomer cement restorations cause an increasing degree of injury to odontoblasts. Deep cavities, therefore, should preferably be lined with calcium hydroxide and overlaid with zinc oxide/eugenol. Resin-modified glass ionomers should also be sublined with calcium hydroxide and their direct contact with dentine in deep cavities avoided.

Reactionary dentine response is important in increasing the dentine thickness postoperatively and is positively related to the size of the cavity, remaining dentine thickness, acid etching and microbial

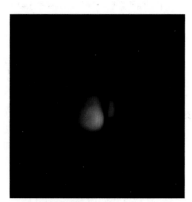

1.40 Incandescence caused by dry cutting of dentine

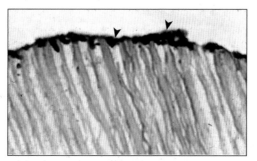

1.41 Bacteria lining the surface of cut dentine

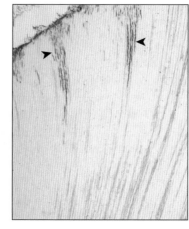

1.42 Bacteria in dentinal tubules (high-power view)

leakage. The greatest reactionary dentine response is seen in cavities with remaining dentine thickness between 0.25 and 0.5 mm and especially in the presence of microbial leakage. It may be that this depth is optimal for the stimulation effects of solubilized growth factors released during restorative procedures and able to reach the pulp. However, when dentine thickness is reduced further the damage to odontoblasts also increases, thereby resulting in a reduced reactionary dentine response. Restorative material plays a minor role in stimulating reactionary dentine but, for obvious reasons, its effect is enhanced by reduced dentine thickness (especially below 0.5 mm). Calcium hydroxide dressing produces the maximum response and zinc polycarboxylate cement no response. This effect is probably mediated via the stimulation of odontoblasts.

Restorations fail and are associated with postoperative complications most frequently as a result of the effects of microbial microleakage (**1.43, 1.44**). The postoperative complications include:

- marginal staining;
- dentine hypersensitivity;
- restoration corrosion or degradation;
- secondary caries;
- pulp inflammation and death.

Microbial leakage is enhanced in larger cavities where there is a greater marginal interface exposed to the oral environment. There is also a greater potential for tooth deformation under load, causing increased strain at the marginal joint and leading to breakdown in the marginal integrity between restoration and cavity. The choice of restorative material also influences the degree of microbial leakage. Zinc oxide/eugenol is the most effective material for preventing microbial leakage although recently introduced resin-modified glass ionomer cements are also useful in this regard. Enamel-bonded or adhesive-bonded composites do not perform well in preventing microbial leakage.

Factors such as restorative material, cavity dimensions, acid-etching and microbial leakage all influence the degree of pulp inflammation. There is a complex interaction between these variables in damaging the pulp. The emphasis on the importance of microbial leakage in no way reduces the potential role of restorative procedures and materials in the demise of the pulp. In clinical practice, teeth undergoing treatment may have a history of previous treatment and, therefore, pulp inflammation, which may go undiagnosed if asymptomatic. It is, therefore, entirely possible that restorative intervention, however minimal, superimposed upon pre-existing pulp inflammation may be sufficient to tip the balance and cause its sudden death and necrosis. The pulp space and tissue could then rapidly become infected if exposed to bacteria.

The approaches to prevention of microbial leakage may be divided into two:

1. Those seeking to reduce the gap between the restoration and the tooth (including attempts at adhesion).
2. Those using the antibacterial properties of materials to inhibit microbial leakage.

Predictable reduction of the gap is dependent upon the properties of the material and its optimal manipulation, taking into account the resilience of teeth and the interfacial interaction between restorative material and tooth tissue. For successful adhesive restoration of teeth, the restoration must deform in phase with the tooth under all loading conditions. Unfortunately, so far no material is able to meet these demands for long periods, consequently all adhesive materials fail at some point in time after placement and allow microbial leakage.

While much emphasis has been placed on reduction or elimination of the gap at the tooth/restoration interface to reduce microleakage, little, if any, emphasis has been placed on the reduction of *microbial leakage*, specifically. The closest approach is the use of zinc oxide/eugenol as a base under amalgam restorations, though the effect of this material if placed directly against the pulp must be considered. Unfortunately the material cannot be used in conjunction with composite (aesthetic) restorative materials because of its potential to interfere with their setting reaction. Another option is to use a resin-modified glass ionomer as a sublining but over a layer of calcium hydroxide. The durability of the antibacterial effect of zinc oxide/eugenol has been questioned, however it need only last as long as the pulp–dentine complex takes to lay down a defence (dentinal sclerosis and secondary dentine formation) against further ingress of bacteria and their products. It could be argued that the same applies to adhesive techniques. The crucial point is that the principle of this approach assumes that the defence of the pulp–dentine complex is foolproof and not compromised by pre-existing inflammation, the depth of cavity or the restorative material. The potential inability to block off all dentinal tubules is the weak link in the ability of the pulp to survive and therefore perpetuate its life to resist further onslaughts. Open dentinal tubules may provide a persistent pathway for bacteria and their products leading to continuing chronic inflammation of the pulp and ultimately to its final demise. Open dentinal tubules associated with a healthy pulp do, however, offer resistance to bacterial invasion compared to that of a non-vital pulp. The period of time it may take for the pulp to die has not been defined but depending on the initial condition, nature of the continuing stimulus, and the pulp response, it may take many years.

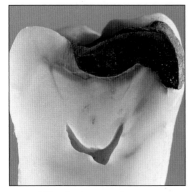

1.43 Microleakage under restorations

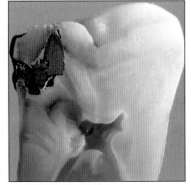

1.44 Microleakage under restorations

Smear layer

Dentine has the characteristic that when it is cut or ground with metal a deformed layer of organic and inorganic dentine matter is formed over its surface called a smear layer (**1.45**). Although the smear layer prevents good adaptation of restorative material in the cavity it may be best to retain it to protect the pulp from the effects of microbial leakage. A reasonable compromise is to remove the smear layer partially so that the surface layer is removed leaving the dentinal plugs intact (**1.46**). Use of 3% hydrogen peroxide may be sufficient for this purpose in most instances. Newer generations of dentine adhesives dictate what happens to the smear layer. In some cases it is retained and reinforced, in others it is partially removed and in others it is removed completely using aggressive acids such as ethylenediamine tetraacetic acid (EDTA) (**1.47**) or phosphoric acid (**1.48**). It is intended that the resin enters the surface layer of dentine to form what has become known as the hybridized layer (**1.49**).

Recommendation for optimal treatment of caries

All of this means that in treating a carious lesion (**1.50**), the following principles should give optimal results: a conservative cavity should be cut to access and remove softened, carious dentine (**1.51**), ensuring that all peripheral caries is removed (**1.52**); if considered necessary the surface of dentine may be scrubbed with 3% hydrogen peroxide to remove only the superficial layer of the smear layer; a sublining of calcium hydroxide should be placed to facilitate repair and kill residual bacteria in the dentine and to harden it (**1.53**); a lining of zinc oxide/eugenol should then be placed to prevent microbial leakage (**1.54**); and finally, a well-adapted amalgam restoration should be placed to ensure no leakage (**1.55**).

SEVERE INFLAMMATORY AND DEGENERATIVE CHANGES IN THE PULP

Spread on pulpal inflammation

If a localized zone of dentinal tubules remains patent following odontoblast injury, only the associated portion of the pulp will be inflamed (**1.56**). The process of spread of inflammation from this localized site to the rest of the pulp is not fully understood. It is presumably related to the ability of the pulp to close off dentinal tubules by the action of replacement odontoblasts from undifferentiated mesenchymal cells. If this fails to wall off the source of inflammation, then it would become persistent and chronic. It can be envisaged that the greater the number of adjacent dentinal tubules involved

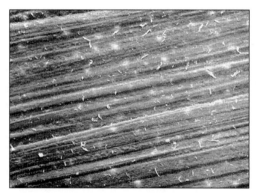

1.45 Smear layer produced by cavity preparation (SEM view)

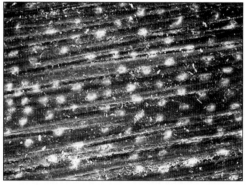

1.46 Partial removal of smear layer using 3% hydrogen peroxide (SEM view)

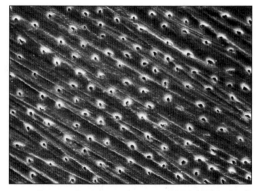

1.47 Removal of smear layer by EDTA (SEM view)

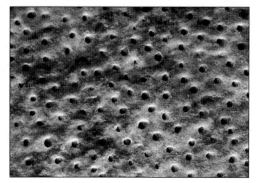

1.48 Removal of smear layer by phosphoric acid to reveal dentinal tubule openings (SEM view)

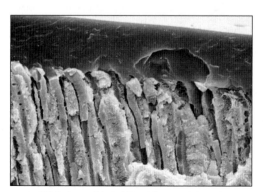

1.49 SEM view of hybridized layer with resin overlying and penetrating the dentinal tubules

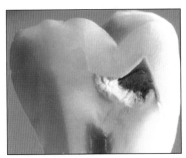

1.50 Carious lesion

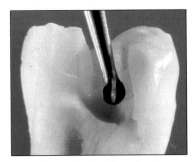

1.51 Removal of carious dentine

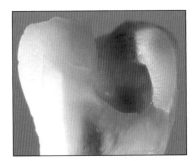

1.52 Completed preparation

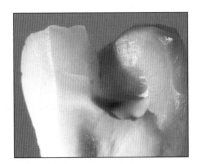

1.53 Sublining with calcium hydroxide

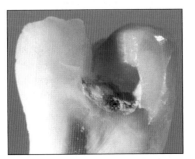

1.54 Lining with zinc oxide/eugenol

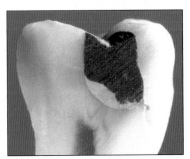

1.55 Placement of amalgam

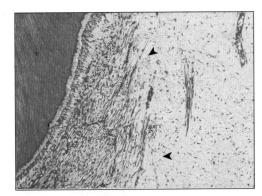

1.56 Localized pulp inflammation

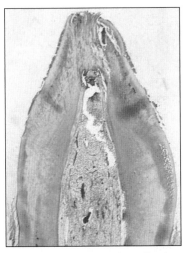

1.57 Severe inflammation affecting most of the pulp

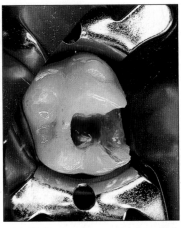

1.58 Pulp chamber containing vital pulp tissue

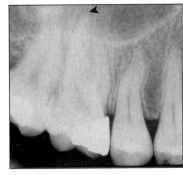

1.59 Radiograph of tooth seen in **1.58**, showing periapical area around palatal root before opening into the pulp

and the greater the degree of odontoblast injury, the larger the volume of pulp tissue embraced by inflammation. The localized response may or may not progress to more severe inflammation depending on stemming of the provoking factors. Progression of the inflammation may produce a range of histological pictures including areas of chronic inflammation coexisting with microabscesses and partial necrosis (**1.57**). Unfortunately all these histological pictures have a poor correlation with clinical signs and symptoms of pulp disease. This makes clinical diagnosis of the state of the pulp extremely difficult as the tissues are hidden from direct view and examination. Added to this picture of uncertainty is the finding that in some cases even in the presence of vital healthy pulp tissue in the roots and perhaps even in the pulp chamber (**1.58**), there may be radiographic evidence of periapical changes (**1.59**) associated with inflammation of the coronal pulp. A reasonably clear distinction between different states of the pulp can only be made between vital (albeit inflamed) and completely necrotic pulps using currently available pulp tests.

Under the specific condition of traumatic impact injuries, sudden severance of the blood supply can result in total necrosis of the pulp without any intervening or subsequent radiographic periapical change. Such change would then only become evident in the event of infection of the necrotic pulp. Such pulps may remain uninfected for up to six years.

Dystrophic pulp calcification

A common finding in the pulp in all age groups is the presence of dystrophic calcification or pulp stones. These are more common in teeth with diseased pulps but may also be found in unerupted teeth. The cause of calcification is unknown. There are two types of calcifications, those, which are smooth and rounded, are formed by concentric laminations and found in the coronal pulp (**1.60**) whereas the irregular calcifications without laminations are found more commonly in the radicular pulp (**1.61**). These may sometimes take the shape of rods or leafs. The laminated stones grow in size by the addition of collagen fibrils to their surface (**1.62**), whereas the irregular type of pulp stones form by calcification of pre-existing collagen fibre bundles (**1.63**). Some regard the calcifications as a dystrophic change, but these calcifications are not always found in association with degenerative changes. The main clinical significance of pulp calcification lies in the difficulty it can cause during root canal treatment. Sometimes the calcification may be extensive enough to almost obliterate the pulp space (**1.64, 1.65**). These changes may make the location and negotiation of canals difficult. Furthermore, dislodged stones may be pushed apically to cause a blockage. Irregular calcification in the canal also has the potential to harbour bacteria and make their elimination more difficult.

TREATMENT OF THE 'COMPROMISED' PULP

From the foregoing discussion, as long as the pulp–dentine complex remains physiologically intact and functional, the pulp is likely to maintain its ability to recover after restorative procedures. The pulp, therefore, becomes compromised when the pulp–dentine complex is damaged beyond functional repair or is anatomically breached. The treatment of the pulp compromised by exposure or near exposure due to deep caries or trauma may either involve attempts at its preservation by pulp therapy or elective sacrifice by pulpectomy and root canal treatment. The choice of approach is based on the operator's perception of the chance of success and long-term prognosis given by the options. This decision is also likely to be significantly

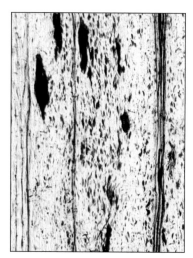

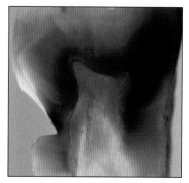

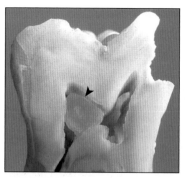

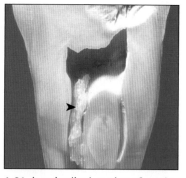

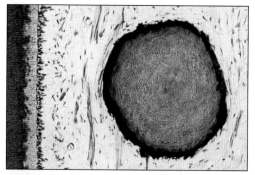

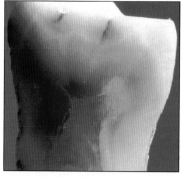

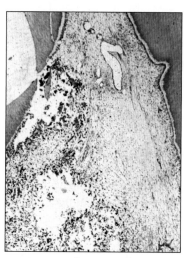

1.60 Longitudinal section of tooth, showing a large round stone in the pulp chamber

1.61 Longitudinal section of tooth: note irregular calcification in the root canal

1.62 Calcified stone in the pulp chamber

1.63 Irregular calcifications in the radicular pulp

1.64 Almost complete obliteration of pulp space by calcification

1.65 Another example of almost complete obliteration of pulp space

1.66 Necrotic/inflamed pulp below pulp exposure

influenced by the overall treatment-planning considerations. A single tooth in an otherwise intact arch, to be restored with a plastic restorative material provides opportunity for convenient review and lends itself to a conservative approach. A tooth scheduled for a cast restoration, on the other hand, provides more limited scope for review and root canal treatment may be more pragmatic.

In a case where there are no overriding restorative considerations, the choice between preservation of the pulp or its extirpation is guided by the clinician's preconceptions about pulp therapy derived from his teachers and their early clinical experience. In this respect two schools of thought appear to have arisen, one believes in the viability of the pulp and its preservation and the other in its inherent susceptibility to long-term failure. Members of the latter school of thought argue that the success rates of primary root canal treatment on teeth with vital pulps are higher (95%). They would further state that irregular calcification and internal resorption in the canal treated by pulp therapy might render root canal treatment more difficult at a later stage. Furthermore, they would claim that the potential for pulp death and infection could reduce the chances of success of delayed root canal treatment down to 85%. The only circumstance in which they would advocate pulp therapy is in the treatment of an incompletely formed root.

Proponents of pulp therapy on the other hand would offer success rates of 85–90% for these procedures if the cases are properly selected and executed and they would counter the evidence for pulp calcification and significant internal resorption. In addition, in its strong favour, a tooth with a preserved vital pulp may be considered to be less susceptible to fracture.

RATIONALE FOR PULP THERAPY

Procedures designed to preserve the pulp have been labelled, *indirect pulp capping, direct pulp capping* and *pulpotomy*. The rationale behind and consequences of these procedures should be properly understood before they are used.

A potentially compromised pulp may present itself in a variety of ways. The pulp may be breached or nearly breached because of caries, tooth surface loss, acute traumatic injury or cavity preparation. In each case the operator has to estimate the pre-existing state of the pulp, the extent of pulp injury and the degree of microbial contamination. In the case of an acute or chronic (tooth surface loss) traumatic injury, the hard tissue wound is clearly seen and its history will reveal the extent of damage at the surface. The nature of the acute injury will give an indication of the probable damage to the pulp and its chances of success. When dealing with a deep carious lesion, the picture is less clear as the extent of the carious lesion in its proximity to the pulp will not be clear. Its acute or chronic nature will provide some insight into the degree of pulp injury as judged by loss of odontoblasts and inflammation. Estimation of the degree of damage is made by a number of clinical assessments. The first assessment is to judge the histological state of the pulp. This judgement is made on the history of pain, examination findings, pulp tests and radiographs. The poor correlation between the histopathology of the pulp and clinical signs and symptoms leaves the operator with an educated guess. Despite this, it has often been stated that teeth exhibiting no history of pain or signs of periapical disease stand a good chance of success following pulpal therapy. The second assessment is to estimate the proximity of the carious lesion to the pulp and lastly to guess the extent to which the superficial pulp may be necrotic and contaminated by bacteria (**1.66**).

The aim of the treatment is to remove all infected hard or soft tissue and to restore the tooth with a bacteria-tight restoration in order to preserve the health of the residual pulp tissue.

Types of pulp therapy

Indirect pulp capping

This clinical procedure (**1.67–1.71**) has drawn some controversy in recent years. The technique is used when excavation of all the

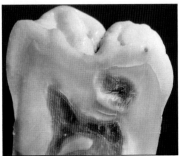

1.67

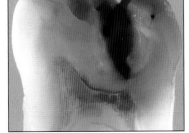

1.68

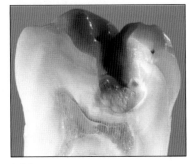

1.69

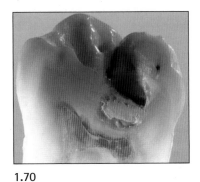

1.70

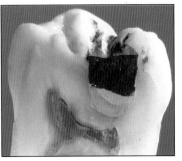

1.71

1.67–1.71
Indirect pulp capping

carious dentine from the pulpal surface might risk a traumatic breach in the pulp through the thin but sound dentine overlying the pulp (**1.67**). When such an eventuality is predicted clinically, some of the carious dentine over the pulp (not peripherally) is left (**1.68**) and dressed with calcium hydroxide to kill residual bacteria and to encourage remineralization and dentine repair (**1.69**). This is followed by the application of a layer of zinc oxide/eugenol to prevent microbial leakage (**1.70**). The tooth is then restored with a permanent material that excludes microbial leakage so that the lesion does not become reactivated (**1.71**). If an adhesive composite material is to be used then resin-reinforced glass ionomer cement may be more suitable. Neither zinc oxide/eugenol nor resin-reinforced glass ionomers should be applied directly to deep dentine because of their potential to cause odontoblast and pulp injury. After this, if there are no clinical symptoms and the tooth shows signs of continuing vitality, two alternatives have been suggested. One is to restore the tooth permanently. The second is to remove the dressing after an arbitrary period of 3 months to excavate the residual carious dentine in the hope that secondary or reactionary dentine formation in the intervening period would prevent exposure. This latter approach is not supported by the rate of secondary dentine formation. At 3 μm per day, only 0.27 mm of dentine would be formed in three months, perhaps an inadequate thickness to prevent a traumatic exposure.

A practical problem with this technique is that it is difficult to gauge the residual depth of the carious lesion. An unacceptable thickness of carious dentine may be left behind together with necrotic pulp tissue adjacent to the lesion (**1.72**). It has been suggested that the accepted guideline that dentine softening and staining precede bacterial invasion may not be completely valid and that bacterial invasion of hard dentine is a distinct possibility. Indirect pulp capping is therefore an unpredictable procedure. Success relies on the correct diagnosis of the pulp condition and leaving only a small amount of carious dentine, covered by an anti-bacterial lining material.

Direct pulp capping

Successful treatment of pulp exposures is guided by the same prerequisites of healthy pulp, low bacterial contamination and absence of subsequent microbial leakage. When excavation of deep caries leads to a traumatic exposure of the pulp, relatively minor bacterial contamination of the pulp tissue is assumed. Pulps left exposed to salivary contamination for several hours following traumatic injury may still be successfully pulp-capped. Minor contamination of the exposure by saliva during the operative procedures is unlikely to affect the outcome. The most important factor in the successful outcome is a healthy pulp (minimally inflamed and capable of replacing lost odontoblasts). The pulp is likely to be healthier in younger teeth and although it has been demonstrated that the success rates may be higher in such teeth, age is not always a good prognostic indicator.

Direct pulp capping (**1.73–1.78**) involves good isolation of the tooth to control the field preferably by rubber dam. The cavity should be carie free and the pulp wound should ideally be fresh and gently exuding blood or serum (**1.75**). This is followed by gentle

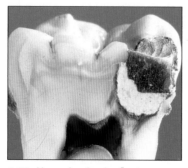

1.72 Necrosis of pulp due to microleakage

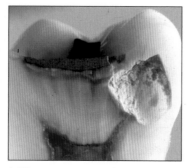

1.73

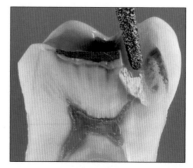

1.74

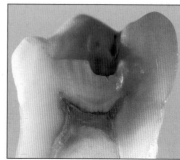

1.75

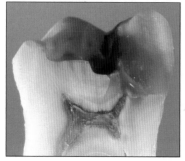

1.76

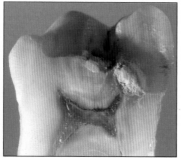

1.77

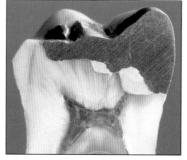

1.78

1.73–1.78
Direct pulp capping

washing of the exposed pulp surface with sterile water or saline to remove any contaminants, debris and dentine chips. The surface may be decontaminated by washing with a 0.5% solution of sodium hypochlorite. This will help to achieve haemostasis but if bleeding persists haemostasis is achieved using wet cotton pellets with most of the moisture removed, dry pellets may cause continued bleeding on removal. Continued profuse bleeding for over approximately five minutes (**1.79**) is a sign of severe pulp inflammation and a more radical approach to treatment should be considered. Once bleeding has stopped the surface of the wound is dressed with a setting or non-setting calcium hydroxide material (**1.76**). It is important that this is placed over vital tissue and not a blood clot. This is then covered with a zinc oxide/eugenol base to eliminate microbial leakage to the exposure (**1.77**). If a composite restorative material is to be used a resin-modified glass ionomer may be considered as an alternative base over the calcium hydroxide. The permanent, well-adapted restorative material is then placed (**1.78**).

There does not appear to be a relationship between the size of the exposure and the success rate, even though it was firmly believed at one time that the larger the exposure the poorer the prognosis. It may be expected that carious exposures would have a lower success rate but studies indicate that in the absence of previous pulpal symptoms, success rates may be similar to those of traumatic exposures. The key elements of successful outcome are good pre-existing potential for replacement of odontoblasts and a good reactionary dentine response in conjunction with an absence of microbial leakage that could compromise healing by causing inflammation.

Pulpotomy

This is the term applied to the removal of coronal pulp tissue when the exposed pulp (**1.80**) is believed to be too severely contaminated by bacteria or inflamed to give a satisfactory prognosis.

The extent of pulp tissue removal is not strictly defined. In the case of fractured teeth with exposed pulps, the pulp surface may exhibit one of two reactions:

- proliferation of the epithelium covered pulp (pulp polyp) where the inflammation is limited to a depth of 2 mm; or
- superficial necrosis with inflammation of the pulp penetrating several millimetres from the exposure site.

The principles of therapy are identical to direct pulp capping except that the exposure is larger and the calcium hydroxide is applied deeper into the root. The aim of the procedure is to remove superficial necrotic pulp tissue down to healthy tissue. Success of the procedure is therefore reliant upon the removal of necrotic and inflamed tissue. It is believed that this is best and most atraumatically achieved with an abrasive diamond bur used at high speed with adequate water cooling in an intermittent light stroking approach to minimize implantation of dentine chips into the exposure (**1.81**). All debris must be removed to achieve a clean wound (**1.82**). After haemostasis is achieved as described above (**1.83**), calcium hydroxide is gently applied without pressure (**1.84**, **1.85**) and is covered with a layer of zinc oxide/eugenol mixed to a thin consistency (**1.86**). Some operators advocate cutting a step in the cavity to support a

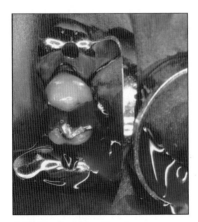

1.79 Profuse bleeding from hyperaemic pulp

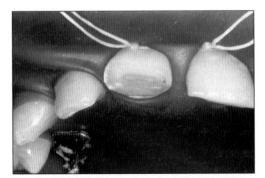

1.80 Pulp exposure due to traumatic fracture

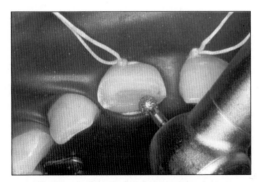

1.81 Removal of superficial necrotic pulp

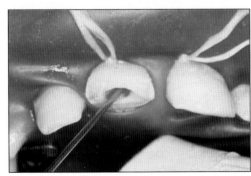

1.82 Irrigating the pulpal wound

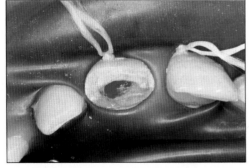

1.83 Haemostasis

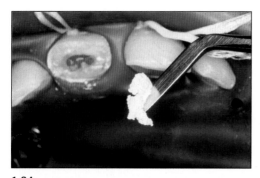

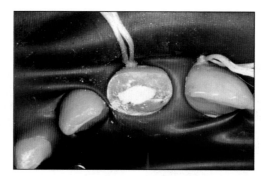

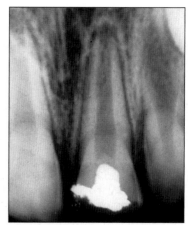

1.86
Zinc oxide/
eugenol
dressing

1.84

1.85

1.84–1.85 Application of calcium hydroxide

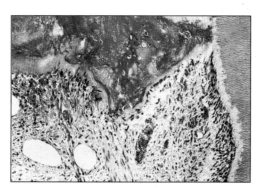

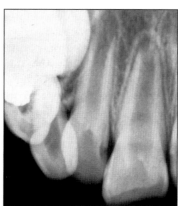

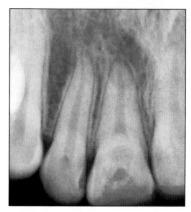

1.88–1.89 Root
formation continues
after successful
pulpotomy

1.87 Calcific bridge formation

1.88

1.89

plastic or Teflon disc on which is placed the zinc oxide/eugenol dressing. As before an alternative is a sub-base of resin-reinforced glass ionomer cement if a composite material is to be used.

ASSESSMENT OF SUCCESS OF PULP THERAPY PROCEDURES

All cases of pulp therapy should be followed up to determine outcome. An initial assessment at between six and twelve weeks is recommended, followed by six- and twelve-monthly reviews. At each examination a history of symptoms is obtained and examination carried out to assess tenderness to palpation of adjacent soft tissues, tenderness to percussion of the tooth, signs of radiographic pulpal and periapical changes and response to vitality tests. However, vitality tests may not be as fruitful in pulpotomized teeth. In the case of pulp capping and pulpotomy additional tests include checking the presence and integrity of the calcific barrier (**1.87**) radiographically and by removal of the dressing and direct probing. Although an initial examination at six weeks has been suggested, this can be modified by the radiographic assessment. If there is no evidence

of a complete bridge formation, the treatment is considered to be a failure and conventional root canal therapy must be considered. In addition in the case of incompletely formed roots there should be radiographic evidence of progressing root formation (**1.88, 1.89**). Once root formation is complete, some believe that it is desirable to carry out root canal treatment in order to avoid the complications of continued calcification of the root canal, which may render the procedure more difficult at a later stage (**1.90, 1.91**). This is not, however, a universally accepted axiom and many consider that the residual pulp would be healthy (**1.92**) and should only be removed if restorative requirements for retention dictate so. **Table 1.2** shows the outcomes of pulp therapy in a number of clinical studies.

Factors affecting outcome of pulp therapy

The most important factors are the pre-existing health of the pulp, adequate removal of infected hard or soft tissues, careful operative technique and elimination of microbial leakage in the final restoration. It can be difficult to gauge the health of the pulp as it is a matter of subjective assessment and relies on experience in pulp

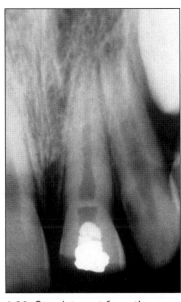

1.90 Complete root formation following pulpotomy

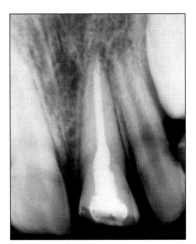

1.91 Elective devitalization following completion of root formation

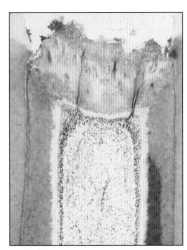

1.92 A pulpotomized tooth with almost normal looking odontoblastic layer and relatively uninflamed pulp. Note the inclusions in the dentine coronal to the pulpotomy.

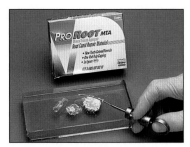

1.93 Mineral trioxide aggregate (MTA)

Table 1.2 Success rates of pulp therapy

Studies	Year of study	Teeth (T)/ cases (C)	Follow-up (years)	Success rate (%)
Shovelton *et al.*	1971	412 (T)	2	69–78 (NP) 50–80 (P)
Haskell *et al.*	1978	149 (C)	5	87
Cvek	1978	60 (T)	3	96
Baume & Holz	1981	110 (C)	4	90
Santini	1983	481 (C)	0.5	75
Horsted *et al.*	1985	510 (T)	5	82
Mejare & Cvek	1993	31 (T)	4	93 (NP)
		6 (T)	4	66 (P)

Key: NP = no pre-existing pain; P = pre-existing pain.

diagnosis. Removal of infected tissue is also a matter of subjective experience but may be aided by various dyes. The final factor is reliant upon the correct choice of restorative material and its adequate manipulation.

Factors such as age and health of the patient, size and nature (carious or traumatic) of pulp exposure, its duration of exposure to the oral environment (up to 48 hours) and the presence of immature root do not in themselves compromise outcomes of pulp therapy.

FUTURE APPROACHES TO PULP THERAPY

Innovation has led to two main new approaches to pulp therapy. One is the extension of adhesive dentistry to pulp capping. It has been suggested that several of the adhesive agents are biocompatible with the pulp tissue which survives following capping. However, these studies are mainly short term and while the approach shows promise there is potential for later failure due to microbial leakage. Given the extensive clinical data currently available for the conventional approaches, described above, it is premature to abandon these procedures in favour of those new methods that, as yet, have little evidence to support them.

Another approach is the use of mineral trioxide aggregate (MTA) (**1.93**) as a pulp capping agent given its biocompatibility with periapical tissues when it is used as a retrograde root-end filling material. The approach is new and shows promise but it may have the disadvantage of staining the tooth and altering its restorative characteristics. MTA needs considerable trial before it can be accepted as a viable routine procedure.

A more promising advent is the recruitment of natural growth factors, harvested from dentine matrix, as agents to encourage the laying down of a more uniform dentine bridge and the formation of the essential replacement pulp–dentine complex. Early experiments show the method may have promise but clinically proven techniques will require some time in development.

References and further reading

Andreason JO, Andreason FM (1994) *Text book and colour atlas of traumatic injuries to the teeth*, 3rd edn. Mosby, Munksgaard, Denmark.

Baume LJ, Holz J (1981) Long term clinical assessment of direct pulp capping. *Int Dent J* **31**, 251–60.

Bender IB, Seltzer S (1972) The effect of periodontal disease on the pulp. *Oral Surg* **33**, 458–74.

Bergenholtz G (2000) Evidence for bacterial causation of adverse pulpal responses in resin-based dental restorations. *Crit Rev Oral Biol Med* **11**(4), 467–80.

Bergenholtz G, Cox CF, Loesche WJ, Syed SA (1982) Bacterial leakage around dental restorations: its effect on the dental pulp. *J Oral Pathol* **11**, 439–50.

Brannstrom M, Lind PO (1965) Pulpal response to early dental caries. *J Dent Res* **44**, 1045–50.

Brannstrom M, Nyborg H (1971) The presence of bacteria in cavities filled with silicate cement and composite resin materials. *Swedish Dent J* **64**, 149–55.

Brannstrom M, Nyborg H (1977) Pulpal reaction to polycarboxylate and zinc phosphate cements used with inlays in deep cavity preparations. *J Am Dent Assoc* **94**, 308–10.

Browne RM, Tobias RS (1986) Microbial microleakage and pulpal inflammation: a review. *Endod Dent Traumatol* **2**, 177–83.

Byers MR, Taylor PE, Khayat BG, Kimberly CL (1990) Effects of injury and inflammation on pulpal and periapical nerves. *J Endod* **16**, 78–84.

Byers MR, Swift ML, Wheeler EF (1992) Reaction of sensory nerves to dental restorative procedures. *Proc Finn Dent Soc* **88** suppl. 1, 73–82.

Cotton WR, Siegel RL (1978) Human pulpal response to citric acid cavity cleanser. *J Am Dent Assoc* **96**, 639–44.

Cox CF (1987) Biocompatibility of dental materials in the absence of bacterial infection. *Oper Dent* **12**(4), 146–52.

Cox CF (1994) Evaluation and treatment of bacterial microleakage. *Am J Dent* **7**, 293–5.

Cox CF, Suzuki S (1994) Re-evaluating pulp protection: calcium hydroxide liners vs cohesive hybridization. *J Am Dent Assoc* **125**, 823–31.

Cox CF, Keall CL, Ostro E, Bergenholtz G (1987) Biocompatibility of surface sealed dental materials against exposed pulps. *J Prosthet Dent* **57**(1), 1–8.

Cvek M (1978) A clinical report on partial pulpotomy and capping with calcium hydroxide in permanent incisors with complicated crown fracture. *J Endod* **4**, 232–7.

Czarnecki RT, Schilder H (1979) A histological evaluation of the human pulp in teeth with varying degrees of periodontal disease. *J Endod* **5**, 242–53.

Dongari A, Lambrianidis T (1988) Periodontally derived pulpal lesions. *Endod Dent Traumatol* **4**, 49–54.

Felton D, Bergenholtz G, Cox CF (1989) Inhibition of bacterial growth under composite restorations following gluma pretreatment. *J Dent Res* **68**(3), 491–5.

Hamilton AI, Kramer IRH (1967) Cavity preparation with and without waterspray. *Br Dent J* **123**, 281–5.

Hartnett JE, Smith WF (1961) The production of heat in the dental pulp by use of the air turbine. *J Am Dent Assoc* **63**, 210–14.

Haskell EW, Stanley HR, Chellemi J, Stringfellow H (1978) Direct pulp capping treatment: a long-term follow-up. *J Am Dent Assoc* **97**, 607–12.

Horsted P, Sondergaard B, Thylstrup A *et al.* (1985) A retrospective study of direct pulp capping with calcium hydroxide compounds. *Endod Dent Traumatol* **1**, 29–34.

Kim S, Edwall L, Trowbridge H, Chien S (1984) Effects of local anaesthetics on pulpal blood flow in dogs. *J Dent Res* **63**, 650–2.

Kramer IRH (1959) Pulp changes of non-bacterial origin. *Int Dent J* **9**, 435–50.

Langeland K (1959) Histologic evaluation of pulp reactions to operative procedures. *Oral Surg, Oral Med, Oral Pathol* **12**, 1235–48.

Langeland K (1961) Effect of various procedures on the human dental pulp. *Oral Surg, Oral Med, Oral Pathol* **14**, 210–33.

Langeland K (1987). Tissue response to dental caries. *Endod Dent Traumatol* **3**, 149–71.

Langeland K, Langeland LK (1965) Pulpal reactions to crown preparations, impression, temporary crown fixation and permanent cementation. *J Prosthet Dent* **15**, 129–42.

Langeland K, Rodrigues H, Dowden W (1974) Periodontal disease, bacteria and pulpal histopathology. *Oral Surg* **37**, 252–70.

Marsland EA, Shovelton DS (1957) The effect of cavity preparation on the human dental pulp. *Br Dent J* **102**(6), 213–22.

Marsland EA, Shovelton DS (1970) Repair in the human dental pulp following cavity preparation. *Arch Oral Biol* **15**, 411–23.

Massler M (1967) Pulpal reaction to dental caries. *Int Dent J* **17**, 441–60.

Mazur B, Kaplowitz B, Massler M (1964) Influence of periodontal disease on the dental pulp. *Oral Surg* **17**, 592–603.

Meister F, Brown RJ, Gerstein H (1980) Endodontic involvement resulting from dental abrasion or erosion. *J Am Dent Assoc* **101**, 651–3.

Mejare B, Mejare I, Edwardsson S (1979) Bacteria beneath composite resotorations – a culturing and histological study. *Acta Odontol Scand* **37**, 267–75.

Mejare I, Mejare B, Edwardson S (1987) Effect of a tight seal on survival of bacteria in saliva-contaminated cavities filled with composite resin. *Endod Dent Traumatol* **3**, 6–9.

Mejare I, Cvek M (1993) Partial pulpotomy in young permanent teeth with deep carious lesions. *Endod Dent Traumatol* **9**, 238–42.

Morrant GA (1977) Dental instrumentation and pulpal injury: Part 1. *J Br Endod Soc* **10**, 3–8 Part 2. *J Br Endod Soc* **10**, 55–62.

Morrant GA, Kramer IRH (1963) The response of the human pulp to cavity preparations using turbine handpieces. *Br Dent J* **115**, 99–110.

Murray PE, Lumley PJ, Smith AJ (2002a) Preserving the vital pulp in operative dentistry: 2. Guidelines for successful restoration of unexposed dentinal lesions. *Dental Update* **29**, 127–35.

Murray PE, Lumley PJ, Smith AJ (2002b) Preserving the vital pulp in operative dentistry: 3. thickness of remaining cavity dentine as a key mediator of pulpal injury and repair responses. *Dental Update* **29**, 172–9.

Murray PE, Lumley PJ, Hafez AA, Cox CF, Smith AJ (2002c) Preserving the vital pulp in operative dentistry: 4. Factors influencing successful pulp capping. *Dental Update* **29**, 225–34.

Nair PNR, Schroeder HE (1995) Number and size spectra of non-myelinated axons of human premolars. *Anat Embryol* **192**, 35–41.

Nixon CE, Saviano JA, King GJ, Keeling SD (1993) Histomorphometric study of dental pulp during orthodontic tooth movement. *J Endod* **19**, 13–16.

Odor TM, Pitt Ford TR, McDonald F (1994) Effect of inferior alveolar nerve block anaesthesia on the lower teeth. *Endod Dent Traumatol* **10**, 144–8.

Ohshima H (1990) Ultrastructural changes in odontoblasts and pulp capillaries following cavity preparation in rat molars. *Arch Histol Cytol* **53**(4), 423–38.

Plamondon TY, Walton R, Graham C, Houston G, Swell G (1990) Pulp response to the combined effects of cavity preparation and periodontal ligament infection. *Oper Dent* **18**, 86–93.

Qvist V (1993) Resin restorations: leakage, bacteria, pulp. *Endod Dent Traumatol* **9**, 127–52.

Reeves R, Stanley HR (1966). The relationship of bacterial penetration and pulpal pathosis in carious teeth. *Oral Surg* **22**(1), 59–65.

Rosenberg PA (1981) Occlusion, the dental pulp, and endodontic treatment. *Dent Clin North Am* **25**, 423–37.

Rubach WC, Mitchell DF (1965) Periodontal disease, accessory canals and pulp pathosis. *J Periodontol* **36**, 34–8.

Rykke M (1992) Dental materials for posterior restorations. *Endod Dent Traumatol* **8**, 139–48.

Santini A (1983) Assessment of the pulpotomy technique in human first permanent mandibular molars. *Br Dent J* **155**, 151–4.

Seltzer S, Bender ID, Ziontz M (1963) The interrelationship of pulp and periodontal disease. *Oral Surg* **16**, 289–301.

Shovelton DS (1976) Pulp Protection. *J Br Endod Soc* **9**, 57.

Shovelton DS, Marsland EA (1958) A further investigation of the effect of cavity preparation on the human dental pulp. *Br Dent J* **103**, 16–27.

Shovelton DS, Friend LA, Kirk EEJ, Rowe AHR (1971) The efficacy of pulp capping materials – a comparative trial. *Br Dent J* **130**, 385–91.

Smith AJ, Murray PE, Lumley PJ (2002) Preserving the vital pulp in operative dentistry: 1. A biological approach. *Dental update* **29**, 64–9.

Spangberg LS, Robertson PB, Levy BM (1982) Pulp effects of electrosurgery involving based and unbased cervical amalgam restorations. *Oral Surg* **59**(6), 678–85.

Stanley HR (1996) Trashing the dental literature – misleading the general practitioners. A point of view. Guest editorial. *J Dent Res* **75**(9), 1624–6.

Stanley HR, Pereira JC, Spiegel E, Broom C, Schultz M (1983) The detection and prevalence of reactive and physiology sclerotic dentine, reparative dentine and dead tracts beneath various types of dental lesions according to tooth surface and age. *J Pathol* **12**, 257–89.

Suzuki M, Goto G, Jordan RE (1973) Pulpal response to pin placement. *J Am Dent Assoc* **87**, 636–40.

Ten Cate AR (1994) *Oral Histology – development, structure and function*, 4th edn. Mosby, St Louis, USA.

Tronstad L, Langeland K (1971) Effect of attrition on subjacent dentin and pulp. *J Dent Res* **51**, 17–30.

Trowbridge HO (1981) Pathogenesis of pulpitis resulting from dental caries. *J Endod* **7**, 52–60.

Turner DF, Marfurt CF, Sattelberg C (1989) Demonstration of physiological barrier between pulpal odotoblasts and its perturbation following routine restorative procedures: a horse-radish tracing study in the rat. *J Dent Res* **68**, 1262–8.

Vojinovic O, Nyborg H, Brannstrom M (1973) Acid treatment of cavities under resin fillings. Bacterial growth in dentinal tubules and pulpal reactions. *J Dent Res* **52**(6), 1189–93.

Chapter 2

Biological and clinical rationale for root canal treatment

K Gulabivala

The boundary between infection of the dying pulp tissue and inflammation of the remaining pulp tissue may progress towards the periradicular tissues via the intercommunicating lateral canals and apical foramina. An understanding of the process of spread of infection and inflammation, their establishment in the periradicular tissues and treatment must begin with knowledge of the normal structure and physiology of the involved tissues.

THE PERIRADICULAR TISSUES

These consist of:

1. Cementum.
2. Periodontal ligament.
3. Alveolar bone.

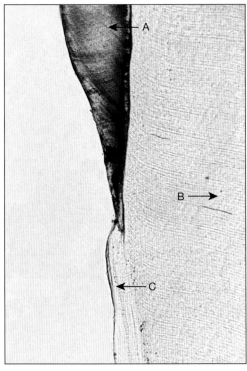

2.1 Ground section showing the relationship between cementum, radicular dentine and enamel:
A = enamel;
B = dentine;
C = cementum

Cementum

Cementum covers the radicular dentine (**2.1**). It abuts the enamel in 70%, overlaps it in 20% and is separated from it by a gap in about 10% of the teeth, which may help explain cervical sensitivity in young teeth without abrasion. The cementum is principally an inorganic tissue which is more impervious than dentine. It is because of this property of cementum that root canal treatment is at all possible. It consists of three types of cemental tissue: (1) cellular; (2) acellular; and (3) intermediate.

Cellular cementum contains cementocytes (**2.2**) that communicate with each other via canaliculi and also with dentine. It is usually found in the apical and furcation regions of the tooth. Sharpey's fibres may be found embedded in cellular cementum (**2.3**).

Acellular cementum (2.4) forms the innermost layer and is devoid of cells. It covers almost the whole root surface in a thin hyaline layer which has incremental lines running parallel to the root surface. It contains closely packed periodontal fibres (Sharpey's fibres) that are mineralized.

Intermediate cementum is found in the region of the cemento–dentinal junction, which has the characteristics of both cementum and dentine. Near the enamel it may have characteristics of aprismatic enamel.

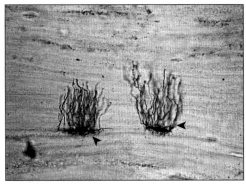

2.2 Cementocytes in cellular cementum (arrowed)

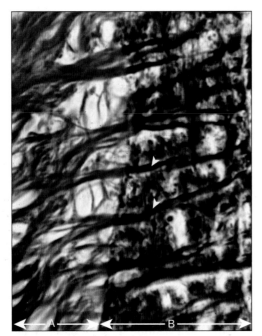

2.3 Sharpey's fibres in cementum (arrowed):
A = unmineralized tissue; B = mineralized tissue

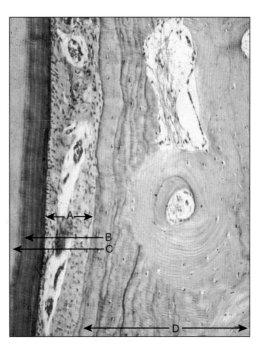

2.4 Cementum; dentine, periodontal ligament
and alveolar bone: A = periodontal ligament;
B = acellular cementum; C = dentine;
D = alveolar bone

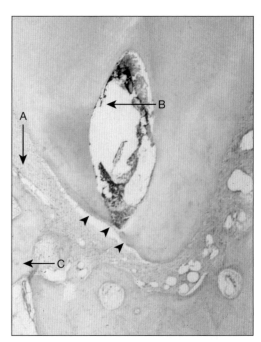

2.5 Healing of periapex with cementum
formation (arrowed): A = periodontal ligament;
B = root canal; C = alveolar bone (courtesy of
Prof. T Pitt Ford)

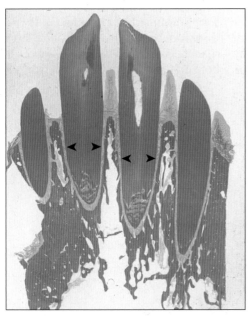

2.6 Periodontal ligament supporting teeth in
alveolar bone (arrowed)

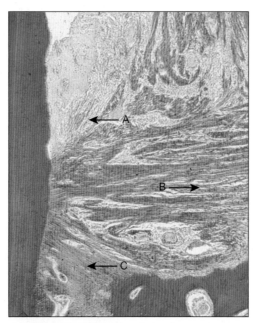

2.7 Gingival, transeptal and alveolar crest
fibres – longitudinal view: A = gingival fibres;
B = transeptal fibres; C = alveolar crest fibres

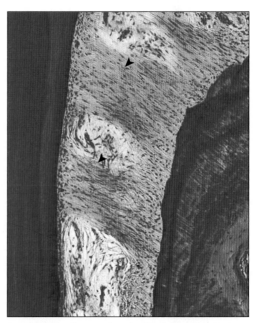

2.8 Oblique fibres – longitudinal view

Functions

Functions of cementum include attachment, tooth wear compensation and repair.

Cementum provides the attachment for the periodontal ligament fibres which suspend the tooth from the alveolar bone. It is laid down through life in compensation for loss of occlusal tooth substance and plays a most important physiologic role in the repair of resorbed cementum and dentine. The breakdown in this normal mechanism may result in external root resorption which may manifest clinically if extensive enough. Cementum formation around the apical foramina is thought to be a desirable end result of successful healing following root canal treatment (**2.5**).

Periodontal ligament

Periodontal ligament is a dense fibrous connective tissue which supports and attaches the tooth to its alveolar socket (**2.6**). Its principle component is collagen, which is embedded in a gel-like matrix. The fibres are arranged in specific groups with individual functions. These include *gingival*, *trans-septal*, *alveolar crest* (**2.7**), *horizontal*, *oblique* (**2.8**, **2.9**) and *apical* fibres. Another important component is the *oxytalan* fibre. Functional adaptation may take place in the broad zone known as the *intermediate plexus* (**2.10**). The main cells are fibroblasts and occasional defence cells. The *root sheath of Hertwig*, which helps in the formation of the root, does not involve completely after completion of root formation but degenerates into what resembles a perforated bag of epithelial cells (**2.11**), called the *rests of Malassez* (**2.12**). The perforations are quite large and the intercommunicating strands of epithelial tissue may not all be seen in a given histological section. These cells can proliferate when stimulated by inflammation to form a cyst. They also produce cytokines and participate in the apical defence response.

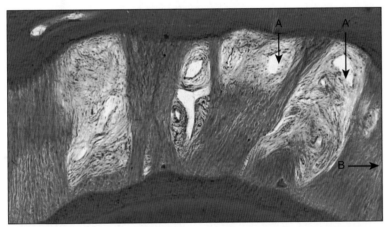

2.9 Oblique fibres – transverse view: A = polyhedric spaces containing blood vessels; B = ligament fibres

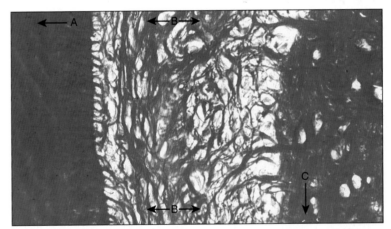

2.10 Intermediate plexus: A = dentine; B = intermediate plexus; C = alveolar bone

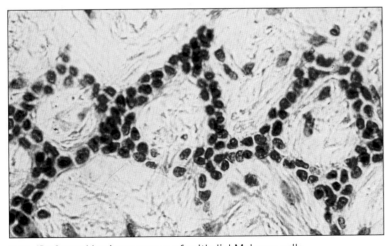

2.11 'Perforated bag' appearance of epithelial Malassez cells

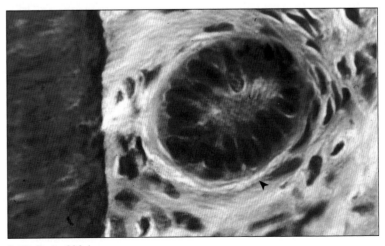

2.12 Rest of Malassez

Blood supply

Blood supply to the periodontal ligament originates from the inferior dental artery. Arterioles enter the ligament near the apex of the root and from the lateral aspects of the alveolar socket and branch into capillaries within the ligament in a polyhedric pattern along the long axis of the root (**2.9**). The collagen fibres run through the polyhedral spaces. The blood vessels are located closer to the bone than to the cementum. Communications between the vasculature of the pulp and periodontal ligament may be evident, especially near the root apex and furcation (**2.13**). Venules drain to the apex or through apertures in the bony wall of the socket and into the marrow spaces.

Nerve supply

Nerve bundles enter the periodontal ligament through numerous foramina in the alveolar bone. They branch and end in small rounded bodies near the cementum. The nerves carry pain, touch and pressure sensations and form an important part of the feedback mechanism of the masticatory apparatus.

Functions

The ligament has a proprioceptive function and acts as a viscoelastic cushion by virtue of its fibres and hydraulic fluid systems (blood vessels and their communications with vessel reservoirs in the bone marrow and the interstitial fluid of the ligament). The ligament has great adaptive capacity. It responds to functional over-loading by widening to relieve the load on the tooth (**2.14–2.17**). The radiographs in **2.14** and **2.15** show the same tooth before and after placement of a crown with a premature occlusal contact: in **2.15** the periodontal ligament space is noticeably wider. **Figure 2.16** shows a histological view of a disused tooth with a lack of proper orientation of fibres in a narrow ligament. **Figure 2.17** shows the periodontal ligament of a tooth under heavy occlusal load, with evidence of adjacent bone resorption causing the ligament to widen; this widening should be distinguished from that which occurs in response to pathological irritation. The periodontal ligament also plays an important part in the eruption of teeth and healing, for example following surgery or trauma. Vascular communications between the pulp and periodontium form pathways for transmission of inflammation and microorganisms between the tissues.

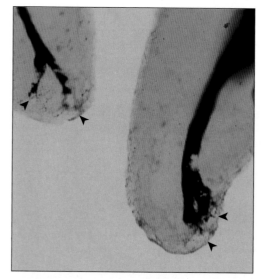

2.13 Vascular communications at the root apex

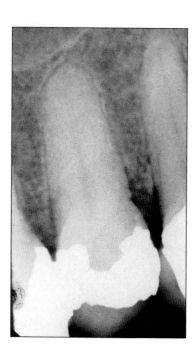

2.14 Normal periodontal ligament

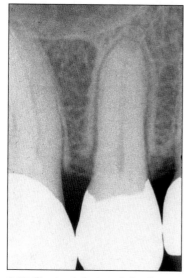

2.15 The tooth in 2.14 following crown placement. Premature occlusal contact caused overloading and widening of periodontal ligament

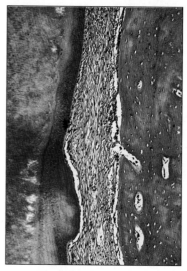

2.16 Disused periodontal ligament. Note the lack of proper orientation of fibres in a narrow ligament

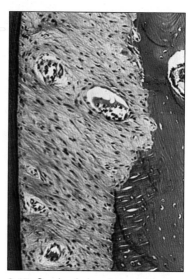

2.17 Overloaded periodontal ligament with oblique fibre orientation and resorption of bone

Alveolar bone

Alveolar bone is that part of the maxilla and mandible which supports the teeth by forming the other attachment for fibres of the periodontal ligament (**2.18**). It consists of two plates of *cortical bone* separated by *spongy bone* (**2.19**). In some areas the alveolar bone is thin with no spongy bone (**2.18**). The alveolar bone and the cortical plates are thickest in the mandible. The spaces between the trabeculae of the spongy bone are filled with marrow, which consists of haematopoietic tissue in early life and of fatty tissue later (**2.19**). The shape and structure of the trabeculae reflect the stress-bearing requirements of the particular site. The surfaces of the inorganic parts of the bone are lined by *osteoblasts* which are responsible for bone formation: those which become incorporated within the mineral tissue are called *osteocytes* and maintain contact with each other via canaliculi; *osteoclasts* are responsible for bone resorption and may be seen in the *Howship's lacunae* (**2.20**). Cortical bone adjacent to the ligament gives the radiographic appearance of a dense white line next to the dark line of the ligament (**2.14, 2.15**). Bone is a dynamic tissue, continually forming and resorbing in response to functional requirements. In addition to such local response to needs, bone metabolism is under hormonal control. It is easily resorbed under the influence of inflammatory mediators at either the periapex or the marginal attachment. In health the crest of the alveolus lies about 2 mm apical to the cemento–enamel junction (**2.21**) but in periodontal disease it may lie much more towards the apex of the root.

AETIOLOGY OF PERIAPICAL DISEASE

A historical perspective

Recognition of the role of bacteria in the pathogenesis of periapical disease was interrupted by many digressions and problems, both scientific and political.

The importance of this heritage is that the 'cultural' attitudes amongst members of this discipline have shaped modern endodontics. Fashions continue to dominate the cycles of change that have seen either biomechanical or biological aspects alternate in apparent importance. Overall though dentists identify more closely with biomechanical reasoning and therefore the biological rationale has been neglected to a greater extent (Noyes 1922, Naidorf 1972).

One aim of this chapter is to correct that balance and side with the biological truth.

In 1697, Anthonie van Leeuwenhoek became the first person to describe bacteria from root canals using one of the earliest versions of the microscope (see Dobell 1960). It was almost 200 years before Willoughby Dayton Miller (1894), working in Robert Koch's laboratory, observed, by the use of a microscope, the presence of a variety of organisms in samples obtained from root canals of diseased teeth. Interestingly, he also noted that cultivation of the samples revealed a much simpler flora leading him to predict that the sampled root canal bacteria would be difficult to cultivate in the

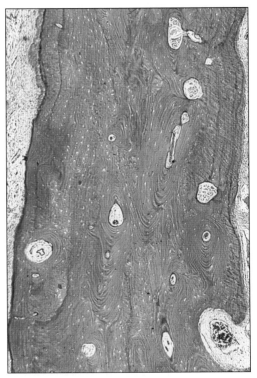

2.18 Alveolar bone

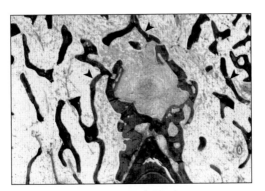

2.19 Trabeculae in spongy bone

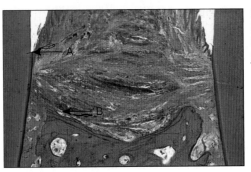

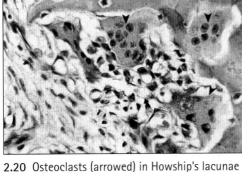

2.20 Osteoclasts (arrowed) in Howship's lacunae

2.21 Relationship between alveolar bone and cementoenamel junction in health: A = cementoenamel junction; B = alveolar bone

laboratory. Over a hundred years later, potentially uncultured bacteria in root canal systems of teeth with periapical disease remain undefined.

The practice of root canal treatment suffered a severe setback for almost 40 years as a result of a hypothesized association between oral focal sepsis and systemic illness. This link, originally made by WD Miller in 1891, was popularized by a British physician, William Hunter addressing the medical faculty of the McGill University (1911). The dental profession presided over the wholesale extraction of teeth in preference to root canal treatment for many years to come. Much research effort has gone into attempting to prove or refute the hypothesis. Paradoxically, incontrovertible proof for both putative relationships; that between bacterial infection of the root canal system and periapical disease and also that between periapical infection and systemic illness, was confounded by shortcomings in the bacterial sampling and cultivation techniques. Even though the sterility of the normal pulp had been established (Henrici & Hartzel 1919), others studying extracted, intact and previously healthy teeth had managed to recover bacteria. This was later attributed to ineffective decontamination procedures and the possible pumping of bacteria from the tooth socket into the vital pulps during tooth extraction. Conversely, those studying the bacterial flora associated with periapical disease were not able to recover bacteria from all teeth. A clear-cut relationship between the presence of bacteria and periapical disease was therefore not obvious and it was concluded that factors other than bacteria might be involved in the pathogenesis of periapical disease.

Aetiological factors implicated

Initial uncertainty about the bacterial origin of periapical disease gave room for other theories to become established first.

Stagnant tissue fluid

The most influential of these theories was the so-called 'hollow tube theory', propounded by Rickert and Dixon (1931) and appears to be propagated even today by some teachers. The theory, based on macroscopic observations of tubes and solid rods implanted in the backs of rabbits (halo of irritation on the skin), suggested that hollow tubes would not be tolerated by the body because circulatory elements and tissue fluid stagnating in the tubes would irritate the tissues. The theory was conclusively disproved using similar methodology that corrected the errors of the previous work. Clinical observations have confirmed the absence of periapical response to tissue fluid in root canals.

Necrotic pulp tissue

Necrotic pulp tissue was also implicated as a cause of periapical disease and further that autolysing pulp tissue in dentinal tubules may cause root resorption. Once again, opposing evidence showed these theories to be untrue: polyethylene tubes with muscle tissue implanted in the backs of rats caused minimal inflammation and was made significantly worse only by bacterial contamination. Clinical evidence from traumatized teeth confirmed the absence of reaction to necrotic pulp tissue, where no periapical disease was noted in the absence of bacteria, despite an interval of two to six years between the traumatic episode that caused pulp necrosis and the root canal sampling. Histological studies have also shown growth of connective tissue and formation of cementum-like hard tissue on root canal walls after a seven-month exposure of apical tissues to necrotic pulp tissue.

Bacterial products

Bacterial products, such as sialic acid, M protein, various enzymes, cell-capsule and cell-wall constituents, and particularly lipopolysaccharide (LPS), have been implicated in initiation of periapical disease. A positive correlation between the presence of LPS and periapical lesions and/or symptoms has been confirmed in many studies.

Viruses

The role of viruses in the pathogenesis of periapical disease has been considered but no definitive evidence found.

Bacteria

The credit for demonstrating a definitive causal association between bacterial infection and periapical lesion development is given to Kakehashi *et al.* (1965), who compared the pulpal and periapical reactions to experimental pulp exposure in germ-free and conventional rats. The teeth in the former case exhibited healing, while the latter showed pulp necrosis and periapical lesion development. The causal relationship between root canal infection and periapical disease was further consolidated when no cultivable bacteria were recovered from traumatized, intact teeth with an absence of periapical disease, using validated, strict anaerobic techniques for sampling and cultivation. In contrast, samples from 18 out of 19 teeth associated with periapical disease gave positive cultures, revealing over 90% strict anaerobes (Sundqvist 1976).

Host factors implicated

Periapical disease is the result of interaction between bacteria (and their products) and the host defences. Both the non-specific and specific branches of host defences are recruited to defend against the potential invasion of the body by bacteria. The periapical lesion is, therefore, the retreat of the bone tissue away from the source of infection, creating space for the body's defensive elements to migrate into the immediate vicinity of the infection to counter it (**2.22**).

Most of the information on the composition of periapical lesions is based on histopathology of long-standing lesions of unknown activity and often undefined clinical status. The full range of immune mechanisms is implicated in the development of the periapical lesion (**2.23**).

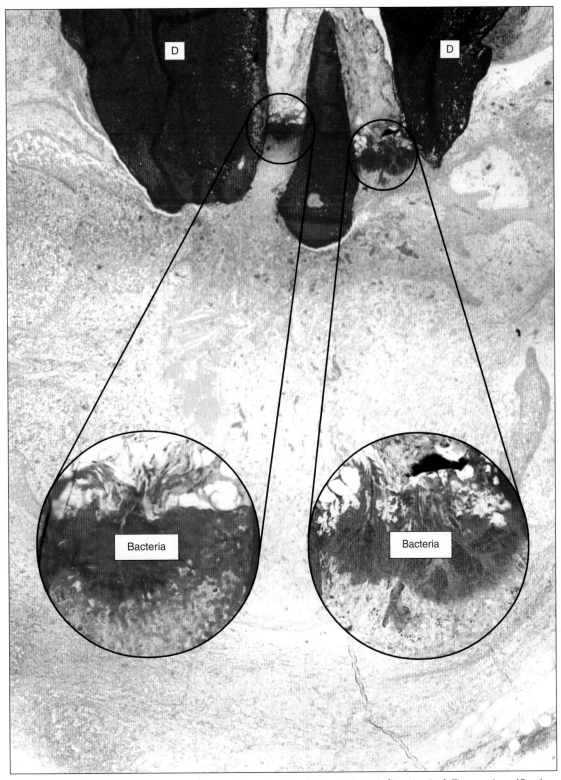

2.22 Bacteria at the apical foramen of a tooth affected with apical periodontitis (D = dentine). The canal ramifications on the right and left, clogged with bacteria, are magnified in the circular insets. Note the strategic location of the bacterial clusters at the apical foramina. The bacterial mass appears to be held back by a distinct wall of neutrophilic granulocytes. Obviously, any surgical and/or microbial sampling procedures of the periapical tissue would contaminate the sample with the intraradicular flora: magnification: × 65, insets × 340 (courtesy of Dr PNR Nair)

The clinical course of the periapical lesion is variable, giving many presentations that have been classified into: acute apical periodontitis; chronic apical periodontitis; acute periapical abscess or suppuration (without sinus tract); chronic periapical abscess or suppuration (with sinus tract); and radicular cysts (World Health Organization 1995). The relative contribution of the normal inflammatory and immune responses varies in these clinical variants. The essential nature of the lesion (except in the incipient lesion) is chronic inflammatory (or granulomatous) tissue, meaning that the two principle elements, inflammation and attempts at healing are coexistent. Depending on the state of the lesion there may be a variable degree of tissue destruction, with the consequent concentration of polymorphonuclear leucocytes (PMNs) and macrophages in the vicinity of the apical foramina (**2.22**).

Chronic inflammation implies a persistence of the irritant stimulus (bacteria and their products), in this case, because of the protective sanctuary of the root canal system, which the host defences can access only to a limited degree. Therefore, in addition to the ubiquitous PMNs and macrophages, a small population of eosinophils and mast cells, various proportions of the immune (lymphocyte and plasma) cells are also evident (**2.24**). Epithelial cells may be present in variable proportions (up to 50%) as arcades of proliferating cells that may help to form a barrier across the apical foramina, as part of sinus tracts or as the lining of developing cysts (**2.25**). Other tissue elements found in the periapical lesion include, endothelial cells and fibroblasts, both being found where there are attempts at healing.

The three-dimensional distribution of these cellular elements is thought by same to fall into zones (**2.26**), based on an animal model of bone infection but others clearly refute this concept, believing the cellular distribution to be too random for discrete zone separation. Perhaps both views are correct and the latter is merely a reflection of repeated acute exacerbations.

Earlier studies concentrated on the proportions of different cell types in the periapical lesions to gain insight into the types of reactions prevalent but there is a limit to the inferences that can be drawn. Later studies focused on the phenotypic evaluation of cell surface markers (CD receptors) using monoclonal antibodies to define the relative proportion of cell subsets giving insight into their roles in the progression of the lesion. The periapical lesion is T-lymphocyte dominated although B lymphocytes are also present. The relative proportions of T and B lymphocytes may be dependent on the nature of the lesion, the T/B cell ratio being significantly higher in lesions containing radicular cysts than granulomas and apical scar lesions. Plasma cells actively producing antibodies locally have been shown by *in situ* hybridization of messenger RNA that codes for protein expression.

The neural and immune systems also interact in controlling the non-specific and specific defensive responses and it is also possible that microorganisms participate in this regulatory function. The ultimate goal is to decipher the mechanisms involved so that a model can be constructed that describes the entire sequence of interactions between the cellular (microbial and host) and neural components leading to the progressive development of the stable but dynamic periapical lesion. This requires synthesis of information from human and animal studies at both cellular and molecular levels. The molecular components implicated include: cytokines (including interleukins, tumour necrosis factors and colony-stimulating factors); interferons; arachidonic acid and metabolites; matrix metallo-proteinases; adhesion molecules; kinins; complement

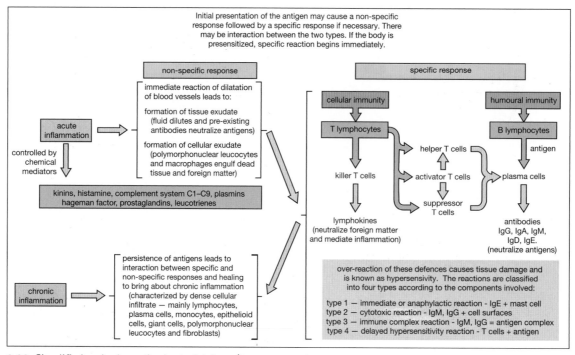

2.23 Simplified and schematic chart of defence/immune reactions

system; fibrinolytic peptides; vasoactive amines; lysosomal enzymes; prostaglandins; leukotrienes; and neuropeptides. The mechanisms coordinating these elements have not yet been elucidated although it is known that some of them function as cascades.

The neuropeptides implicated include: calcitonin gene-related peptide (CGRP); substance P; vasoactive intestinal polypeptides; dopamine hydrolase; and neuropeptide Y. The most interesting among these is the possible role of CGRP, which has been implicated both in the response to pulp and periapical injury (**2.27**).

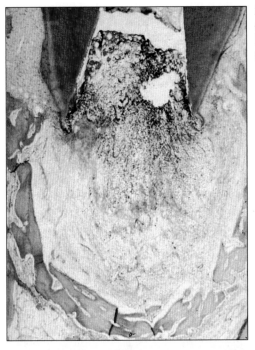

2.24 Gross structure of a periapical lesion. Note zonal distribution of cellular types

MODEL OF PATHOGENESIS AND NATURAL HISTORY OF PERIAPICAL DISEASE

The precise pathological mechanisms involved in the genesis of the periradicular lesion are unclear, so a *'synthesized' model of the possible sequence of events is proposed from the available information*. Initially it is assumed that an undefined, polymicrobial infection stimulates the host response, the relevance of its composition and pathogenicity are discussed later.

The pathogenesis of periapical lesions has been studied in a variety of animal models by artificial induction. The models include: rats; rabbits; dogs; ferrets; cats; and monkeys (**2.28, 2.29**). The findings are interpreted with caution because the microbial flora and host responses may be different from the human condition.

As the root canal infection develops and matures, it progresses apically in the root canal until certain, as yet undefined, elements either bacterial products or bacteria themselves are in a position to stimulate the periapical tissues via the apical foramina (**2.30**). In a previously unexposed host, the initial response will be a non-specific acute inflammation, consisting of a fluid exudate followed by a cellular exudate (principally PMNs). The PMNs are attracted to the site by a number

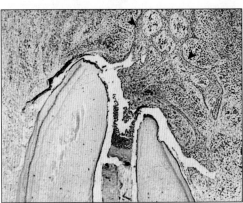

2.25 Proliferation of epithelial tissue adjacent to the apical foramen

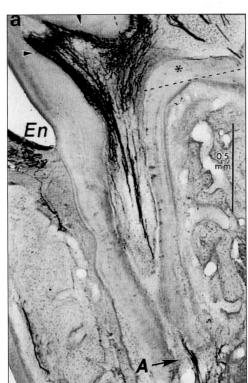

2.27 Immunocytochemical section showing calcitonin gene–related peptide (CGRP) nerve fibres in pulp horns and also extending to the apical (A) part of the root canal: En = enamel (Byers *et al.* 1990)

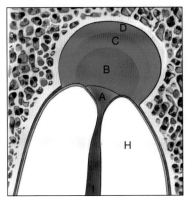

2.26 Zones of Fish: A = zone of infection; B = zone of contamination; C = zone of irritation; D = zone of stimulation; E = alveolar bone; F = periodontal ligament; G = cementum; H = dentine; I = root canal

of bacteria-derived chemo-attractants, such as the peptide F-Met-Leu-Phe that constitutes the amino terminus of many bacterial proteins. In a previously exposed host, this initial exudate will also bring with it any circulating antibodies that may be present. The PMN migration would also then be further stimulated by activation of complements C3b and C5a via antigen–antibody-complex formation. The overall effect of pre-existing immunity is better confinement of the bacteria to their source (apical foramina), requiring only a sparse cellular infiltrate to deal with them and a fibro-encapsulation of the rich granulation tissue (**2.31**). In contrast, lack of pre-existing immunity results in poorer bacterial confinement as well as that of the cellular infiltrate, which is

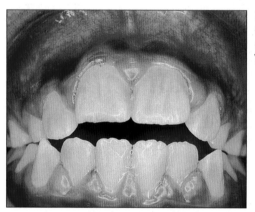

2.28 Monkey's oral cavity used in experiments by Valderhaug (1974)

more diffuse and spread into the trabecular system. These histological pictures translate into radiographic views of well circumscribed, smaller, and better-demarcated periapical radiolucencies compared to more diffuse and extensive lesions, respectively. The acute response may be accompanied by the usual clinical signs of pain, tenderness on percussion and tooth elevation, but it may also be too transient and minimal to be noticed. So far little bone resorption is likely to have taken place and no radiographic changes would be discernible.

Since the bacteria and their products are not removed, because of their seclusion in the root canal system, a delayed immune response is mounted and the specific immune response commences. These responses are mediated by direct stimulation of the host cells by the bacteria and their products as well as cascade triggers from subsequent responses.

Depending upon the nature of the stimulus and host susceptibility, a whole range of effects may be manifested, including Type 1–4 hypersensitivity reactions (**2.23**). The magnitude of the response varies from individual to individual, depending upon both the stimulus and the host characteristics. In some cases the host response may be exaggerated causing greater damage than the bacterial assault.

The clinical progression of the lesion may take one of several paths, including: acute apical abscess formation, an intensely painful event until bone resorption relieves some of the tissue pressure; chronic suppuration with sinus tract formation; or conversion to a chronic, stable but dynamic state.

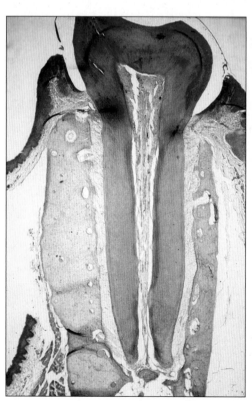

2.29 Monkey model of apical periodontitis (Valderhaug 1974)

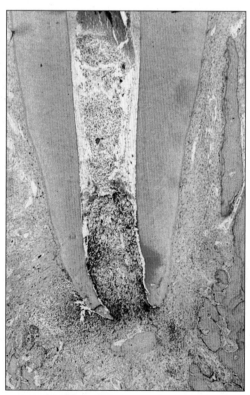

2.30 Apical progression of root canal infection and establishment of apical granuloma (Valderhaug 1974)

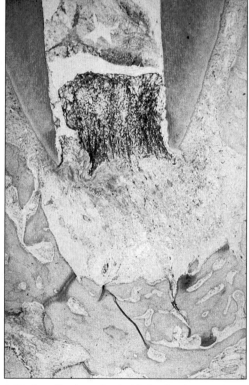

2.31 Localization of apical infection by a well-defined granuloma

In the event of bacteria entering the periapical tissues, they would normally be removed rapidly by PMNs and macrophages; the latter release leukotrienes and prostaglandins. The former class of these molecules attract more macrophages to the site and the latter contribute to bone resorption, creating space for invasion by more immune cells. The activated macrophages also continue to produce a variety of other mediators of inflammation, including interleukin 1 (IL-1), tumour necrosis factor-α (TNF-α) and chemotactic factors such as interleukin 8 (IL-8). These cytokines intensify the local vascular response, osteoclastic bone resorption, and can provoke a general alert by endocrine stimulation of fever and output of acute phase proteins and other serum factors. The IL-1 and TNF-α act in concert with IL-6 to up-regulate the production of haemopoietic colony stimulating factors that are able to mobilize more PMNs and pro-macrophages from bone marrow. Death of bacteria, PMNs and macrophages in this encounter can result in suppuration, which may follow an acute or a chronic course (**2.32a–c**). In the latter case, cytokines and lipopolysaccharide from bacterial breakdown products

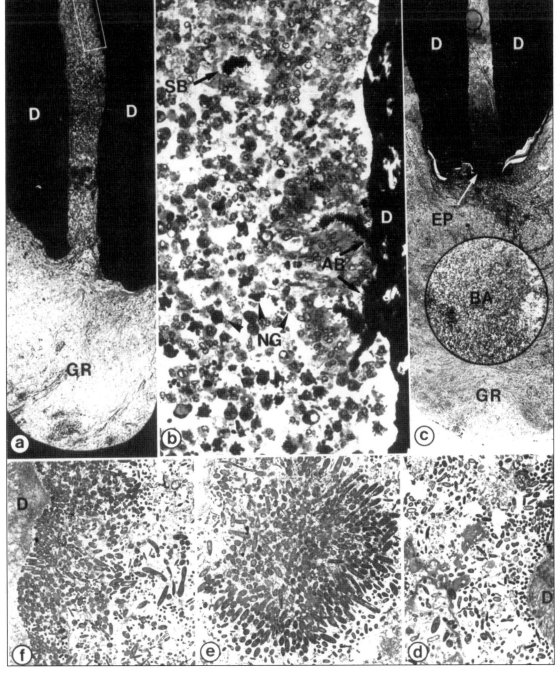

2.32 The endodontic flora in the apical third of a periapically affected human root. The flora appears to be blocked by a wall of neutrophils (NG in **b**) or an epithelial plug (EP in **c**). Note the dense aggregates of bacteria sticking to the dentine wall (AB in **b**) and similar ones (SB in **b**) along with loose connections of bacteria (insert in **c**) remaining suspended in the root canal among neutrophils. A cluster of an apparently monobacterial colony is magnified in **e**. Electron micrographs show bacterial condensation on the surface of the dentine wall, forming thin (**d**) or thick (**f**) layered bacterial plaques. The rectangular demarcated portion in **a** and the circular one in **c** are magnified in **b** and the inset in **c**, respectively: GR = granuloma, D = dentine. Original magnification: **a** × 50; **b** × 400; **c** × 40 (inset × 400); **d** × 2440; **e** × 3015; **f** × 3215 (from Nair 1987)

may stimulate the epithelial cells in the rests of Malassez to proliferate and line a tissue path for pus to escape to a body surface (usually intraoral). Roughly half of all induced periapical lesions (in a monkey study) developed sinus tracts. The prevalence of various clinical presentations in the disease process (natural history), that is the numbers that follow acute or chronic abscess (with or without sinus tract) or become chronic asymptomatic granulomas, is unknown. It is likely that the majority follow an asymptomatic chronic progression.

The most rapid phase of lesion expansion takes place between the 7th and 15th days, followed by a slower expansion in the following 30 days when the lesion will become apparent by radiography. From 15 days onwards, the lymphocytes predominate in the cellular infiltrate (50–60%), followed by PMNs (25–40%), then macrophage-monocytes, plasma cells and blasts. The lymphocytes are mobilized by the pro-inflammatory IL-1 and TNF-α. The T-helper (T_H) cells predominate in the active phase of the lesion expansion, whereas the T-suppressor (T_S) cells predominate in the more chronic lesions. The relative balance of these two cell types therefore appears to be involved in modulation of lesion growth. In molecular terms, the T_H-mediated mechanisms involve production of γ-interferon which activates macrophages to produce bone-resorptive mediators IL-1β, IL-1α, IL-4, IL-5, and IL-6 which stimulate antibody production and ultimately form immune complexes. Sixty per cent of the total bone-resorbing activity of interleukins is attributed to IL-1β, whilst the rest is due to IL-1α, TNFα and LT. Arachadonic acid and its metabolites also participate in bone-resorbing activity as do numerous other mediators but the precise synchronization of events is far from clear. The macrophages may also be stimulated to produce the same factors by phagocytosis of bacteria and activation by LPS while the T_H cells may also participate in direct bacterial killing and produce lymphotoxin (LT).

An interesting phenomenon in chronic inflammatory periapical lesions is the observation that PMNs are chemo-attracted to the apical foramina, where they congregate to form an almost continuous 'barrier' to the egress of bacteria. In other cases this barrier is surprisingly formed by proliferation of epithelial cells by mechanisms already mentioned (2.32a–c).

The chronic lesions may undergo acute exacerbations as a result of changes in the balance between the bacteria and host responses or due to the proliferation of specific bacteria. Such acute phases, accompanied by invasion of the periapical lesion by viable bacteria (many of which will die there) may also result in increase in the size of the periapical lesion.

The change in the relative balance between the bacteria (and their products) and the host defences causes variations not only in the histological but also the clinical picture, although there is no strict correlation between the histological and clinical pictures. The range of conditions may be classified as follows.

Acute periapical inflammation

This entity as an incipient event is uncommon and arises if the transition from pulpal inflammation to a periapical inflammation occurs more rapidly than periapical bone resorption. The result is an accumulation of PMNLs and oedema due to the vascular response in the periapical periodontal ligament, giving rise to pain. The tooth may feel raised in the socket and this would be accompanied by acute tenderness to touch. At this early stage, there may not be any obvious periapical tenderness to palpation but it soon becomes apparent (2.33). There would be no demonstrable radiographic periapical change (2.34). Subsidence of the pain is accompanied by the appearance of a periapical area and the transition of the inflammation to a chronic state.

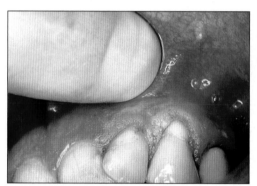

2.33 Tenderness to palpation over maxillary left lateral incisor and canine

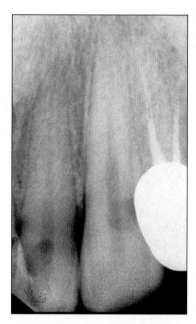

2.34 Definite evidence of radiographic periapical change is lacking

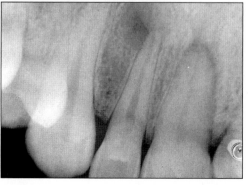

2.35 Radiographic appearance of chronic periradicular inflammation

Chronic periapical inflammation

The histological picture of this entity is as described in detail above. It is clinically asymptomatic and presents as a radiographic periapical radiolucency (**2.35**).

Chronic suppurative periapical inflammation

In some cases the conflict between the bacteria and the defence cells which are primarily the PMNLs, results in the death of many bacteria and host cells without either side gaining the upper hand. The accumulation of dead cells and the consequent release of lysosomal enzymes results in the formation of pus. This is usually conveyed to the nearest body surface by the formation of a sinus tract which over time becomes lined by epithelium (**2.36**). Clinically, there may be a draining sinus tract which may sometimes be raised to form a 'gumboil' (**2.37**). The patient may complain of bad taste in the mouth but rarely pain, there may sometimes be some mild discomfort especially on palpation of the area. The radiographic picture (**2.38**) would be similar to the previous category, however the sinus tract presents the opportunity of placing a gutta-percha point in it, to locate its source if there is any doubt (**2.37**).

Acute periapical abscess/cellulitis

This entity may arise from any of the other categories described so far. When it arises directly from acute periapical inflammation without any other transition, it is an exquisitely painful condition. The pain usually subsides as soon as a periapical lesion forms and pressure is relieved. Opening access to such a tooth is difficult and is aided by applying pressure to the tooth with a finger while drilling as the vibration causes the discomfort. The abscess is caused by an influx of large numbers of bacteria into the periapical area that overwhelm the defences (**2.39**). This causes a rapid influx of large numbers of PMNLs. The rapid death of large numbers of cells and the release of lysosomal enzymes causes an accumulation of pus called an abscess. The highly acidic environment causes the further death of surrounding tissues and may lead to further exacerbation. Clinically there would be various degrees of swelling and pain (**2.40–2.50**). The position of the swelling depends on the tissue planes (themselves determined by muscle and fascia attachments) through which pus spreads and accumulates. The tooth would feel elevated in the socket. If severe, and accompanied by an allergic response, there is a large exudative component leading to a build-up of fluid pressure. The viable bacteria, cellulitis and pus may spread through the tissue planes causing a spreading cellulitis with pyrexia, and causing the patient to feel unwell. If it is associated with a maxillary tooth, swelling may cause the ipsilateral eye to close (**2.50**). Cellulites manifest as a diffuse firm swelling and can lead to life-threatening conditions. If a maxillary tooth is involved, cavernous sinus thrombosis may develop. If a mandibular tooth is involved, Ludwig's angina may develop. Patients with Ludwig's angina (**2.45, 2.46**) become seriously ill, with marked pyrexia, and swallowing, speaking and

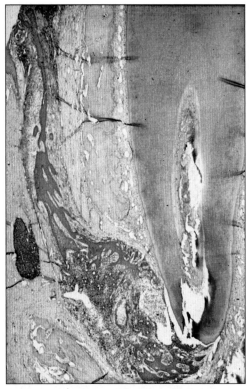

2.36 Epithelium-lined sinus tract (Valderhaug 1974)

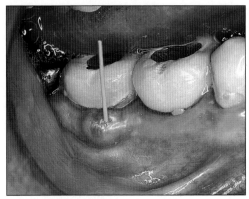

2.37 Chronic suppurative periradicular inflammation (gutta-percha point in sinus)

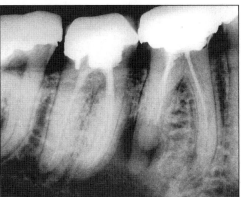

2.38 Radiograph of tooth in **2.37**

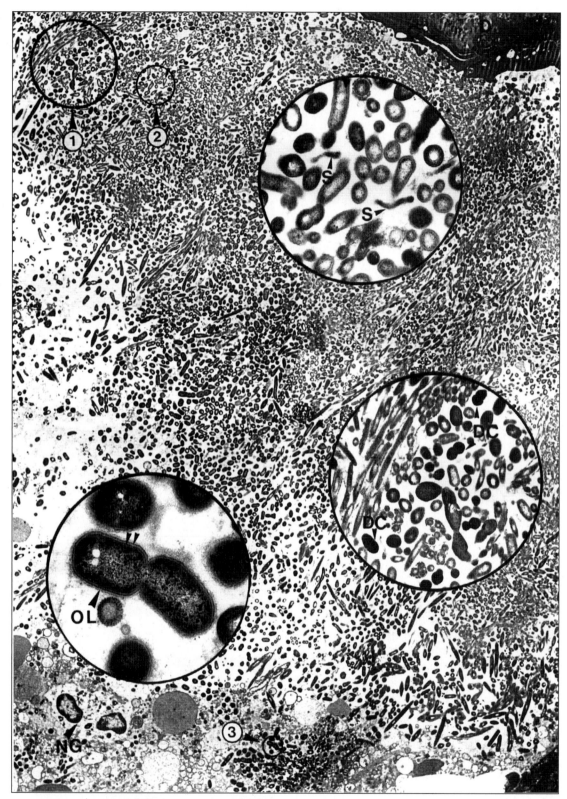

2.39 A massive periapical plaque associated with an acute lesion. Note the mixed nature of the flora. Numerous dividing cocci (DC, middle inset), rods (lower inset), filamentous bacteria and spirochaetes (S, upper inset) can be seen. Rods often reveal a Gram-negative cell wall (double arrowhead), some of them showing a third outer layer (OL). The circular areas 1, 2 and 3 are magnified in the middle, upper and lower insets, respectively: D = dentine; C = cementum; NG = neutrophils. Original magnification × 2680; upper inset × 19 200; middle inset × 11 200; lower inset × 36 400 (from Nair 1987)

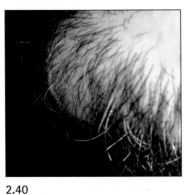

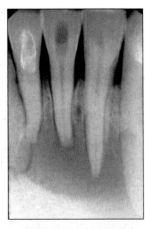

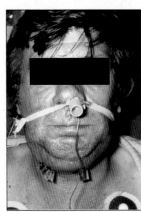

2.42 Large mandibular radiolucency related to the incisor teeth

2.40

2.41

2.40–2.41 Swelling of chin associated with mandibular anterior teeth

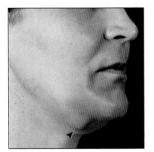

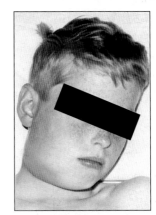

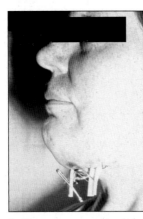

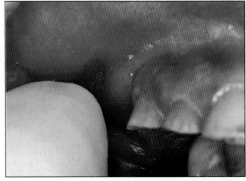

2.45–2.46 Treatment of Ludwig's angina

2.43 Localized submandibular swelling (arrowed)

2.44 Spreading submandibular swelling

2.45

2.46

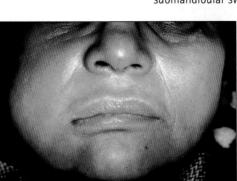

2.47 Right facial and infraorbital swelling associated with maxillary canine

2.48 Intraoral view of swelling in **2.47**

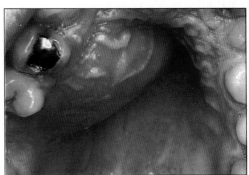

2.49 Palatal swelling associated with maxillary lateral incisor

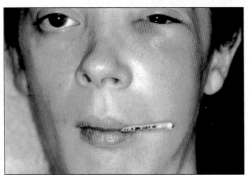

2.50 Closure of eye associated with infection thought to arise from maxillary canine

breathing become difficult. If the glottis becomes involved the patient may die within 12 to 24 hours. The condition should be identified early and the patient referred urgently for medical attention. Management involves extracting the tooth, draining the abscess and antibiotic therapy.

Periapical osteomyelitis

This is a very rare but serious progression of a periapical infection. The local infection spreads in a diffuse manner through the medullary spaces causing the necrosis of bone. The spread may be limited or extensive. PMNLs fill the medullary spaces and destroy osteoblasts lining the bony trabeculae, starting the process of bone resorption. The patient's temperature is elevated, lymph nodes are swollen and pain is severe. The teeth may be loosened but there may not be obvious swelling in the early stage. Untreated, the acute osteomyelitis can progress to a chronic stage which is less symptomatic but just as serious and merits prompt treatment.

Periapical osteosclerosis or condensing osteitis

Information is scarce on this uncommon entity. It is thought to be a low-grade response of the body to mild irritation. This usually occurs when the coronal part of a pulp is necrotic and infected while the apical portion is still vital. The intervening pulp tissue reduces the potency of the infection and, therefore, its direct impact on the periapical tissues. It stimulates bone deposition as opposed to erosion causing increased bone density with mild chronic inflammation in the marrow spaces. Clinically, the lesion is asymptomatic and presents as a radiopacity surrounding a severely widened periodontal ligament (**2.51**). In rare instances the inflammation is sufficient to cause apical resorption at the same time (**2.52, 2.53**).

Granulomas epithelial proliferation and cysts

The epithelial rests of Malassez may be stimulated by inflammation to proliferate. The pattern of proliferation is variable, with formation of strands, arcades or rings at the junction of the uninflamed connective tissue and granulation tissue. Proliferation may also occur within the body of the granuloma, where it helps to plug the apical foramen and limit egress of bacteria and their toxins (**2.25, 2.32**). In some instances these epithelial plugs bulge out into the periapical lesion, forming a sac connected to the root and continuous with the root canal, termed a 'Bay or pocket cyst' (**2.54, 2.55**). In these cases, microorganisms from the root canal have direct access to the 'cyst' cavity and may invade it (**2.56**).

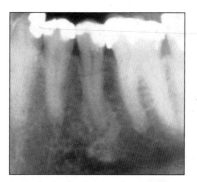

2.51 Periradicular condensing osteitis associated with 35

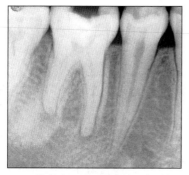

2.52 Apical resorption associated with condensing osteitis

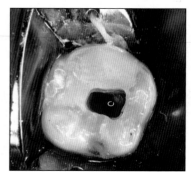

2.53 Access cavity into the tooth in **2.52** shows vital but inflamed pulp tissue

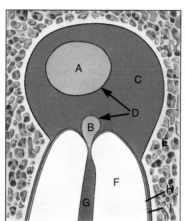

2.54 Bay and true cysts: A = true cyst; B = bay cyst; C = granuloma; D = epithelium; E = alveolar bone; F = dentine; G = root canal; H = cementum; I = periodontal ligament

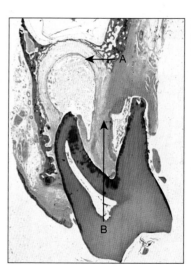

2.55 Histological section showing a bay cyst (A): B = granuloma

A true cyst has been defined as a separate pathological, epithelium-lined cavity usually containing fluid or semi-solid material. It does not communicate with the root canal or any other opening (**2.54, 2.57**) and develops in periapical lesions with a prevalence of about 15%. It was once believed that large circumscribed radiographic lesions with a sclerotic border were likely to be cysts but such a correlation has not been proven. However, lesions of the size shown in **Figure 2.58** are likely to show cystic change. The bay cyst would by inference heal by

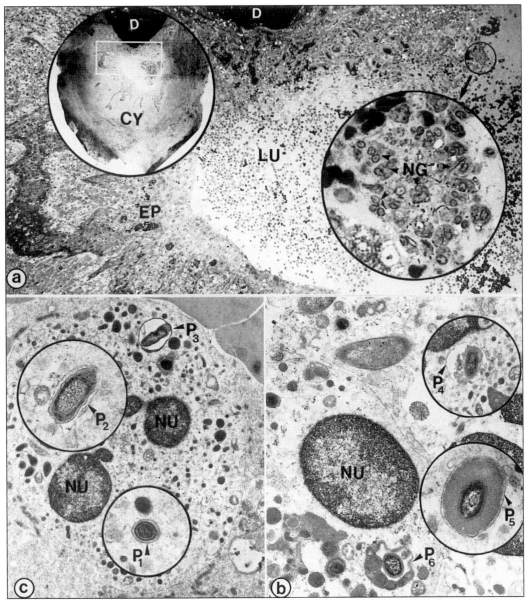

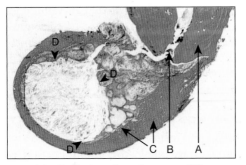

2.57 Histological section of true cyst (D). A = root apex; B = root canal; C = granuloma

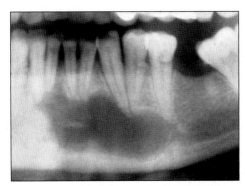

2.58 Large periradicular cyst associated with mandibular incisors

2.56 Bacteria in a radicular cyst. Note the distinct epithelial lining (EP) of the cyst lumen (LU) and a cluster of neutrophils (NG) showing phagocytosed bacteria. The upper inset in **a** shows an overview of the well-encapsulated cyst (CY). The electron micrographs in **b** and **c** show the several types of membrane-delimited phagosomes (P_1 to P_6) containing bacteria. Note the close adherence of bacteria and the phagosome membrane in P_1 and P_2, although a clear space is visible between them in P_3. An electron-dense coating of varying thickness may be distinguished on the bacterial surface in P_4 and P_5. Note the bacterium in P_6 is devoid of such a coating but the phagosome contains several membrane-delimited granule-like structures: D = dentine; NU = nucleus. Original magnification a × 100: (left inset × 10, right inset × 850); b × 12 800 (upper inset × 8900, lower inset × 17 500); c (lower inset × 8 900, upper inset × 17 500) (from Nair 1987)

elimination of the bacterial contamination of the root canal. Successful treatment of the true cyst may require surgery after conventional root canal treatment has failed to resolve it.

The exact aetiology and mechanisms of cyst formation are not clear. The epithelium may surround an abscess or granuloma cutting off the tissues within from their nutrient source and causing their degeneration. Alternatively, dividing epithelial cells may grow until the central cells are starved of their nutrient sources, causing their degeneration. The method of cyst enlargement is also speculative. Theories involve selective absorption of fluids and an active biochemical interaction between the cyst wall and adjacent tissues. Whatever the explanation, it is clear that cysts tend to grow. The cyst is therefore an independent pathological entity within another pathological entity, the granuloma (**2.57**). The relative proportions of granulomatous and cystic tissue may vary. As such it could be argued that while the granulomatous lesion may be treatable by removal of the aetiological agents from the canal, the cyst having become independently established continues to flourish until specifically inhibited. The successful treatment of the cyst has been thought to require its enucleation, its deflation by puncture or induction of acute inflammation in the vicinity. Enucleation has been reliably tested without significant recurrence but the effectiveness of the decompression method is debatable, as healing is slow and unpredictable, and allows no opportunity for biopsy. However, it is a valuable means of reducing the cyst's size before surgical enucleation. The last method, of inducing acute inflammation in the cyst's vicinity, requires instrumentation through the apical foramen as advocated by Bhaskar (1972). This rather unpredictable procedure did not gain wide support and is not recommended. Despite the overall lack of clarity about the pathogenesis and treatment of a cyst, the therapeutic regime for all periapical lesions associated with compromised pulps, is relatively clear. In view of the inability to differentiate a granuloma from a cyst clinically and the high rate of success of conventional non-surgical root canal treatment, this approach is the preferred method of treatment of all periapical lesions associated with necrotic and infected pulps in the first instance. If upon follow-up, a technically adequate root canal treatment does not lead to resolution, then a surgical approach should be considered.

NATURE OF THE PERIAPICAL LESION ASSOCIATED WITH TREATED TEETH

Much of the research on human periapical tissue has been conducted on undefined samples, that is, it is not known whether the sample was associated with treated or untreated teeth. Many investigators have assumed that the responses would be the same. Only a few studies have focused on specified tissue samples, either from treated teeth or untreated teeth. A quantitative comparison of lymphocytes and their subsets in periapical lesions harvested from treated or untreated teeth has shown differences in the inflammatory infiltrate and relative proportions of T, B and T_H cells.

The short-term (7–14 days) response of apical tissues to different root canal treatment procedures may result in atypical lesions with total cellular destruction in the centre and PMNs aggregated at the periphery, possibly as a result of sodium hypochlorite extrusion.

Periapical lesions persistent over a longer term may represent persistent chronic inflammation as a result of residual intraradicular infection (**2.59**) established extra-radicular infection (**2.60, 2.61**), a foreign body response (**2.62**) or a radicular cyst (**2.63–2.66**).

ASSOCIATION BETWEEN ROOT CANAL BACTERIA AND PERIAPICAL LESION DEVELOPMENT

A range of periapical responses to the root canal microbial flora has been described above. The question raised is whether this is primarily a function of variation in host response or a function of fundamentally different types of microbial flora. It is a clinically attractive proposition to be able to segregate different types of flora that not only have different pathogenicity but also different susceptibilities to treatment and therefore merit specific treatment protocols.

The fundamental reason for accurate identification of bacteria from root canals is to disclose those bacteria or combinations that may play key roles in the progress of the disease or its acute exacerbation and especially those that may be resistant to conventional therapy or implicated in treatment failure.

The counter-view has also been expressed that it would be difficult to segregate the effect of individual species because of the polymicrobial nature of the infection. The concept of non-specific polymicrobial infection holds that it would be difficult to attribute specific roles to individual species, as even subspecies variation could account for increased pathogenicity.

The possible association between the type of root canal flora or individual species and periapical lesion development has been studied by several groups of investigators. It is found that the number of bacterial colonies does not increase between days 7 and 15, when the critical periapical lesion expansion takes place. The proportion of strict anaerobes doubles from 25% to 50% during this time and the proportion of Gram negative bacteria also doubles. The mean number of species (~ 3.5) per tooth remains the same between these time points but the overall diversity increases on day 15. The critical period of lesion expansion correlates with the change in the root canal flora to one that is more anaerobic and Gram negative.

A series of classical studies evaluated the periapical responses to indigenous bacterial infections in a monkey model, using an experimental design that comes as close as it is possible to get to testing Koch's postulates for a polymicrobial infection, as normally these apply to a mono-infection.

Non-infected teeth were not found to develop periapical radiolucencies or inflammation while most of the infected teeth developed periapical lesions and the proportion of facultative anaerobic species decreased and strict anaerobic species increased during the experimental period.

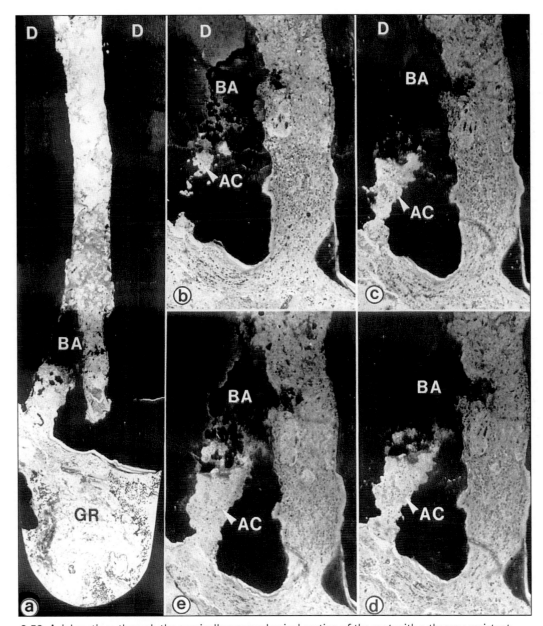

2.59 Axial sections through the surgically removed apical portion of the root with a therapy-resistant periapical lesion (GR). Note the cluster of bacteria visible in the root canal (BA). Parts **b–e** show serial semi-thin sections taken at varying distances from the section plane of **a** to reveal the emerging (**b**) and gradually widening (**c–e**) profiles of an accessory root canal (AC). Note that the accessory canal is clogged with bacteria (BA). Original magnification: **a** × 52; **b–e** × 62 (From Nair *et al.* 1990)

Another study evaluated the distribution of bacteria (between main canal, dentine and apical 3–4 mm of the canal) in similarly infected root canals after varied times of closure (90, 180, 1060 days). The ratio of obligate anaerobic to facultative anaerobic bacteria increased from 1.7 (7 days) to 3.9 (90 days) to 6.5 (180 days) and finally to > 11.3 (1060 days). The major site of infection was the main canal followed by dentine and then the apical part of the canal. The flora in the apical part of the canal was thought to be the most likely to have interacted with the host tissues.

To account for the possible contribution of unsampled or uncultivated bacteria in the pathogenesis of lesions, eleven isolated strains (including eight strains from one tooth, representing its

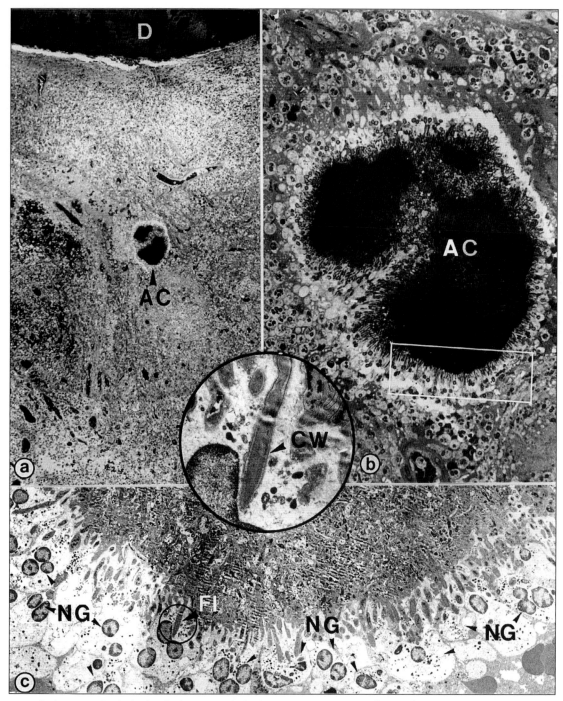

2.60 Actinomyces in the body of a human periapical granuloma. The colony (AC in **a**) is magnified in **b**. The rectangular area demarcated in **b** is magnified in **c**. Note the starburst appearance of the colony with needle-like peripheral filaments surrounded by few layers of neutrophilic granulocytes (NG), some of which contain phagocytosed bacteria. A dividing peripheral filament (FI) is magnified in the inset. Note the typical Gram-positive wall (CW): D = dentine. Original magnification: **a** × 60; **b** × 430; **c** × 1680; inset × 6700 (From Nair & Schroeder 1984)

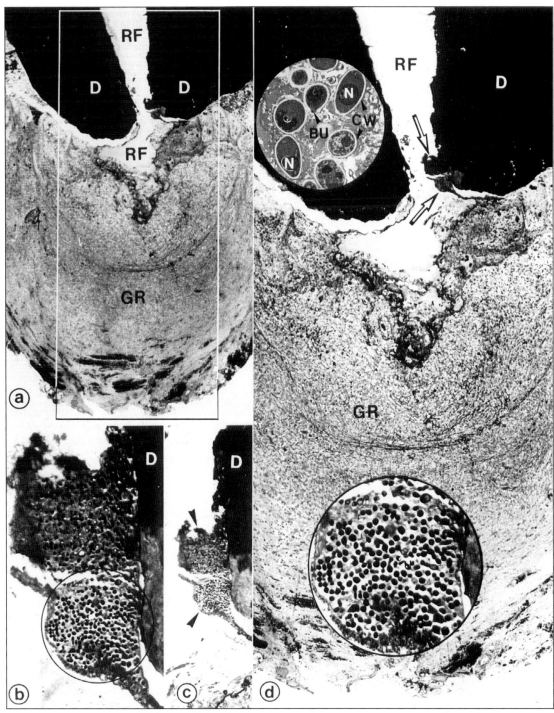

2.61 Fungus in the root canal and apical foramen of a root-filled (RF in **a** and **d**) tooth with a therapy-resistant periapical lesion (GR in **a** and **d**). The rectangular demarcated area in **a** is magnified in **d**. Note the two clusters of microorganisms located between the dentinal wall (D) and the root filling (arrows in **d**). Those microbial clusters are stepwise magnified in **c** and **d**. The circular demarcated area in **b** is further magnified in the lower inset in **d**. The upper inset is an electron microscopic view of the orgnisms. They are about 3–4 μm in diameter and reveal distinct cell wall (CW), nuclei (N) and budding forms (BU). Original magnifications: **a** × 33; **b** × 330; **c** × 132; **d** × 59; lower inset × 530; upper inset × 3400 (from Nair *et al.* 1990a)

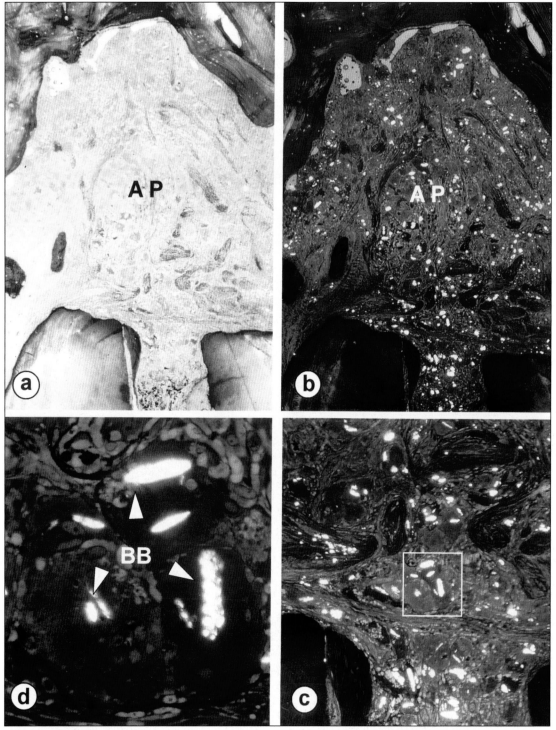

2.62 Apical periodontitis (AP) characterized by foreign body giant cell reaction to gutta-percha cones contaminated with talc (a). The same field when viewed in polarized lights (b). Note the birefringent bodies distributed throughout the lesion (b). The apical foramen is magnified in (c) and the rectangular demarcated area in (c) is further enlarged in (d). Note the birefringence (BB) emerging from slit-like inclusion bodies in multinucleated giant cells. Magnifications: **a, b** × 25; **c** × 66; **d** × 300 (from Nair 1998)

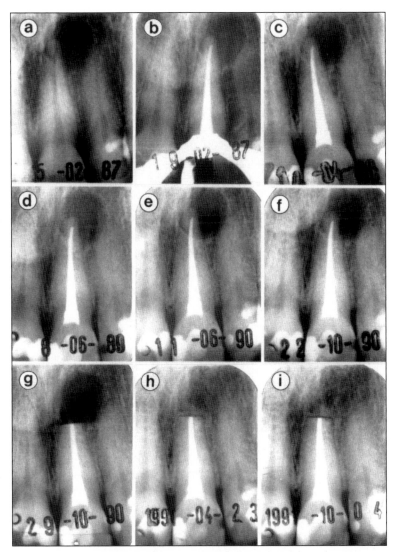

2.63 Longitudinal radiographs of a periapically affected left central incisor of a 37-year-old woman over a period of 4 years and 9 months of clinical management. Note the large eccentrically located apical radiolucency observed before (a) and immediately after (b) root filling. The lesion did not show any reduction in size in control radiographs taken 14, 28, 40 and 44 months (c–f) after endodontics. Apical surgery was performed (g) and the periapical area shows distinct bone healing (h, i) within 1 year of surgery (from Nair *et al.* 1993)

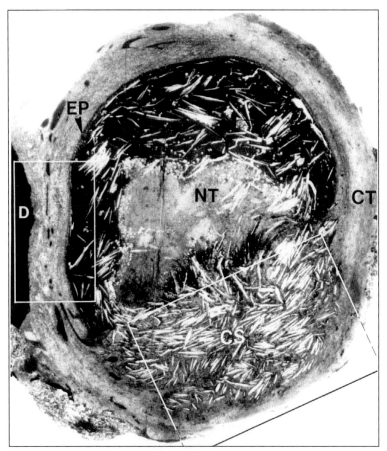

2.64 Axial section through the apical biopsy removed from the radiolucent area visible in **2.63 (g)**. The large lesion is encapsulated with a narrow rim of dense capsular connective tissue (CT) and contains a distinct lumen lined with stratified squamous epithelium (EP). Note the vast number of cholesterol clefts (CS) concentrated in the connective tissue at the distocervical aspect of the lesion. The luminal centre contains pale staining necrotic tissue (NT) and the rest of the lumen is filled with dark staining erythrocytes among which cholesterol spaces can be seen. The large rectangular demarcated area is further magnified in **2.66** (from Nair *et al.* 1993)

total cultivable infection) from previous studies were inoculated in freshly necrotized monkey teeth, in various combinations, but always in equal proportions. The 'eight-strain collection' consisted of *Bacteroides oralis, Fusobacterium, necrophorum, Fusobacterium nucleatum, Streptococcus milleri, Streptococcus faecalis* (*Enterococcus faecalis*), *Peptostreptococcus anaerobius, Actinomyces bovis* and *Propionibacterium acnes*. After six months, the 'eight-strain collection' was recovered from all teeth, and interestingly, in the same proportions that it had been recovered from the original tooth. This

suggested that selective pressures were at play in the root canal system that reproduced the 'same infection'. Other combinations did not survive as effectively, some species were not recovered at all.

Periapical destruction was consistently associated with the mixed infections but not with the single-strain infections, where some periapical inflammation was evident depending upon the extent and type of bacterial survival. Of the single strains inoculated, only *Enterococcus faecalis* survived in every case. *Bacteroides oralis*, which dominated all mixed infections, did not survive as a monoinfection.

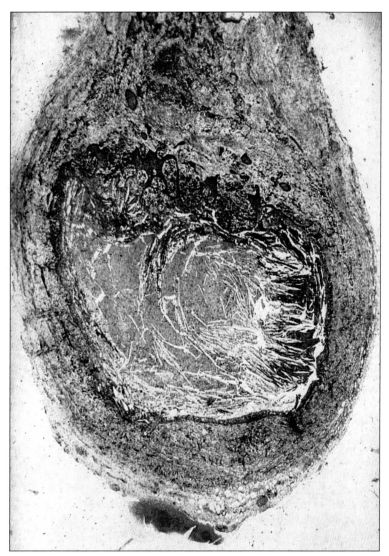

2.65 Section of a true apical radicular cyst

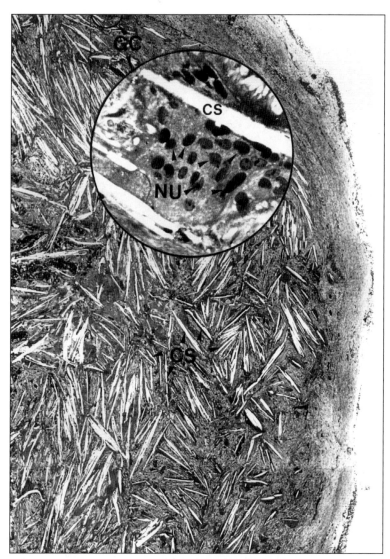

2.66 Presence of vast numbers of cholesterol clefts (CS) in the lesion. The cholesterol spaces are surrounded by multinucleated giant cells (GC), of which a selected one is magnified in the inset. Note the large number of nuclei (NU). Original magnification × 98 (inset × 322) (from Nair *et al.* 1993)

Inoculation of *Staphylococcus aureus*, *Streptococcus sanguis*, *Pseudomonas aeruginosa* and *Bacteroides fragilis* as monocultures in root canals could elicit periapical responses.

In summary, periapical disease is caused by a polymicrobial infection of the root canal system. There appears to be a direct relationship between the size of the periapical lesion and the number and type of bacterial strains present.

The relationship between specific bacteria and the presence of acute signs and symptoms is still confusing. Black-pigmented *Bacteroides* species, especially *Bacteroides melaninogenicus* as well as *Peptostreptococcus micros* were originally implicated in purulent infections. The presence of black-pigmented *Bacteroides* species does not, however, consistently result in acute abscesses. Other species have also become associated with acute signs and symptoms, including: *Actinomyces* species; *Peptostreptococcus magnus*; other *Bacteroides* species; *Peptococcus* species; *Eubacterium* species; *Porphyromonas* species; *Propionibacterium* species; spirochaetes; and *Fusobacterium* species. The relatively weak associations sometimes reported between symptoms and species have been explained by the small number of bacterial cells, strain variants and other as yet undeciphered microbial and host factors in those cases. The true basis for acute exacerbation of periapical lesions is still unknown.

NATURE OF THE ROOT CANAL FLORA

Qualitative analysis

Studies before the 1960s, which did not have the advantage of advanced culturing techniques, found mainly aerobic and facultative organisms and some strict anaerobes. The typical flora would include streptococci, lactobacilli, Gram-negative cocci, and a range of anaerobic bacteria. As culturing techniques improved, particularly for strict anaerobic bacteria, it was possible to isolate and identify many more strains and species. The picture of root canal infection has therefore undergone tremendous change. Almost all of these bacteria originate from the oral cavity and only rarely from other parts of the body or the general environment. The unique milieu of the root canal system only allows the survival of certain bacteria and hence the different proportional composition of the flora compared to that of the oral and periodontal sites. The advent of molecular techniques for detection and identification of bacteria has resulted in the further expansion of the diversity of bacteria implicated in root canal infections. This is because for the first time they are able to reveal uncultivable bacteria which are estimated to comprise between 50 and 90% of the environmental flora and somewhat less of the oral flora.

Future microbial ecological studies will reveal the true extent of the uncultivable component of the flora. The bacteria found in the root canal system so far are listed in **Table 2.1**.

Quantitative analysis

The bacteria listed in **Table 2.1** are not all present in every infected tooth. The mean total number of bacteria present in infected teeth is estimated to the $10^{7.7}$ CFU/mL of sample. A mean of six species per tooth may be found and the mean number of bacterial species exceeding 10^5 CFU/mL is 4.8. Anaerobic bacteria account for a mean 64% of the species in concentrations exceeding 10^5 CFU/mL. According to quantitative analysis, the total concentration of aerobes and anaerobes is nearly equal. The relative proportions vary from study to study and from tooth to tooth. The bacterial quantity of 10^5 cells per millilitre of sample is consistent with that in other infections. The total range is 10^1–10^8 CFUs per sample. In contrast, canals under treatment have a residual flora with a cell concentration of between 10^1–10^3 CFUs per sample. It has been noted that when staphylococci are present, they occur at very high counts.

Table 2.1　Showing bacteria isolated from previously untreated teeth associated with periapical disease

Aerobes	Facultative anaerobes	Anaerobes
Gram-positive cocci	**Gram-positive cocci**	**Gram-positive cocci**
Dietzia maris	*Enterococcus faecalis*	*Peptococcus* sp.
Micrococcus luteus	*Enterococcus faecium*	*Peptostreptococcus anaerobius*
Micrococcus lylae	*Enterococcus hirae*	*Peptostreptococcus assacharolyticus*
	Gemella haemolysans	*Peptostreptococcus magnus*
Gram-positive rods	*Gemella morbillorum*	*Peptostreptococcus micros*
Arthrobacter sp.	*Leuconostoc* sp.	*Peptostreptococcus prevotii*
Brachybacterium sp.	*Pediococcus acidilactici*	*Ruminococcus* sp.
	Rothia sp.	
Gram-negative cocci	*Staphylococcus aureus*	**Gram-positive rods**
Neisseria sp.	*Staphylococcus epidermidis*	*Bifidobacterium*
	Staphylococcus hominis	*Eubacterium brachy*
Gram-negative rods	*Staphylococcus warneri*	*Eubacterium lentum*
Acinetobacter lwolfii	*Stomatococcus mucilaginosus*	*Eubacterium nodatum*
Campylobacter sputorum	*Streptococcus anginosus*	*Eubacterium* spp.
Kingella sp.	*Streptococcus constellatus*	*Eubacterium timidum*
Pseudomonas aeruginosa	*Streptococcus gordonii*	*Slackia exigua*
Wolinella curva	*Streptococcus infantis*	
Wolinella recta	*Stretococcus intermedius*	**Gram-negative cocci**
	Streptococcus mitior	*Acidaminococcus* sp.
	Streptococcus mitis	*Veillonella dispar*
	Streptococcus mutans	*Veillonella parvula*
	Streptococcus oralis	
	Streptococcus pyogenes	
	Streptococcus salivarius	
	Streptococcus sanguinis	
	Streptococcus sobrinus	
	Streptococcus suis	

Table 2.1 continued

Aerobes	Facultative anaerobes	Anaerobes
	Gram-positive rods	**Gram-negative rods**
	Actinomyces meyeri	Acidaminobacter sp.
	Actinomyces naeslundii	Bacteroides sp
	Actinomyces odontolyticus	Clostridium sp.
	Actinomyces radicidentis	Fibrobacter sp.
	Actinomyces viscosus	Fusobacterium necrophorum
	Bacillus flexus	Fusobacterium nucleatum
	Bacillus megaterium	Fusobacterium varium
	Bacillus pumilus	Leptotrichia sp.
	Corynebacterium diphtheriae	Megamonas sp.
	Lactobacillus fermentum	Mitsuokella sp.
	Lactobacillus gasseri	Porphyromonas asaccharolyticus
	Lactobacillus casei	Porphyromonas endodontalis
	Lactobacillus rhamnosus	Porphyromonas gingivalis
	Propionibacterium acnes	Prevotella buccae
	Propionibacterium propionicum	Prevotella intermedia
		Prevotella loeschia
	Gram-negative cocci	Prevotella melaninogenicus
	—	Prevotella oralis
		Prevotella oris
	Gram-negative rods	Selenomonas sputigena
	Actinobacillus sp.	Treponema spp.
	Citrobacter sp.	
	Eikenella corrodens	
	Enterobacter sp.	
	Escherichia sp.	
	Haemophilus influezae	
	Klebsiella pneumonia	
	Pasteurella sp.	
	Proteus sp.	

The number of genera per tooth range from 0 to 16 with mean range between 6 and 9.2. The range of number of species per tooth is currently estimated at 1–12. The mean ranges from 2.0 to 5.7 per tooth. There is a general trend towards later studies showing higher numbers of species per tooth but this is not universally true. The numbers probably reflect better cultivation and identification techniques. Molecular studies show more than 40 taxa per tooth.

DISTRIBUTION OF INTRARADICULAR BACTERIA

Bacteria gain access to the root canal system by a number of routes. The commonest is probably through the crown by means of a carious exposure, through open dentinal tubules in the crown or root, through lateral canals either before devitalization via blood vessels communicating with the periodontium or after exposure to the oral environment due to periodontal disease. Cracks in the tooth also allow root canal infection. Another less common route is by anachoresis.

This is the term used to denote infection of a chronically inflamed area by a blood-borne infection or a bacteraemia. The pulp in this case has to be inflamed but it is unlikely that an empty canal would be infected in this way. The point of entry of the bacteria is likely to dictate the subsequent development of the infection and its distribution.

Cultivation and molecular studies on the nature of the bacterial flora in root canals far out-number morphological or culture studies seeking to reveal the distribution of bacteria. Our knowledge is based on light, dark-field and electron microscopic (SEM, TEM) studies, cultivation studies and analysis of distribution of bacterial toxins.

Microscopic studies

Several microscopic surveys (light, dark-field, TEM and SEM) of teeth have shown the pattern of bacterial invasion and associated pulp necrosis. A 'synthesized view' is presented below based on the observations from these studies.

Bacterial invasion usually begins in the coronal part of the tooth and root and is concentrated there. Bacteria appear in smaller numbers in the root canals as the apical foramen is reached in teeth with closed pulp chambers but where the teeth are cariously exposed the canals are evenly coated with a bacterial plaque. Vital pulp tissue may be present apically and, if so, the intensity of the infection tapers off towards it.

A significantly greater percentage of coccoid and rod forms are noted in the coronal rather than the apical parts of canals, whereas the distribution of motile rods does not differ. In contrast, the percentage of filaments and spirochaetes are slightly higher in the apical than the coronal parts of the canal. A significant correlation is noted between the size of the apical radiolucency and the percentage of spirochaetes present.

TEM observation of carious teeth confirms that the bulk of the flora in the apical part of the root exists as a loose collection of a variety of morphologically distinct but taxonomically unidentifiable bacteria consisting of cocci, rods and filamentous forms (**2.32**). Most of the flora in the apical 5 mm of the root canal remains suspended in an apparently moist canal lumen. Less frequently, dense aggregates of bacteria are observed sticking to the dentinal wall of the root canal or existing free among vast numbers of PMNs in the canal lumen. The dense aggregates are clusters of morphologically uniform cells. The interbacterial spaces are filled with an amorphous extracellular matrix. Independent of these tooth-adhering monobacterial aggregates, the dentinal wall is covered by single or multilayered bacterial condensations containing various types of bacteria. The filamentous forms are often adherent perpendicular to the canal wall with coccoid forms arranged in strings in the same direction. Cocci occasionally attach to the filaments to give a corncob appearance.

Deposits resembling bacterial plaque are also evident in the apical 2 mm of the root canal. Epithelial cells or a wall of PMNs often plugs the apical canal. In those cases where the floral front extends into the periapical lesion, there may be limited to extensive tissue necrosis and acute PMN response. In the latter instance, the chronic granulomatous tissue immediately around the tooth apex may be lysed and occupied by an apparently young apical plaque. SEM views reveal scalloped root resorption with multilayered bacterial plaque embedded in an extracellular matrix. Such extraradicular extension of bacteria is, however, rare.

Bacterial penetration into dentine is only evident in the presence of pulp necrosis. The predentine is easily and commonly infected but the calcified dentine less so. Bacterial penetration into dentine around the root canal is confined to the close proximity of the root canal. In some teeth, bacteria may be evident penetrating up to a third or a half of the depth of dentinal tubules where they end in a vital periodontal membrane. Only in cases where the tubules end in necrotic periodontal tissue, are the bacteria observed along the entire length of the dentinal tubules (**2.67**). Dentine tubule infection is deeper in the apical part, particularly in cariously exposed teeth. Cementum is rarely infected except in the presence of extraradicular infection.

Cultivation studies

Morphological studies do not give the identity of bacteria and so require supplementation by cultivation studies. In common with the morphological studies, these also focus on the coronal-apical distribution of bacteria in root canals and the penetration of bacteria into dentine. The earliest studies were interested to determine the existence of

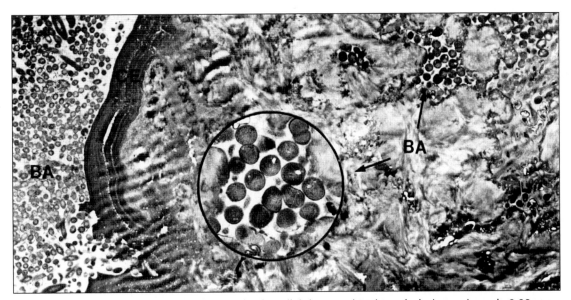

2.67 Presence of bacterial clusters in the root dentine, slightly coronal to the periapical area shown in **2.39**. Note part of the apical plaque is visible peripheral to the cementum (CD) and clusters of bacteria (BA) existing in apparently disintegrating dentinal tubules. Original magnification × 5300; inset × 12 800 (from Nair 1987)

infection in periapical tissues because of the controversy caused by the focal infection theory. The prevalence and truth about periapical infection remains unresolved. The chronic periapical lesion can remain sterile even when the root canal is infected. The fact that the majority of periapical lesions heal upon tooth extraction suggests that only rarely do infections become established extraradicularly.

Cultivation of bacteria from samples similar to those described by Nair (1987) showed the presence of *Actinomyces*, *Lactobacillus*, black-pigmented *Bacteroides*, *Peptostreptococcus*, non-pigmented *Bacteroides*, *Veillonella* species, *Enterococcus faecalis*, *Fusobacterium nucleatum* and *Streptococcus mutans*. The majority (68%) were anaerobes.

The bacterial flora invading the deep layers (0.5–2.0 mm) of dentine in root canals of carious teeth is mostly (80%) composed of strict anaerobes. The predominant bacteria are Gram positive rods (68%) and Gram positive cocci (27%). *Lactobacillus* (30%), *Streptococcus* (13%) and *Propionibacterium* species (9%) are dominant. A similar study of teeth with undefined coronal status but evaluating the full thickness of dentine found a more diverse flora consisting of a mix of Gram positive and Gram negative types including: *Prevotella*, *Porphyromonas*, *Fusobacterium*, *Peptostreptococcus*, *Actinomyces*, *Streptococcus*, *Propionibacterium*, *Lactobacillus* and *Bifidobacterium* species. The presence of Gram negative bacteria in the inner layers of root canal dentine has been confirmed by the finding of lipopolysaccharide in dentine up to 300 µm in depth.

Cementum from apical portions of roots harvested during apical surgery may show the presence *Prevotella*, *Fusobacterium*, *Peptostreptococcus*, *Eubacterium* and *Campylobacter* species. This observation can be reconciled with previous studies if the teeth are associated with sinus tracts. Some researchers have investigated the penetration of bacteria and their products into cementum from the periodontal surface but the positive findings remain controversial. The reason is that they imply that such bacteria could coexist with vital, perhaps healthy, pulps and others have shown that vital pulps resist invasion by bacteria.

In summary, the overall picture is one of a variable distribution of bacteria within the root canal system and dentine. The state at any given time may represent the stage of infection with bacteria extending up to and sometimes beyond the apical foramina. The depth of penetration into dentine is also variable but generally appears to be confined within the area close to the root canal and is probably dominated by Gram positive bacteria, mostly streptococci. The distribution of morphotypes also appears to be variable.

In rare instances in chronic lesions the bacteria may proliferate beyond the apical foramen and into the periapical lesion. Mainly anaerobic bacteria have been demonstrated in the periapical tissues, perhaps associated with foreign or dead (cellular or dentinal) material, to which the defence cells have no access. The bacteria may also be found embedded in an extracellular plaque-like matrix covering the external surface of the root. The bacteria in this plaque have been observed to be mainly cocci and rods but fibrillar forms may be present too. The main species implicated in periapical tissue invasion include *Actinomyces* species and *Propionibacterium propionica*. Many others from the root canal flora have also been implicated but their true presence in the periapical tissues remains controversial because of the difficulties of obtaining an uncontaminated sample. In the majority of chronic periapical lesions no bacteria may be found, although bacterial invasion of the periapical tissues is a common event in acute exacerbation where, for unknown reasons, the root canal bacteria overwhelm the local periapical defences.

IMPORTANCE OF MICROBIAL ECOLOGY AND BIOFILMS IN THE TREATMENT OF ROOT CANAL INFECTION

Microbial ecology

Periapical lesion development is dependent upon the nature of the mixed infection, the succession of bacterial species within it and its ultimate survival. It is influenced by, as yet, undiscovered ecological factors in the root canal system. Studies, therefore, focused on the nature of bacterial interactions with their environment.

Interactions between microorganisms and their biotic (living) and abiotic (non-living) surroundings are important in enabling their survival. The restricted nature of the root canal flora suggests selective pressures. A study (Sundqvist 1992a) of associations between bacteria in root canal systems by isolating all cultivable bacteria from a large number of root canals associated with periapical disease and calculating the likelihood of pairs of bacteria occurring together has confirmed:

● positive associations between some species:
  Fusobacterium nucleatum and *Peptostreptococcus micros*; *Porphyromonas endodontalis*, *Selenomonas sputigena* and *Wolinella recta*; *Prevotella intermedia* and *Peptostreptococcus micros*; *Peptostreptococcus anaerobius* and *Eubacterium* species.

● negative associations between other species:
  Propionibacterium propionicum, *Capnocytophaga ochracea* and *Veillonella parvula*.

The positive and negative associations are thought to be due to nutritional interactions, local physiological conditions (Eh, pH), bacteriocins and bacterial coaggregation or physical attraction and binding (**2.68**).

Microbial interactions within communities enable them to evolve, depending on the local environmental variations, thus supragingival and subgingival plaque, only a few millimetres apart develop vastly differently depending on their salivary and serum nutritional sources, respectively. A similar model is proposed for the root canal flora: coronal leakage may allow salivary ingress and facultative organisms to grow in the coronal part of the canal, whereas serum from the apical part of the canal may favour the growth of proteolytic bacteria at the root apex.

The root canal environment has a unique natural history in terms of a nutritional source in the human body, though it has not been characterized adequately in its necrotic, infected state from an ecological point of view. It begins with a very rich supply of vital tissue during the stages of pulpal inflammation but once it becomes necrotized, the nutritional supply is rapidly exhausted as the environment is secluded by the dentine shell. As the habitat is altered by the primary colonizers, secondary invaders join and may replace them. According to classical ecological theory, succession ends when a relatively stable assembly of populations, called a climax community is achieved. This concept has been difficult to apply to microbial communities in the general environment as random disturbances prevent the community from ever reaching equilibrium although this may well be achieved in the secluded root canal environment in chronic cases. Additional nutritional sources are limited to coronal seepage of saliva or apical seepage of serum. In the later stages of an enclosed root canal infection, therefore the bacteria presumably enter some sort of a starvation or dormant phase, although this aspect has not specifically been investigated in root canal sites. If dormancy does play a significant part, then it may help contribute to the chronic nature of periapical disease. The overall ecological picture is one of a complex polymicrobial community that may function as one in response to its environment and presumably to treatment as well.

The interdependence of different bacterial species and with their environment is the key to the success of root canal treatment. The treatment procedures (mechanical and chemical) essentially interfere with the environment, killing some bacteria and by a domino effect, indirectly killing other species by altering the nutritional and toxic balance. The surviving bacteria are usually those hardy enough to resist the treatment and capable of living independently of other species in the unique nutrition-depleted conditions. This means that a poor first attempt at root canal treatment may result in a more resistant and hardy infection to eradicate at the next attempt. It is therefore best to launch the most comprehensive effort at eradicating the infection at the first attempt.

Biofilms

The aggregations of microorganisms into communities at surface interfaces, which exhibit well-defined structures and succession, are called biofilms. Indeed, the only reliable *in situ*, observation of the root canal flora, revealed both attached root canal biofilms and bacteria suspended in a column of apical root canal fluid (Nair 1987). It is not known whether the suspended bacteria were simply shed from the root canal surface or were growing independently. The relative distribution of biofilm and planktonic phenotypes in the root canal system is not yet known but these may dictate the properties of the infection, in particular those that allow biofilm persistence after treatment. Until recently, the concept of the root canal flora as a biofilm has not been given serious consideration.

Root canal infection is essentially a bacterial biofilm coating the dentine surface, including the tubules to variable depths and extending to the apical foramina and sometimes beyond. This biofilm may be continuous (**2.69**) or broken (**2.70**), and different populations of bacteria may communicate with each other through fluid films or columns by the medium of molecular messengers. Individual cells within this cooperative may respond to their immediate surroundings and neighbours by switching on or off relevant genes for survival. Nutrition depletion may slow their metabolism and allow some to enter a dormant state. This may also make them uncultivable if sampled. In certain situations only the presence of adequate numbers of bacteria enables certain genes to be expressed, a fact communicated among the bacteria by so called quorum-sensing molecules.

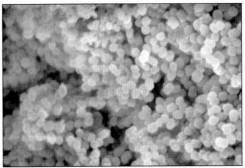

2.69 SEM of a continuous mono-species biofilm

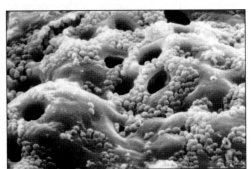

2.70 SEM of a discontinuous mono-species biofilm

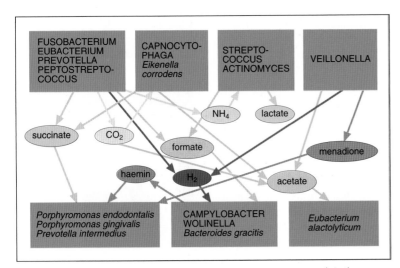

2.68 Nutritional interactions between some common root canal pathogens

The bacterial population is therefore diverse in terms of species and phenotypes (both biofilm and planktonic). This interreliance of the bacterial species is both therapeutically useful and also potentially problematic in helping to resist and induce resistance to treatment.

Given the complexity of the root canal anatomy, it is highly unlikely that bacterial killing agents would reach all aspects of the root canal system. Reliance is placed on using higher concentrations of antibacterial agents so that adequate amounts reach bacteria along a diffusion gradient. It is probably because of the interreliance among bacteria that the more fastidious species are killed in a chain sequence because of deprivation of their nutrients and stimulants from their neighbours. Root canal treatment therefore probably works by a combination of direct and indirect killing effects. The importance of indirect killing is underestimated in modern endodontics.

Recognition that root canal infection is a biofilm is important in devising strategies for treatment because bacteria in biofilms can be more resistant to killing. This may be because of several mechanisms, including the following:

- the exopolysaccharide in which the bacteria are embedded may restrict diffusion of the antibacterial agents to the cells;
- different layers of cells may similarly act as barriers to diffusion;
- some bacterial cells may be slower-growing or be dormant and therefore be more resistant to killing;
- cells may exhibit specific resistance mechanisms; or
- biofilm phenotypes may be inherently resistant.

Effective treatment techniques should recognize these problems and be sufficiently efficacious at the first attempt (visit) to prevent the infection from becoming dominated by surviving resistant strains.

TREATMENT OF PERIAPICAL DISEASE

Based on the fact that periapical lesions develop as a result of the *interaction between* bacteria (and their products) and the host defences, it is clear that their resolution depends upon terminating this interaction. A number of approaches have been used to achieve this general aim. The healing process after root canal treatment has not been deeply researched but can be conceptualized using 'Fish's zones' (**2.26**) in a chronic inflammatory lesion. The removal of bacteria and their products results in the elimination of the zones of infection and contamination. This allows the macrophages in the zone of irritation to invade the areas previously occupied by the zones of infection and contamination in order to remove dead cells and debris. This process also makes way for the osteoblasts and fibroblasts, together with new in-growing blood vessels and nerve fibres from the outermost and active zone of stimulation to proliferate into the zone of irritation. In this way, gradual healing takes place from the boundary of the lesion inwards until a normal periodontal ligament is established. Provided that the periodontal tissues and cells, in particular, have not been irreversibly damaged, ideal healing would eventually result in the formation of cementum over the apical foramen isolating the root canal system completely from the periapex

(**2.71**) but this is not an inevitable end result. Incomplete removal of the infection may reduce but not eliminate the inflammatory area. Healing may be modified and delayed by the treatment procedures and materials used.

Periapical disease is treated by a series of procedures (mechanical and chemical) termed root canal treatment. It consists of obtaining coronal access to the pulp chamber under aseptic conditions, followed by mechanical preparation of the main root canals (radicular access) to gain access to the entire root canal system. The radicular access or the mechanical canal preparation (as it has been more commonly known) is then used to irrigate the root canal system using an antiseptic or antibacterial solution. Chemical debridement and antibacterial killing is continued between visits in infected teeth by sealing a chemical agent in the canal system over this period of time, to kill residual bacteria and to prevent them from recolonizing the root canal system. Historically, a culture sample was taken from the canal at the end of the chemo- mechanical debridement visit to check how effective the procedures had been. The access is sealed and the tooth left for a period of at least a week. At the next appointment (when the result of the culture test is available), the tooth is re-entered under similar aseptic conditions and the canal system reirrigated to remove the antibacterial dressing and any residual bacteria. If obvious clinical signs and symptoms of disease have subsided and the culture test is negative, then the root canal system is considered ready for root filling. The stages prior to root filling are usually sufficient to achieve periapical healing (**2.72, 2.73**). The purpose of root filling is to fill the root canal system with an inert material (usually

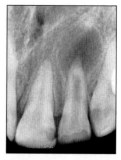

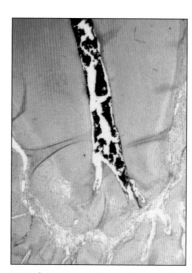

2.72

2.71 Low-power view of healing by cementum formation when Sealapex is used. (Black particles are residual Sealapex and root filling material) (courtesy of Prof. M Tagger)

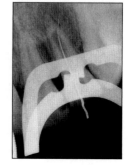

2.73
2.72–2.73 Periapical healing by cleaning alone

gutta-percha and a sealer) to seal off the periapical tissues from the canal system and in turn from the oral environment. It also helps incarcerate residual infection in the root canal system. The permanent access cavity restoration or the permanent tooth restoration provides the definitive coronal seal preventing reinfection of the root canal system.

The culture test during root canal treatment has fallen out of favour in contemporary practice for a variety of reasons. The issue, though, remains controversial and there are some who still practice it. The outcome measures at the end of root canal treatment are absence of clinical signs and symptoms of persistent periapical disease and curiously the radiographic appearance of the root filling (its shape and homogeneity). The definitive outcome measure, however, is periapical healing, since the treatment is aimed at resolution of the periapical tissues (**2.74, 2.75**). This can take anything up to four years or longer and is measured by sequential radiographs which follow the diminution in the size of the periapical radiolucency until normal architecture is restored.

BACTERIA THAT CAN SURVIVE ROOT CANAL TREATMENT PROCEDURES

Numerous studies have evaluated the effect of different stages of root canal treatment on the intraradicular bacterial flora, both qualitatively and quantitatively. Some studies merely report positive culture tests whereas others have identified and quantified intraradicular bacteria before and after stages of treatment.

The effect of 'mechanical preparation' on the bacterial flora has been tested using only water or saline as the irrigant. Taking the studies together, negative cultures were achieved in 4.6–53% of teeth (mean 25%).

When sodium hypochlorite (concentration range 0.5–5.0%) irrigation supplemented the 'mechanical preparation', the frequency of negative cultures immediately after debridement increased to 25–98% of teeth (mean 73%).

Most studies report culture reversals during the interappointment period when active antibacterial dressing is not used in the root canal system between appointments. The reversals are due to regrowth of residual bacteria or recontamination by bacterial leakage around the access cavity dressing.

Other chemical irrigants and dressings have the following effect on negative cultures:

- Biosept (a quaternary ammonium compound) –32–40% negative cultures;
- Nebacin antibiotic –60% negative cultures;
- Cresatin/CMCP/polyantibiotic paste –76% negative cultures.

The most well-controlled studies (from Sundqvist's group) evaluated the effect of various root canal treatment procedures on the bacterial flora both qualitatively and quantitatively. They tested the effect of mechanical preparation, sodium hypochlorite irrigation (0.5%, 5.0%, 5.0% with EDTA), the addition of ultrasonic activation and calcium hydroxide dressing; each increment in chemical canal

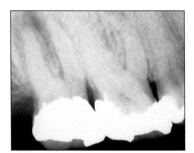 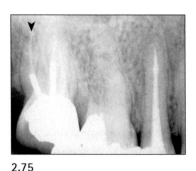

2.74 **2.75**

2.74–2.75 Delayed healing caused by extruded filling material from the distobuccal canal of a maxillary second molar (arrowed)

preparation improved the antibacterial effect on residual bacteria further. They found the antibacterial action to reduce the number of bacteria from an initial range of 10^2–10^8 cells to 10^2–10^3 fewer cells after initial debridement, further reducing down to no recoverable cells after interappointment dressing with calcium hydroxide. Calcium hydroxide dressing is also effective after mechanical preparation and irrigation with water. Only one recent study has found no obvious benefit of dressing with calcium hydroxide between visits.

The collective antibacterial action during root canal treatment has not been shown to cause persistence of any particular species. Specific bacteria, therefore, were not implicated in persistent infections during primary (first attempt) root canal treatment. In contrast, data from secondary (second attempt) root canal treatment showed that certain species were more prevalent after biomechanical procedures than others suggesting that they may be more resistant to treatment protocols, contrary to the previous view. The persistent species were:

- *Enterococcus faecalis*;
- *Streptococcus* species;
- *Staphylococcus* species;
- *Lactobacillus* species;
- *Propionibacterium* species;
- *Actinomyces* species;
- yeasts;
- other Gram-positive bacteria.

Even though most longitudinal studies of the root canal flora do not definitively show resistance of particular species, other studies suggest that Gram-positive bacteria are found with an unexpectedly high frequency in post-treatment cultures.

THE EFFECT OF PERSISTENT BACTERIA ON ROOT CANAL TREATMENT OUTCOME

A preobturation negative culture result can increase treatment success by an average of 12% (range 0–26%). A mixture of many factors led to the gradual abandoning of the culture test in clinical practice. One criticism was that numerous factors could potentially account for treatment outcome but were not all considered in these studies.

One large study (Seltzer *et al.* 1963) in particular contributed to the demise of the culture test but even their study showed a 10% difference in success in favour of the negative culture test when periapical disease was present. The outcome is even worse when a positive culture combines with the presence of a periapical lesion.

The bacteria in preobturation cultures include: *Enterococcus*, *Streptococcus*, *Staphylococcus*, *Lactobacillus*, *Veillonella*, *Pseudomonas*, *Fusobacterium* species and yeasts. Some studies have found no relationship between individual species and treatment failure but others have. While the overall failure rate for cases with positive cultures was 31%, that for teeth with *Enterococcus* species was 55% and for teeth with *Streptococcus* species was 90% (Frostell 1963); in another study, good quality root canal treatment on 54 teeth with asymptomatic periapical disease gave an overall success rate of 74%, but teeth with *Enterococcus faecalis* had a success rate of 66% (Sundqvist *et al.* 1998). These associations cannot be regarded as cause–effect and a relationship should also be sought between numbers of bacteria and treatment outcome. The success rate for teeth with no bacteria was 80% while that for teeth with bacteria in the canal before obturation was 33%.

Regardless of the technique for obtaining a culture, the use of a negative culture to inform progress of treatment has a positive impact on treatment outcome. The association of specific species with treatment failure is not well established but the identity of the small group of species isolated from positive cultures is relatively constant and may hold answers to treatment resistance and failure. It is, however, important to account for the other factors that influence root canal treatment outcome.

FACTORS AFFECTING OUTCOME OF ROOT CANAL TREATMENT

Clinical judgement of the outcome of treatment is dependent upon the absence of signs of infection and inflammation, such as pain, tenderness to percussion of the tooth, tenderness to palpation of the related soft tissues, absence of swelling and sinus and radiographic demonstration of healing of the periapical lesion, with a completely normal periodontal ligament space.

Absence of signs and symptoms of periapical disease but a persistence of a periapical radiographic radiolucency may indicate either healing by fibrosis (2.76) or persistent chronic inflammation. Only

time and an acute exacerbation will identify the latter, whereas the former should remain asymptomatic.

A systematic review and meta-analysis of the factors affecting root canal treatment outcome based on an analysis of 117 studies has revealed the following: the mean success rate is 95% when a vital pulpectomy is carried out as there is no established infection; this reduces to 85% when the root canal treatment procedure is aimed at eradicating an established infection associated with a periapical lesion.

The factors having a major impact on root canal treatment outcome are:

- presence and size of periapical lesion;
- apical extent of root canal treatment in relation to radiographic apex;
- outcome of culture test;
- quality of root canal treatment judged by radiographic appearance of root filling;
- quality of the final coronal restoration.

The factors having minimal effect on root canal treatment outcome are:

- age of patient;
- gender of patient;
- general health of patient;
- treatment technique (preparation, irrigation and obturation material and technique) other than length control.

The improvements in techniques of mechanical and chemical canal preparation have not resulted in increases in success rates over the last century (**Table 2.2**).

A comparison of success rates in studies from Sweden (38%) (known for their biological approach) with the studies from USA (73%) (known for their chemo-mechanical approach) showed the former to have a higher mean success rate (by strict criteria); further highlighting the importance of changing the emphasis in treatment objectives.

It is notable that all the factors having a strong influence on treatment outcome are associated in some way with root canal infection. Further improvements in root canal treatment outcomes may therefore be obtained by understanding the nature of the root canal infection (especially apical) and the manner in which the microflora is altered by treatment.

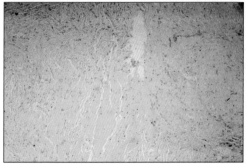

2.76 Fibrous healing (histological view)

Table 2.2 Root canal treatment success rates

Period (Year)	Number of studies	Mean success rate (%)
1900–1950	10	78
1951–1960	12	84
1961–1970	21	82
1971–1980	10	81
1981–1990	11	83
1991–1999	5	83

BACTERIA ASSOCIATED WITH FAILED ROOT CANAL TREATMENT

Bacterial species recovered from root-treated teeth with persistent periapical disease are presented in **Table 2.3**, which shows a different spectrum compared to that in untreated teeth. The flora is dominated by Gram-positive bacteria (**2.77**), many of which are coccoid facultative anaerobes. The retrieval of bacterial samples from obturated root canal systems is compromised by the need to remove root-filling material first, which may kill the bacteria present. The most frequently identified species are:

- *Enterococcus faecalis*;
- *Propionibacterium* species;
- *Streptococcus* species;
- *Lactobacillus* species;
- yeasts;
- *Peptostreptococcus* species.

The species recovered from root treated teeth reside in accessory canals, in dentinal tubules or in the main canal alongside the root filling. They are a subset of those found in untreated teeth though the diversity and quantity is reduced. The recovered bacteria include: *Eubacterium*; *Lactobacillus*; *Propionibacterium*; *Actinomyces*; *Peptostreptococcus*; *Streptococcus*; *Bacteroides*; *Fusobacterium*; *Selenomonas*; and *Veillonella* species. Unlike untreated teeth, treated teeth appear to contain few mixed cultures, often only three, two or one species are found with a mean of only 1.7 species per tooth.

Table 2.3   Showing diversity of bacteria in treated teeth with persistent periapical disease

Aerobes	Facultative anaerobes	Anaerobes
Gram-positive cocci	**Gram-positive cocci**	**Gram-positive cocci**
Dietzia maris	*Enterococcus faecalis*	*Peptococcus* sp.
Micrococcus luteus	*Enterococcus faecium*	*Peptostreptococcus assacharolyticus*
	Gemella morbillorum	*Peptostreptococcus magnus*
Gram-positive rods	*Leuconostoc* sp.	*Peptostreptococcus micros*
Brachybacterium sp.	*Staphylococcus aureus*	
	Staphylococcus epidermidis	**Gram-positive rods**
Gram-negative cocci	*Streptococcus anginosus*	*Eubacterium lentum*
Neisseria sp.	*Streptococcus gordonii*	*Eubacterium timidum*
	Streptococcus mutans	*Eubacterium* spp.
Gram-negative rods	*Streptococcus pyogenes*	
Campylobacter sputorum	*Streptococcus sanguinis*	**Gram-negative cocci**
Pseudomonas aeruginosa		*Acidaminococcus* sp.
	Gram-positive rods	*Veillonella* sp.
	Actinomyces naeslundii	
	Actinomyces odontolyticus	**Gram-negative rods**
	Actinomyces radicidentis	*Bacteroides* sp
	Actinomyces viscosus	*Fusobacterium* sp.
	Bacillus megaterium	*Leptotrichia* sp.
	Corynebacterium diphtheriae	*Porphyromonas endodontalis*
	Lactobacillus fermentum	*Prevotella intermedia*
	Lactobacillus gasseri	*Prevotella melaninogenicus*
	Lactobacillus casei	*Selenomonas sputigena*
	Lactobacillus rhamnosus	
	Propionibacterium acnes	
	Propionibacterium propionicum	
	Gram-negative cocci	
	—	
	Gram-negative rods	
	Citrobacter sp.	
	Eikenella corrodens	
	Enterobacter sp.	
	Escherichia sp.	
	Klebsiella pneumonia	
	Proteus sp.	

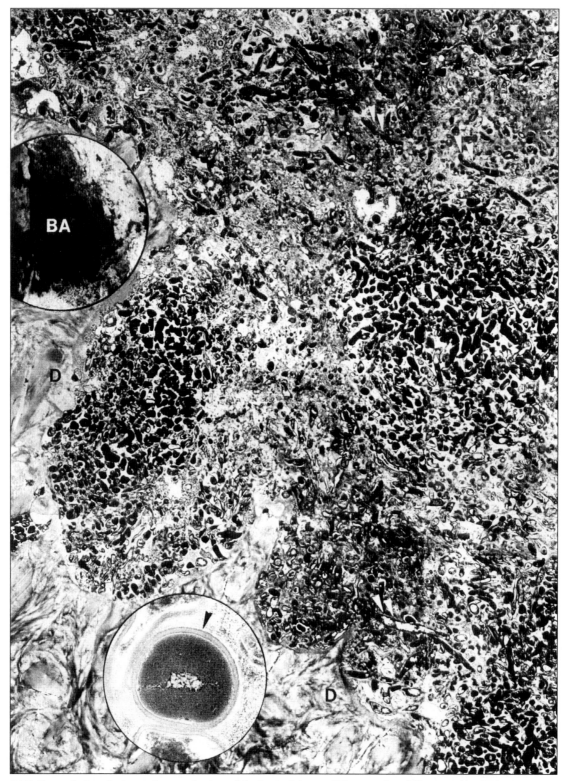

2.77 Transmission electron microscopic view of the bacterial mass (BA, upper inset) illustrated in **2.59a**. Morphologically the bacterial population appears to be composed only of Gram-positive, filamentous organisms (arrowhead). Note the distinct Gram-positive wall in the lower inset. The upper inset is a magnification of the bacterial cluster (BA) in **2.59a**. Original magnification: × 3400; upper inset × 132; lower inset × 21 300 (from Nair *et al.* 1990)

Teeth with poor root fillings have the highest bacterial counts (10^3–10^5) with a maximum of 3–6 species per canal and a diversity that resembles that of untreated teeth, perhaps reflecting poor treatment technique. *Enterococcus faecalis* is the commonest species and when it is present in small numbers in the primary infection it is easily eliminated, but if it infects in large numbers it is difficult to eradicate.

Although specific bacterial species have not been implicated as being resistant to treatment in longitudinal studies, the presence of specific groups of bacteria in root-treated teeth suggests that other than being survivors from the pre-existing infection they may be contaminants introduced during treatment. This may be due to:

- inadequate tooth isolation;
- poor asepsis;
- leakage of the access dressing;
- access cavity being left open for drainage.

OUTCOME OF ROOT CANAL RETREATMENT OF FAILED PREVIOUS TREATMENT

When root canal treatment fails to resolve periapical disease, it is often considered appropriate to retreat the tooth using conventional approaches, especially when the previous treatment is technically deficient (**2.78**). This requires removal of the previous root-filling material and any other material placed for restorative reasons. Correction of any iatrogenic procedural errors may also be required, if possible. All material must be removed in its entirety to ensure delivery of antibacterial agents to all surfaces of the root canal dentine (**2.79**). The success rates of retreatment are generally lower compared to primary treatment because of:

- obstructed access to the apical infection;
- a more resistant bacterial flora.

Table 2.4 gives the outcomes from a range of studies and shows that the mean weighted success rate is 66%, almost 20% lower than in the case of primary treatment.

PERIAPICAL SURGERY AND RETROGRADE SEAL

In a proportion of cases, the conventional chemo-mechanical approach alone does not resolve the problem because it may not allow access to the site of infection in the apex of the tooth (**2.59**), in apical dentinal tubules (**2.80–2.83**) or perhaps because the infection is established extraradicularly (**2.60, 2.61**). In these instances, a surgical approach to the periapex may be required in addition to the conventional approach (**2.81**). Extraradicular infection cannot be diagnosed before primary treatment. It is rather a differential diagnosis arrived at by initial conventional treatment of the intraradicular infection. The healing process in such cases follows a more complicated pathway. Initially there may be attempts at healing because of the removal of the primary source of infection, so there may be a reduction in the size of the periapical lesion. The persistent extraradicular infection would, however, frustrate attempts at complete healing.

Table 2.4 Retreatment outcomes

Study	Number of teeth	Success rate (%)
Strindberg (1956)	123	84
Grahnen & Hansson (1961)	104	74
Engstrom et al. (1964)	85	74
Selden (1974)	52	88
Bergenholtz et al. (1979)	234	48
Molven & Halse (1988)	98	71
Sjogren et al. (1990)	94	62
Friedman et al. (1995)	86	56
Hepworth & Friedman (1997)	Weighted average	66

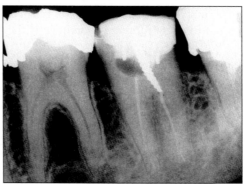

2.78 Technically deficient root canal treatment

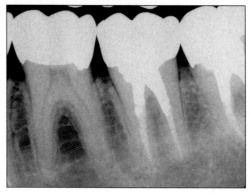

2.79 Tooth in **2.78**, after root canal retreatment

The surgical procedure consisting of the incisional and dissectional wounds concluding with the apical resection of the root (**2.82**) would then inflict additional trauma to the site and change the picture altogether. The procedure would hopefully remove the causative factors leaving a complicated wound to heal by a process which is different from that in response to conventional root canal treatment. The healing essentially involves epithelial and connective tissue resolution processes that are interdependent. The first step is the formation of an epithelial seal which matures with the nutrient support from the developing underlying connective tissue. Reattachment of the mucoperiosteal flap may be compromised by the presence of periodontal disease. Further connective tissue healing consists of removal and organization of the clot into periosteum, alveolar bone, cementum and periodontal ligament. The apical root resection creates a surface of exposed dentine with a root canal outline which is large and filled with a material of variable toxicity. The exposed dentinal surface may become covered with cementum if the tubules are not infected but none forms over the root canal over which fibrous tissue develops. If a retrograde filling material, such as mineral trioxide aggregate (MTA) is used, its osteogenic potential may allow better coverage of the root-end by regeneration of tissues as opposed to repair.

ALTERNATIVE APPROACHES TO ROOT CANAL TREATMENT

The philosophy adopted by some operators has been that the root canal system anatomy is so complex that adequate biomechanical debridement is impossible and time-consuming. Consequently they

advocate the use of chemical agents to destroy and fix the organic pulp tissue together with the bacteria with a reduced emphasis on asepsis and mechanical preparation. A variety of materials (N2, Endomethasone, Spad) all containing formaldehyde as the fixative agent has been recommended. When used together with some degree of mechanical preparation, and the material is confined within the root canal system, the technique may, in some instances, provide successful results. However, there is no scientific body of evidence to substantiate this practice as a predictable procedure. Furthermore, it has been demonstrated that the fixed pulpal tissue is antigenically altered and can stimulate an immune response on its own, whereas unfixed necrotic tissue cannot.

When such material is inadvertently extruded (**2.84**), there are serious consequences. The toxicity of the material can cause necrosis and can alter nerve function. The clinical manifestations of these include severe pain and paraesthesia, especially when the material is extruded into the inferior dental canal (**2.85**). Of course, the same sequelae are likely if other materials are extruded into the nerve canal, but most of these resolve spontaneously over time, whereas this is less likely with the formaldehyde-containing materials.

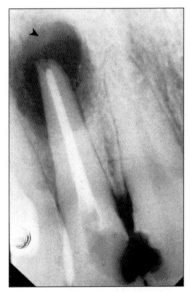

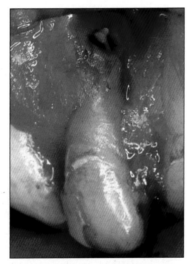

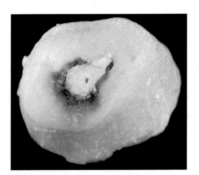

2.80 Adequate root filling demonstrated on radiograph

2.81 Periapical surgery and root resection of the tooth shown in **2.80** (arrowed) shows stained root dentine

2.82 Resected root showing stained/infected dentine

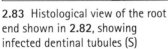

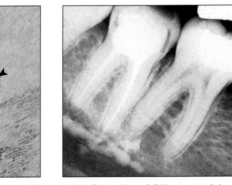

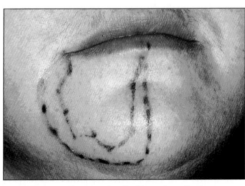

2.83 Histological view of the root end shown in **2.82**, showing infected dentinal tubules (S)

2.84 Extrusion of filling material into the inferior dental canal

2.85 Zones of anaesthesia (inner) and paraesthesia (outer)

Bibliography

Abou-Rass M, Bogen G (1998) Microorganisms in closed periapical lesions. *Int Endod J* **31**, 39–47.

Alavi AM, Gulabivala K, Speight PM (1998) Quantitative analysis of lymphocytes and their subsets in periapical lesions. *Int Endod J* **31**, 233–41.

Allard U, Nord CE, Sjoberg L, Stromberg T (1979) Experimental infections with *Staphylococcus aureus. Streptococcus sanguis. Pseudomonas aeruginosa* and *Bacteroides fragilis* in the jaws of dogs. *Oral Surg, Oral Med, Oral Path* **48**, 454–62.

Allard U, Stromberg U, Stromberg T (1987) Endodontic treatment of experimentally induced apical periodontitis in dogs. *Endod Dent Traumatol* **3**, 240–4.

Ando A, Hoshino E (1990) Predominant obligate anaerobes invading the deep layers of root canal dentine. *Int Endod J* **23**, 20–7.

Andreasen JO, Rud J (1972) A histobacteriologic study of dental and periapical structures after endodontic surgery. *Int J Oral Surg, Oral Med, Oral Pathol* **1**, 272–81.

Assed S, Ito IY, Leonardo MR, Silva L, Lopatin DE (1996) Anaerobic microorganisms in root canals of human teeth with chronic apical periodontitis detected by indirect immuno-fluorescence. *Endod Dent Traumatol* **12**, 66–9.

Atlas RM, Bartha R (1993) *Microbial ecology – fundamentals and applications*, 3rd Edn. Benjamin/Cummings Publishing Company, Inc.

Babal P, Soler P, Brozman M, Jakubovsky J, Beyly M, Basset F (1987) *In situ* characterization of cells in periapical granuloma by monoclonal antibodies. *Oral Surg, Oral Med, Oral Pathol* **64**, 348–52.

Baumgartner JC, Falker WA Jr (1991) Bacteria, in the apical 5 mm of infected root canals. *J Endod* **17**, 380–3.

Baumgartner JC, Falkler WA Jr, Beckerman T (1992) Experimentally induced infection by oral anaerobic microorganisms in a mouse model. *Oral Microbiol Immunol* **7**, 253–6.

Baumgartner JC, Watkins BJ, Bae KS, Xia T (1999) Association of black-pigmented bacteria with endodontic infections. *J Endod* **25**, 413–15.

Bence R, Madonia JV, Weine FS, Smulson MH (1973) A microbiologic evaluation of endodontic instrumentation in pulpless teeth. *Oral Surg, Oral Med, Oral Pathol* **35**, 676–83.

Bergenholtz C (1974) Microorganisms from necrotic pulp of traumatized teeth. *Odontol Revy* **25**, 347–58.

Bergenholtz G, Lekholm U, Milthon R, Heden G, Odesjo B, Engstrom B (1979) Retreatment of endodontic fillings. *Scand J Dent Res* **87**, 217–24.

Bergenholtz G, Lekholm U, Liljenberg B, Lindhe J (1983) Morphometric analysis of chronic inflammatory periapical lesions in root-filled teeth. *Oral Surg, Oral Med, Oral Pathol* **55**, 295–301.

Bhaskar SN (1972) Non-surgical resolution of radicular cysts. *Oral Surg* **34**, 458–76.

Bogen G, Slots J (1999) Black-pigmented anaerobic rods in closed periapical lesions. *Int Endod J* **32**, 204–10.

Brauner AW, Conrads G (1995) Studies into the microbial spectrum of apical periodontitis. *Int Endod J* **28**, 244–8.

Brogden KA, Guthmiller JM (2003) Polymicrobial diseases, a concept whose time has come. *ASM News* **69**, 2.

Brown LR, Rudolph CE (1957) Isolation and identification of micro-organisms from unexposed canals of pulp-involved teeth. *Oral Surg, Oral Med, Oral Pathol* **10**, 1094–99.

Byers MR, Taylor PE, Khayat BG, Kimberley (1990) Effects of injury and inflammation on pulpal and periapical nerves. *J Endod* **16**, 78–84.

Bystrom A, Sundqvist G (1981) Bacteriologic evaluation of the efficacy of mechnical root canal instrumentation in endodontic therapy. *Scand J Dent Res* **89**, 321–8.

Bystrom A, Sundqvist G (1983) Bacteriologic evaluation of the effect of 0.5% sodium hypochlorite in endodontic therapy. *Oral Surg, Oral Med, Oral Pathol* **55**, 307–12.

Bystrom A, Sundqvist G (1985) The antibacterial action of sodium hypochlorite and EDTA in 60 cases of endodontic therapy. *Int Endod J* **18**, 35–40.

Bystrom A, Claesson R, Sundqvist G (1985) The antibacterial effect of camphorated paramonochlorophenol, camphorated phenol and calcium hydroxide in the treatment of infected root canals. *Endod Dent Traumatol* **1**, 170–5.

Cavalleri G, Cuzzolin L, Urbani G, Benoni G (1989) Root canal microflora: qualitative changes after endodontic instrumentation. *J Chemother* **1**, 101–2.

Cheung GSP, Ho MWM (2001) Microbial flora of root canal treated teeth associated with asymptomatic periapical radiolucent lesions. *Oral Microbiol Immunol* **16**, 332–7.

Chirnside (1957) A bacteriologic and histologic study of traumatized teeth. *New Zealand Dent J* **53**, 176–90.

Conrads G, Gharbia SE, Gulabivala K, Lampert F, Shah LN (1997) The use of 16S rDNA directed PCR for the detection of endodontopathogenic bacteria. *J Endod* **23**, 433–8.

Cooper M, Batchelor SM, Prosser JI (1995) Is cell density-signalling applicable to biofilms? Pg 93–6. In Wimpenny J, Nichols W, Stickler D, Lappin-Scot H (eds) *The life and death of a biofilm*, pp. 93–6. Bioline.

Crawford JJ, Shankle JR (1961) An application of newer methods to study the importance of root canal and oral microbiota in endodontics. *Oral Surg, Oral Med, Oral Pathol* **14**, 1109–23.

Cvek M, Hollender L, Nord CE (1976a) Treatment of non-vital permanent incisors with calcium hydroxide. *Odontol Revy* **27**, 93–108.

Cvek M, Nord CE, Hollender L (1976b) Antimicrobial effect of root canal debridement in teeth with immature roots. A clinical and microbiological study. *Odontol Revy* **27**, 1–10.

Dahle UR, Tronstad L, Olsen I (1996) Characterisation of new periodontal and endodontic isolates of spirochaetes. *Eur J Oral Sci* **104**, 41–7.

Dahlen G, Bergenholtz G (1980) Endotoxic activity in teeth with necrotic pulps. *J Dent Res* **59**, 1033–40.

Dahlen G, Haapasalo M (2000) Microbiology of apical periodontitis. Chapter 5. In Pitt Ford T, Ørstavik D (eds), *Essential endodontology*, Blackwell Scientific, Oxford.

Dahlen G, Moller AJR (1992) Microbiology of endodontic infections. Chapter 24. In Slots J, Taubman MA (eds), *Contemporary oral microbiology and immunology*, Mosby-Year Book, Inc.

Dahlen G, Samuelsson W, Molander A, Reit C (2000) Identification and antimicrobial susceptibility of enterococci isolated from the root canal. *Oral Microbiol Immunol* **15**, 309–12.

Dahlen G, Magnusson BC, Moller AJR (1981) histological and histochemical study of the influence of lipopolysaccharide extracted from *Fusobacterium nucleatum* on the periapical tissues in the monkey *Macca Fascicularis*. *Arch Oral Biol* **26**, 591–8.

Dahlen G, Fabricius L, Heyden G, Holm SE, Moller AJR (1982) Apical periodontitis induced by selected bacterial strains in root canals of immunized and non-immunized monkeys. *Scand J Dent Res* **90**, 207–16.

Dahlen G, Fabricius L, Holm SE, Moller A (1987) Interactions within a collection of eight bacterial strains isolated from a monkey dental root canal. *Oral Microbiol Immunol* **2**, 164–70.

Dalton CB, Orstavik D, Phillips C, Pettiette M, Trope M (1998) Bacterial reduction with nickel-titanium rotary instrumentation. *J Endod* **24**, 763–7.

De Paz Villanueva LE (2002) *Fusobacterium nucleatum* in endodontic flare-ups. *Oral Surg, Oral Med, Oral Pathol, Oral Radiol, Endodontics* **93**, 179–83.

Dobell C (1960) *Antony van Leeuwenhoeck and his 'little animals'*. Dover, New York. [Facsimile edition of original work of 1932.]

Dougherty WJ, Bae KA, Watkins BJ, Baumgartner JC (1998) Black-pigmented bacteria in coronal and apical segments of infected root canals. *J Endod* **24**, 356–8.

Egan MW, Spratt DA, Ng YL, LAM JM, Moles DR, Gulabivala K (2002) Prevalence of yeasts in saliva and root canals of teeth associated with apical periodontitis. *Int Endod J* **35**, 321–9.

Engstrom B (1964) The significance of enterococci in root canal treatment. *Odontol Revy* **15**, 87–106.

Engstrom B, Frostell G (1961) Bacteriological studies of the non-vital pulp in cases with intact pulp cavities. *Acta Odontol Scand* **19**, 23–39.

Engstrom B, Frostell G (1964) Experiences of bacteriological root canal control. *Acta Odontol Scand* **22**, 43–69.

Engstrom B, Segerstad LHA, Ramstrom G, Frostell G (1964) Correlation of positive cultures with the prognosis for root canal treatment. *Odontol Revy* **15**, 257–70.

Eriksen HM (1991) Endodontology – Epidemiologic considerations. *Endod Dent Traumatol* **7**, 189–95.

Fabricius L, Dahlen G, Holm G, Moller AJR (1982a) Influence of combination of oral bacteria on periapical tissues of monkeys. *Scand J Dent Res* **90**, 200–6.

Fabricius L, Dahlen G, Ohman AE, Moller AJR (1982b) Predominant indigenous oral bacteria isolated from infected root canals after varied times of closure. *Scand J Dent Res* **90**, 134–44.

Fouad AF, Walton RE, Rittman BR (1992) Induced periapical lesions in ferret canines: histologic and radiographic evaluation. *Endod Dent Traumatol* **8**, 56–62.

Fouad AF, Barry J, Caimano M, Lawson C, Zhu Q, Carver R, Hazlett K, Radolf JD (2002) PCR-based identification of bacteria associated with endodontic infections. *J Clin Microbiol* **40**, 3223–31.

Friedman S, Lost C, Zarrabian M, Trope M (1995) Evaluation of success and failure after endodontic therapy using a glass ionomer cement sealer. *J Endod* **21**, 384–90.

Frostell G (1963) *Clinical significance of the root canal culture*. Transactions of the Third International Conference on Endodontics. University of Pensylvania, Philadelphia, pp. 112–22.

Fukushima H, Yamamoto K, Hirohata K, Sagawa H, Leung KP, Walker CB (1990) Localisation and identification of root canal bacteria in clinically asymptomatic periapical pathosis. *J Endod* **16**, 534–8.

Gohean RJ, Pantera EE, Shuster GS (1990) Indirect imuno-fluorescence for the identification of *Actinomyces* sp. in endodontic disease. *J Endod* **16**, 318–22.

Goldman M, Pearson AH (1969) Post-debridement bacterial flora and antibiotic sensitivity. *Oral Surg, Oral Med, Oral Pathol* **28**, 897–905.

Gomes BPFA, Drucker DB, Lilley JD (1994) Association of specific bacteria with some endodontic signs and symptoms. *Int Endod J* **27**, 291–8.

Gomes BPFA, Lilley JD, Drucker DB (1996a) Clinical significance of dental root canal microflora. *J Dent* **24**, 47–55.

Gomes BPFA, Lilley JD, Drucker DB (1996b) Variations in the susceptibility of components of the endodontic microflora to bio-mechanical procedures. *Int Endod J* **29**, 235–41.

Goncalves RB, Mouton C (1999) Molecular detection of *Bacteroides forsythus* in infected root canals. *J Endod* **25**, 336–40.

Goodman AD (1977) Isolation of anaerobic bacteria from root canal systems of necrotic teeth by use of transport solution. *Oral Surg, Oral Med, Oral Pathol* **43**, 766–70.

Grahnen H, Hansson H (1961) The prognosis of pulp and root canal therapy. *Odontol Revy* **12**, 146–65.

Grahnen H, Krasse B (1963) The effect of instrumentation and flushing of non-vital teeth in endodontic therapy. *Odontol Revy* **14**, 167–77.

Griffee MB, Patterson SS, Miller CH, Kafrawy AH, Newton CW (1980) The relationship of *Bacteroides melaninogenicus* to symptoms associated with pulpal necrosis. *Oral Surg, Oral Med, Oral Pathol* **50**, 457–61.

Grossman LI (1953) the use of antibiotics in endodontic practice. *Br Dent J* **95**, 281–5.

Gutmann JL (1992) Clinical, radiographic, and histologic perspectives on success and failure in endodontics. *Dent Clinic North Am* **36**, 379–92.

Haapasalo MB (1986) *Bacteroides buccae* and related taxa in necrotic root canal infections. *J Clin Microbiol* **24**, 940–4.

Haapasalo M (1989) *Bacteriodes* spp. in dental root canal infections. *Endod Dent Traumatol* **5**, 1–10.

Haapasolo M (1993) Black-pigmented gram-negative anaerobes in endodontic infections. *FEMS Immunol Med Microbiol* **6**, 213–17.

Haapasalo M, Ranta H, Ranta KT (1983) Facultative gram-negative enteric rods in persistent periapical infections. *Acta Odontol Scand* **41**, 19–22.

Haapasalo M, Ranta H, Ranta K, Shah H (1986) Black pigmented *Bacteriodes* spp. in human apical periodontitis. *Infect Immunol* **53**, 149–53.

Haapasalo M, Ranta K, Ranta H (1987) Mixed anaerobic periapical infection with sinus tract. *Endod Dent Traumatol* **3**, 83–5.

Hahn CL, Falker WA, Minah GE (1991) Microbiological studies of carious dentine from human teeth with irreversible pulpitis. *Arch Oral Biol* **36**, 147–53.

Hahn CL, Falker WA, Minah GE (1993) Correlation between thermal sensitivity and microorganisms isolated from deep carious dentine. *J Endod* **19**, 26–30.

Hampp EG (1957) Isolation and identification of spirochaetes obtained from unexposed canals of pulp-involved teeth. *Oral Surg, Oral Med, Oral Pathol* **10**, 1100–4.

Hancock HH, Sigurdsson A, Trope M, Moiseiwitsch J (2001) Bacteria isolated after unsuccessful endodontic treatment in a North American population. *Oral Surg, Oral Med, Oral Pathol, Oral Radiol, Endodontics* **91**, 579–86.

Handley PS, McNab R, Jenkinson HF (1999) Adhesive surface structures on oral bacteria. In Newman HN, Wilson M (eds), pp. 145–70. *Dental plaque revisited – oral biofilms in health and disease*. (editors), Bioline.

Happonen RP, Soderling E, Viander M, Elliniemi LK (1985) Immunocytochemical demonstration of *Actinomyces* species and *Arachnia propionica* in periapical infections. *J Oral Pathol* **14**, 405–13.

Harty FJ, Parkins BJ, Wengraf AM (1970) Success rate in root canal therapy. *Br Dent J* **128**, 65–70.

Heintz CE, Deblinger R, Oliet S (1975) Antibiotic sensitivities of enterococci isolated from treated root canals. *J Endod* **1**, 373–6.

Heithersay G, Bjerken E (1962) Incidence of *Staphylococcus albus* and *Streptococccus salivarius* in root canal cultures. *Odontol Revy* **13**, 152–7

Heling B, Shapira J (1978) Roentgenologic and clinical evaluation of endodontically treated teeth, with or without negative culture. *Quintessence Int* **11**, 79–84.

Heling I, Morag-Hezroni M, Marva E, Hochman N, Zakay-Rones Z, Morag A (2001) Is herpes simplex virus associated with pulp/periapical inflammation? *Oral Surg, Oral Med, Oral Pathol, Oral Radiol, Endodontics* **91**, 359–61.

Henderson B (1999) Bacterial/host interactions in the periodontal diseases: clues to the development of novel therapeutics for the periodontal diseases. In Newman HN, Wilson M (eds) *Dental plaque revisited – oral biofilms in health and disease*. Proceedings of a conference held at the Royal College of Physicians, London. Bioline, Cardiff.

Henrici AT, Hartzell TB (1919) The bacteriology of vital pulps. *Res J* **1**, 419–22.

Hepworth MJ, Friedman S (1997) Treatment outcome of surgical and non-surgical management of endodontic failures. *J Can Dent Assoc* **63**, 364–71.

Hirai K, Tagami A, Okuda K (1991) Isolation and classification of anaerobic bacteria from pulp cavities of non-vital teeth in man. *Bull Tokyo Dent Coll* **32**, 95–8.

Hobson P (1959) An investigation into the bacteriological control of infected root canals. *Br Dent J* **106**, 63–70.

Horiba N, Maekawa Y, Matsumoto T, Nakamura H (1990) A study of the distribution of endotoxin of infected root canals. *J Endod* **16**, 331–4.

Horiba N, Maekawa Y, Abe Y, lto M, Matsumoto T, Nakamura H (1991) Correlations between endotoxin and clinical symptoms or radiolucent areas in infected root canals. *Oral Surg, Oral Med, Oral Pathol* **71**, 492–5.

Hoshino E, Ando N, Sato M, Kota K (1992) Bacterial invasion of non-exposed dental pulp. *Int Endod J* **25**, 2–5.

Hoshino E, Ando-Kurihara N, Sato I, Vematsu H, Sto M, Kota K, Iwaku M (1996) *In vitro* antibacterial susceptibility of bacteria taken from infected root dentine to a mixture of ciprofloxacin, metronidazole and minocycline. *Int Endod J* **29**, 125–30.

Hunter W. (1911) The role of sepsis and antisepsis in medicine. *Lancet* **January 14**, 79–86.

Ingle JI, Zeldow BJ (1958) An evaluation of mechanical-instrumentation and the negative culture in endodontic therapy. *J Am Dent Assoc* **57**, 471–6.

Kakehashi S, Stanley HR, Fitzgerald W (1965) The effects of surgical exposures of dental pulps in germ free and conventional laboratory rats. *Oral Surg, Oral Med, Oral Pathol* **20**, 340–9.

Kalfas S, Figdor D, Sundqvist G, (2001) A new bacterial species associated with failed endodontic treatment. Identification and description of *Actinomyces radicidentis*. *Oral Surg, Oral Med, Oral Pathol, Oral Radiol, Endodontics* **92**, 208–14.

Kantz WE, Henry CA (1974) Isolation and classification of anaerobic bacteria from intact pulp chambers of non vital teeth in man. *Arch Oral Biol* **19**, 91–5.

Kerekes K, Tronstad L (1979) Long-term results of endodontic treatment performed with a standardised technique. *J Endod* **5**, 83–90.

Kessler S (1972) Bacteriological examination of root canals. *J Dent Assoc South Africa* **27**, 9–13.

Kettering JD, Torabinejad M (1993) Presence of natural killer cells in human chronic periapical lesions. *Int Endod J* **26**, 344–7.

Keudell K, Conte M, Fujimoto L, Ernest M, Berry HG (1976) Microorganisms isolated from pulp chambers. *J Endod* **2**, 146–8.

Khemaleelakul S, Baumgartner JC, Pruksakorn S (2002) Identification of bacteria in acute endodontic infections and their antimicrobial susceptibility. *Oral Surg, Oral Med, Oral Pathol, Oral Radiol, Endodontics* **94**, 746–55.

Kiryu T, Hoshino E, Iwaku M (1994) Bacteria invading periapical cementum. *J Endod* **20**, 169–72.

Kobayashi T, Hayashi A, Hoshikawa R, Okuda K, Hara K. (1990) The microbial flora from root canals and periodontal pockets of non-vital teeth associated with advanced periodontitis. *Int Endod J* **23**, 100–6.

Kohsaka T, Kumazawa M, Yamasaki M, Nakamura H (1996) Periapical lesions in rats with streptozotocin-induced diabetes. *J Endod* **2**, 418–21.

Kolenbrander PE (2000) Oral microbial communities: biofilms, interaction, and genetic systems. *Ann Rev Microbiol* **54**, 413–37.

Kontiainen S, Ranta H, Lautenschlager I (1986) Cells infiltrating human periapical inflammatory lesions. *J Oral Pathol* **15**, 544–6.

Kumar T, Spratt DA, Ng Y-L, Gulabivala K (2002) A preliminary evaluation of a new method for sampling the intra-radicular bacterial flora. *Int Endod J* **35**, 85.

Leavitt JM, Naidorf IJ, Shugaevsky P (1958) Bacterial flora of root canals as disclosed by a culture medium for endodontics. *Oral Surg, Oral Med, Oral Pathol* **11**, 302–8.

Lewsey JD, Gilthorpe MS, Gulabivala K (2001) An introduction to meta-analysis within the framework of multi-level modelling using the probability of success of root canal treatment as an illustration. *Comm Dent Health* **18**, 131–7.

Lomcali G, Sen BH, Cankaya H (1996) Scanning electron microscopic observations of apical root surfaces of teeth with apical periodontitis. *Endod Dent Traumatol* **12**, 70–6.

Longman LP, Preston AJ, Martin MV, Wilson NHF (2000) Endodontics in the adult patient: the role of antibiotics. *J Dent* **28**, 539–48.

Love RM, McMillan MD, Jenkinson HF (1997) Invasion of dentinal tubules by oral streptococci is associated with collagen recognition mediated by the antigen I/II family of polypeptides. *Infect Immun* **65**, 5157–64.

MacDonald JB, Hare GC, Wood AWS (1957) The bacteriologic status of the pulp chambers in intact teeth found to be non-vital following trauma. *Oral Surg, Oral Med, Oral Pathol* **10**, 318–22.

Mah T-FC, O'Toole GA (2001) Mechanisms of biofilm resistance to antimicrobial agents. *Trends Microbiol* **9**, 34–9.

Marton IJ, Kiss C (2000) Protective and destructive immune reactions in apical periodontitis. *Oral Microbiol Immunol* **15**, 139–50.

Meghji S, Qureshi W, Henderson B, Harris M (1996) The role of endotoxin and cytokines in the pathogenesis of odontogenic cysts. *Arch Oral Biol* **41**, 523–31.

Melville TH, Slack GL (1961) Bacteria isolated from root canals during endodontic treatment. *Br Dent J* **110**, 127–30.

Melville TH, Birch RH (1967) Root canal and periapical floras of infected teeth. *Oral Surg, Oral Med, Oral Pathol* **23**, 93–8.

Miller WD (1894) An introduction to the study of the bacterio-pathology of the dental pulp. *Dent Cosmos* **36**, 505–28.

Molander A, Reit C, Dahlen G (1990) Microbiological evaluation of clindamycin as a root canal dressing in teeth with apical periodontitis. *Int Endod J* **23**, 113–8.

Molander A, Reit C, Dahlen G (1996a) Microbiological root canal sampling: diffusion of a technology. *Int Endod J* **29**, 163–7.

Molander A, Reit C, Dahlen G (1996b) Reasons for dentists' acceptance or rejection of microbiological root canal sampling. *Int Endod J* **29**, 168–72.

Molander A, Reit C, Dahlen G, Kvist T (1998) Microbiological status of root-filled teeth with apical periodontitis. *Int Endod J* **31**, 1–7.

Moller AJR (1966) Microbiological examination of root canals and periapical tissues of human teeth. *Odontol Tidskrift* **74** (Special Issue), 1–380.

Moller AJR, Fabricius L, Dahlen G, Ohman AE, Heyden G (1981) Influence on periapical tissues of indigenous oral bacteria and necrotic pulp tissue in monkeys. *Scand J Dent Res* **89**, 475–84.

Molven O, Halse A (1988) Success rates for gutta-percha and kloro-percha N-O root fillings made by undergraduate students: radiographic findings after 10–17 years. *Int Endod J* **21**, 243–50.

Molven O, Olsen I, Kerekes K (1991) Scanning electron microscopy of bacteria in the apical part of root canals in permanent teeth with periapical lesions. *Endod Dent Traumatol* **7**, 226–9.

Morse DR (1971) The endodontic culture technique: an impractical and unnecessary procedure. *Dent Clin North Am* **15**, 793–806.

Morse DR (1981) Endodontic microbiology in the 1970s. *Int Endod J* **14**, 69–79.

Munson MA, Pitt Ford T, Chong B, Weightman A, Wade WG (2002) Molecular and cultural analysis of the microflora associated with endodontic infections. *J Dent Res* **81**, 761–6.

Myers JW, Marshall FJ, Rosen S (1969) The incidence and identity of microorganisms present in root canals at filling following culture reversals. *Oral Surg, Oral Med, Oral Pathol* **28**, 889–96.

Naidorf I (1972) Inflammation and infection of pulp and periapical tissues. *Oral Surg, Oral Med, Oral Pathol* **34**, 486–97.

Naidorf IJ (1974) Clinical Microbiology in endodontics. *Dent Clin North Am* **18**, 329–44.

Nair PN, Sjogren U, Krey G, Kahnberg KE, Sundqvist G (1990a) Intraradicular bacteria and fungi in root-filled, asymptomatic human teeth with therapy-resistant periapical lesions: a long-term light and electron microscopic follow-up study. *J Endod* **16**, 580–8.

Nair PN, Sjogren U, Krey G, Sundqvist G (1990b) Therapy-resistant foreign body giant cell granuloma at the periapex of a root-filled human tooth. *J Endod* **16**, 589–95.

Nair PN, Sjogren U, Schumacher E, Sundqvist G (1993) Radicular cyst affecting a root-filled human tooth: a long-term post-treatment follow-up. *Int Endod J* **26**, 225–33.

Nair PNR (1987) Light and electron microscope studies of root canal flora and periapical lesions. *J Endod* **13**, 29–39.

Nair PNR (1997) Apical periodontitis: a dynamic encounter between root canal infection and host response. *Periodontol 2000* **13**, 121–48.

Nair PNR (1998) Review – new perspectives on radicular cysts: do they heal? *Int Endod J* **31**, 155–60.

Nair, PNR (1998) Pathology of apical periodontitis. In Ørstavik D, Pitt Ford TR (eds) *Essential endodontology*. Blackwell, Oxford

Nair PNR, Schroeder HE (1984) Periapical actinomycosis. *J Endod* **10**, 567–70.

Nelson IA (1982) Endodontics in general practice – a retrospective survey. *Int Endod J* **15**, 168–72.

Nicholls E (1962) The efficacy of cleansing of the root canal. *Br Dent J* **112**, 167–70.

Noyes (1922) In Blayney JR (1922) The clinical results of pulp treatment. *J Nat Dent Assoc* **16**, 198–208.

Nygaard-Ostby B, Schilder H (1972) Inflammation and infection of the pulp and periapical tissues: a synthesis. *Oral Surg, Oral Med, Oral Pathol* **34**, 498–501.

Oguntebi BR (1994) Dentine tubule infection and endodontic therapy implications. *Int J Endod* **27**, 218–22.

Olgart LG (1969) Bacteriological sampling from root canals directly after chemo-mechanical treatment: a clinical and bacteriological study. *Acta Odontol Scand* **27**, 91–103.

Oliet S, Sorin S (1969) Evaluation of clinical results based upon culturing root canals. *J Br Endod Soc* **3**, 3–6.

Ørstavik D, Pitt Ford TR (eds) (1998) *Essential endodontology*. Blackwell, Oxford.

Ørstavik D, Kerekes K, Molven O (1991) Effects of extensive apical reaming and calcium hydroxide dressing on bacterial infection during treatment of apical periodontitis: a pilot study. *Int Endod J* **24**, 1–7.

Peciuliene V, Balciuniene I, Eriksen HM, Haapasalo M (2000) Isolation of *Enterococcus faecalis* in previously root-filled canals in a Lithuanian population. *J Endod* **26**, 593–5.

Peciuliene V, Reynaud AH, Balciuniene I, Haapasalo M (2001) Isolation of yeasts and enteric bacteria in root-filed teeth with chronic apical periodontitis. *Int Endod J* **34**, 429–34.

Peters LB, Wesselink PR, Bujis JF, van Winkellhoff AJ (2001) Viable bacteria in root dentinal tubules of teeth with apical periodontitis. *J Endod* **27**, 76–81.

Peters LB, van Winklehoff AJ, Buijs JF, Wesselink PR (2002) Effects of instrumentation, irrigation and dressing with calcium hydroxide on infection in pulpless teeth with periapical bone lesions. *Int Endod J* **35**, 13–21.

Peters LB, Wesselink PR, Moorer WK (1995) The fate and role of bacteria left in root canal dentinal tubules. *Int Endod J* **28**, 95–9.

Phillips JM (1967) Rat connective tissue response to hollow polyethylene tube implants. *J Can Dent Assoc* **33**, 59–64.

Pinheiro ET, Gomes BP, Ferraz CC, Sousa EL, Teixeira FB, Souza-Filho FJ (2003) Microorganisms from canals of root-filled teeth with periapical lesions. *Int Endod J* **36**, 1–11.

Pitts DL, Williams B Morton TH (1982) Investigation of the role of endotoxin in periapical inflammation. *J Endod* **8**, 10–8.

Reit C, Dahlen G (1988) Decision-making analysis of endodontic treatment strategies in teeth with apical periodontitis. *Int Endod J* **21**, 291–9.

Reit C, Molander A, Dahlen G (1999) The diagnostic accuracy of microbiologic root canal sampling and the influence of antimicrobial dressings. *Endod Dent Traumatol* **15**, 278–83.

Ribeiro Sobrinho AP, de Melo Maltos SM, Farias LM, de Carvalho MA, Nicoli JR, de Uzeda M, Vieira LQ (2002) Cytokine production in response to endodontic infection in germ-free mice. *Oral Microbiol Immunol* **17**, 344–53.

Rickert U, Dixon CM (1931) The controlling of root surgery. *Int Dent Cong (8th)* Supp. 111A, 15.

Rocas IN, Siqueira JF, Santos KRN, Coelho AMA (2001) 'Red complex' (*Bacteroides forsythus, Porphyromonas gingvalis*, and *Tresponema denticola*) in endodontic infections: a molecular approach. *Oral Surg, Oral Med, Oral Pathol, Oral Radiol, Endodontics* **91**, 468–71.

Rolph HJ, Lennon A, Riggio MP, Saunders WP, MacKenzie D, Coldero L, Bagg J (2001) Molecular identification of microorganisms from endodontic infections. *J Clin Microbiol* **39**, 3282–9.

Sato I, Ando-Kurihara N, Kota K, Iwaku M, Hoshino E (1996) Sterilization of infected root-canal dentine by topical application of a mixture of ciprofloxacin, metronidazole and minocycline *in situ*. *Int Endod J* **29**, 118–24.

Sato T, Hoshino E, Uematsu H, Noda T (1993) Predominant obligate anaerobes in necrotic pulps of human deciduous teeth. *Microb Ecol Health Dis* **6**, 269–75.

Schein B, Schilder H (1975) Endotoxin content in endodontically involved teeth. *J Endod* **1**, 19–21.

Selden HS (1974) Pulpoperiapical disease: diagnosis and healing. *Oral Surg* **37**, 271–83.

Seltzer S, Bender I, Turkenkopf S (1963) Factors affecting successful repair after root canal therapy. *J Am Dent Assoc* **67**, 651–62.

Sen BH, Piskin B, Demrici T (1995) Observations of bacteria and fungi in infected root canals and dentinal tubules by SEM. *Endod Dent Traumatol* **11**, 6–9.

Shindell E (1962) Studies on the possible presence of a virus in subacute and chronic periapical granulomas. *Oral Surg, Oral Med, Oral Pathol* **15**, 1382–4.

Shinoda S, Murayama Y, Okada H (1986) Immunopathological role of pulpal tissue components in periapical pathosis. *J Endod* **12**, 528–33.

Shovelton DS (1964) The presence and distribution of microorganisms within non-vital teeth. *Br Dent J* **117**, 101–7.

Shovelton DS, Sidaway S (1960) Infection in root canals. *Br Dent J* **108**, 115–18.

Sims W (1973) Some comments on the microbiological examination of root canals. *J Dent* **2**, 2–6.

Siqueira JF (2001) Aetiology of root canal treatment failure: how well-treated teeth can fail. *Int Endod J* **34**, 1–10.

Siqueira JF, de Uzeda M (1996) Disinfection by calcium hydroxide pastes of dentinal tubules infected with two obligate and one facultative anaerobic bacteria. *J Endod* **22**, 674–6.

Siqueira JF, Lopes HP (2001) Bacteria on the apical root surfaces of untreated teeth with periradicular lesions: a scanning electron microscopy study. *Int Endod J* **34**, 216–20.

Siqueira JF, Rôças IN (2002) *Dialister pneumosintes* can be a suspected endodontic pathogen. *Oral Surg, Oral Med, Oral Pathol, Oral Radiol, Endodontics* **94**, 494–8.

Siqueira JF, Rôças IN, Favieri A, Lima KC (2000a) Chemomechanical reduction of the bacterial population in the root canal after instrumentation and irrigation with 1%, 2.5% and 5.0% sodium hypochlorite. *J Endod* **26**, 331–4.

Siqueira JF, Rôças IN, Souto R, de Uzeda M, Colombo AP (2000b) Checkerboard DNA–DNA hybridization analysis of endodontic infections. *Oral Surg, Oral Med, Oral Pathol, Oral Radiol, Endodontics* **89**, 744–8.

Siqueira JF, Rôças IN, Favieri A, Oliveira JCM, Santos KRN (2001a) Polymerase chain reaction detection of *Treponema denticola* in endodontic infections within root canals. *Int Endod J* **34**, 280–4.

Siqueira JF, Rôças IN, Oliveri JCM, Santos KRN (2001b) Detection of putative oral pathogens in acute periradicular abscesses by 16S rRNA-directed polymerase chain reaction. *J Endod* **27**, 164–7.

Siqueira JF, Rôças IN, Oliveira JCM, Santos KRN (2001c) Molecular detection of black-pigmented bacteria in infections of endodontic origin. *J Endod* **27**, 563–6.

Siqueira JF, Rôças IN, Lopes HP (2002a) Patterns of microbial colonization in primary root canal infections. *Oral Surg, Oral Med, Oral Pathol, Oral Radiol, Endodontics* **93**, 174–8.

Siqueira JF, Rôças IN, Moraes SR, Santos KRN (2002b) Direct amplification of rRNA gene sequences for identification of selected oral pathogens in root canal infections. *Int Endod J* **35**, 345–51.

Siren EK, Haapasalo M, Ranta K, Salmi P, Kerosuo ENJ (1997) Microbiological findings and clinical treatment procedures in endodontic cases selected for microbiological investigation. *Int Endod J* **30**, 91–5.

Sjogren U, Sundqvist G (1987) Bacteriologic evaluation of ultrasonic root canal instrumentation. *Oral Surg, Oral Med, Oral Pathol* **63**, 366–70.

Sjogren U, Happonen RP, Kahnberg KE, Sundqvist G (1988) Survival of *Arachnia propionica* in periapical tissue. *Int Endod J* **21**, 277–82.

Sjogren U, Hagglund G, Sundqvist G, Wing K (1990) Factors affecting the long-term results of endodontic treatment. *J Endod* **16**, 498–504.

Sjogren U, Figdor D, Sangberg L, Sundqvist G (1991) The antimicrobial effect of calcium hydroxide as a short-term intracanal dressing. *Int Endod J* **24**, 119–25.

Sjogren U, Figdor D, Persson S, Sundqvist G (1997) Influence of infection at the time of root filling on the outcome of endodontic treatment of teeth with apical periodontitis. *Int Endod J* **30**, 297–306.

Slack GL (1953) The bacteriology of infected root canals and in vitro penicillin sensitivity. *Br Dent J* **95**, 21–4.

Sobrinho APR, Barros MHM, Nicoli JR, Carvalho MAR, Farias LM, Bambira EA, Bahia MGA, Vieira EC (1998) Experimental root canal infections in conventional and germ-free mice. *J Endod* **24**, 405–8.

Sommer J, Crowley M (1940) Bacteriologic verification of Roentgenographic findings in pulp involved teeth. *J Am Dent Assoc* **27**, 723–34.

Spratt DA, Pratten J, Wilson M, Gulabivala K (2001) The *in vitro* effect of antiseptic agents on bacterial biofilms generated from selected root canal isolates. *Int Endod J* **34**, 300–7.

Stabholz A, McArthur WP (1978) Cellular immune response of patients with periapical pathosis to necrotic dental pulp antigens determined by release of LIF. *J Endod* **9**, 282–7.

Stabholz A, Sela MN (1983) The role of oral microorganisms in the pathogenesis of periapical pathosis. I. Effect of *Streptoccocus mutans* and its cellular constituents on the dental pulp and periapical tissue of cats. *J Endod* **9**, 171–5.

Stashenko P, Wang CY, Tani-Ishii N, Yu SM (1994) Pathogenesis of induced rat periapical lesions. *Oral Surg, Oral Med, Oral Pathol* **78**, 494–502.

Stashenko P, Teles R, D'Souza R (1998) Periapical inflammatory responses and their modulation. *Crit Rev Oral Biol Med* **9**, 498–521.

Stewart GG, Cobe HM, Rappaport H (1961) A study of a new medicament in the chemomechanical preparation of infected root canals. *J Am Dent Assoc* **63**, 33.

Stobberingh EE, Eggink CO (1982) The value of the bacteriological culture in endodontics. II. The bacteriological flora of endodontic specimens. *Int Endod J* **15**, 87–93.

Storoe W, Haug RH, Lillich TT (2001) The changing face of odontogenic infections. *J Oral Maxillofacial Surg* **59**, 739–48; discussion 748–9.

Strindberg LZ (1956) The dependence of the results of pulp therapy on certain factors – an analytical study based on radiographic and clinical follow-up examinations. *Acta Odontol Scand* **14**, 1–175.

Sulitzeanu A, Bender EH, Epstein LJ (1964) Bacteriological studies of pulp-involved teeth by cultural and microscopic methods. *J Am Dent Assoc* **69**, 300.

Sunde PT, Tronsatd L, Eribe ER, Lind PO, Olsen I (2000) Assessment of periradicular microbiota by DNA–DNA hybridization. *Endod Dent Traumatol* **16**, 191–6.

Sundqvist G (1976) *Bacteriologic studies of necrotic dental pulps*. Dissertation. University of Umea, Sweden.

Sundqvist G (1992a) Associations between microbial species in dental root canal infections. *Oral Microbiol Immunol* **7**, 257–62.

Sundqvist G (1992b) Ecology of the root canal flora. *J Endod* **18**, 427–30.

Sundqvist G (1994) Taxonomy, ecology and pathogenicity of the root canal flora. *Oral Surg, Oral Med, Oral Pathol* **78**, 522–30.

Sundqvist GK, Eckerbom MI, Larsson AP, Sjogren UT (1979) Capacity of anaerobic bacteria from necrotic dental pulps to induce purulent infections. *Infect Immun* **25**, 685–93.

Sundqvist G, Johansson E, Sjogren U (1989) Prevalence of black-pigmented *Bacteroides* species in root canal infections. *J Endod* **15**, 13–9.

Sundqvist G, Figdor D, Hanstrom L, Sorlin S, Sandstrom G (1991) Phagocytosis and virulence of different strains of *Porphyromonas gingivalis. Scand J Dent Res* **99**, 117–29.

Sundqvist G, Figdor D, Persson S (1998) Microbiological analysis of teeth with failed endodontic treatment and outcome of conservative re-treatment. *Oral Surg, Oral Med, Oral Pathol* **85**, 85–93.

Takahashi K (1998) Microbiological, pathological, inflammatory, immunological and molecular biological aspects of periradicular disease. *Int Endod J* **31**, 311–25.

Taklan S (1974) A bacteriological study of the pulp of intact non-vital teeth. *J Br Endod Soc* **7**, 75–7.

Tani-Ishii N, Wang CY, Tanner A, Stashenko P (1994) Changes in root canal microbiota during the development of rat periapical lesions. *Oral Microbiol Immunol* **9**, 129–35.

Ten Cate AR (1994) *Oral histology – development, structure and function*, 4th edn, Chapter 10, pp. 169–217. Mosby, St Louis, USA.

Thilo BE, Baelini P, Holtz J (1986) Dark field observation of the bacterial distribution in root canals followed pulp necrosis. *J Endod* **12**, 202–5.

Torabinejad M (1994) Mediators of acute and chronic periradicular lesions. *Oral Surg, Oral Med, Oral Pathol* **78**, 511–21.

Torabinejad M, Bakland LK (1978) Immunopathogenesis of chronic periapical lesions: a review. *Oral Surg, Oral Med, Oral Pathol* **46**, 685–99.

Torneck CD (1966) Reaction of rat connective tissue to polyethylene tube implants. Parts 1 & 2. *Oral Surg, Oral Med, Oral Pathol* **21**, 379–87 & 674–83.

Tronstad L, Barnett F, Riso K, Slots J (1987) Extra-radicular endodontic infections. *Endod Dent Traumatol* **3**, 86–90.

Tsatsas B, Tzamouranis, Mitsis F (1974) A bacteriological examination of root canals before filling. *J Br Endod Soc* **7**, 78–80.

Valderhaug J (1974) a histologic study of experimentally induced periapical inflammation in primary teeth in monkeys. *Int J Oral Surg* **3**, 111–23.

van Winklehoff A, van Steenbergen M, de Graaff J (1992) *Porphyromonas (Bacteroides) endodontalis*: its role in endodontal infections. *J Endod* **18**, 431–4.

Vigil GV, Wayman BE, Dazey SE, Fowler CB, Bradley DV (1997) Identification and antibiotic sensitivity of bacteria isolated from periapical lesions. *J Endod* **23**, 110–4.

Waltimo TMT, Siren EK, Torkko HLK, Olsen I, Haapasalo MPP (1997) Fungi in therapy-resistant apical periodontitis. *Int Endod J* **30**, 96–101.

Walton RE, Garnick JJ (1986) The histology of periapical inflammatory lesions in permanent molars in monkeys. *J Endod* **12**, 49–53.

Ward D, Brassell S, Eglinton G (1985) Archebacterial lipids in hot-spring microbial mats. *Nature* **318**, 656–9.

Wasfy MO, McMahon, Minah GE, Falker WA (1992) Microbiological evaluation of periapical infections in Egypt. *Oral Microbiol Immunol* **7**, 100–5.

Waterman PA Jr, Torabinejad M, McMillan PJ, Kettering JD (1998) Development of periradicular lesions in immunosuppressed rats. *Oral Surg, Oral Med, Oral Pathol, Oral Radiol, Endodontics* **85**, 720–5.

Watts A (1981) Cellular responses in the dental pulp: a review. *Int Endod J* **14**, 10–21.

Watts A, Paterson RC (1993) Atypical apical lesions detected during study of short term tissue responses to three different endodontic instrumentation techniques. *Endod Dent Traumatol* **9**, 200–10.

Weiger R, Manncke B, Werner H, Lost C (1995) Microbial flora of sinus tracts and root canals of non-vital teeth. *Endod Dent Traumatol* **11**, 15–19.

World Health Organization (1995) *Application of the International Classification of Diseases to Dentistry and Stomatology*, 3rd edn. WHO, Geneva, pp. 66–7.

Wilson M, Pratten J (1999) Laboratory assessment of antimicrobials for plaque-related diseases. In Newman HN, Wilson M (eds) *Dental plaque revisited – oral biofilms in health and disease*. Proceedings of a conference held at the Royal College of Physicians, London. Bioline, Cardiff.

Wilson MI, Hall J (1968) Incidence of yeasts in root canals. *J Br Endod Soc* **2**, 56–9.

Wilson MJ, Weightman WJ, Wade WG (1997) Applications of molecular ecology in the characterisation of uncultured micro organisms associated with human diseases. *Rev Med Microbiol* **8**, 91–101.

Wittgow WC, Sabiston CB (1975) Microorganisms from pulpal chambers of intact teeth with necrotic pulps. *J Endod* **1**, 168–71.

Yamasaki M, Nakane A, Kumazawa M, Hashioka K, Horiba N, Nakamura H (1992) Endotoxin and Gram-negative bacteria in the rat periapical lesions. *J Endod* **18**, 501–4.

Yared GM, Bou Dagher FE (1994) Influence of apical enlargement on bacterial infection during treatment of apical periodontitis. *J Endod* **20**, 535–7.

Yoshida M, Fukushima H, Yamamoto K, Ogawa K, Toda T, Sagawa H (1987) Correlation between clinical symptoms and microorganisms isolated from root canals of teeth with periapical pathosis. *J Endod* **13**, 24–8.

Yu SM, Stashenko P (1987) Identification of inflammatory cells in developing rat periapical lesions. *J Endod* **13**, 535–40.

Zavistocki J, Dzink JBS, Onderdonk A, Bartlett J (1980) Quantitative bacteriology of endodontic infections. *Oral Surg, Oral Med, Oral Pathol* **49**, 171–80.

Zielke DR, Heggers JP, Harrison JW (1976) A statistical analysis of anaerobic versus aerobic culturing in endodontic therapy. *Oral Surg, Oral Med, Oral Pathol* **42**, 830–7.

Chapter 3

Patient assessment

C J R Stock

At the first appointment the dentist must assess both the patient and the dental problem before commencing treatment because many factors affect the management of the patient and the method of treatment chosen. Accurate, clear records must be kept of all treatment undertaken and all relevant information taken from the patient. What is written on a patient's treatment card will be used as evidence in any legal disputes.

The operator will be examining the patient for a variety of disorders in an endodontic assessment. In many cases the patient seeks treatment because of pain, but many conditions are discovered only by clinical examination. Common disorders, which may be revealed during an endodontic assessment, include:

- inflamed pulp;
- concussed pulp;
- necrotic pulp;
- acute periapical inflammation;
- acute periapical abscess;
- chronic periapical inflammation;
- resorption of the tooth,
    internal;
    external;
- fractured tooth,
    crown (vital/non-vital pulp);
    root (vital/non-vital pulp);
    horizontal fracture;
    vertical fracture;
- periodontal disease;
- traumatic occlusion;
- iatrogenic problems (operator induced);
- local non-dental pathology,
    soft tissues;
    hard tissues;
- systemic disease;
- atypical facial pain.

HEALTH HISTORY

A medical history is taken to find out whether the patient has any medical condition or is taking medication that could affect the treatment. The most convenient way of recording such information is to use a checklist that is kept in the patient's file, such as that shown in **Table 3.1**.

No medical conditions specifically contraindicate endodontic treatment, although patients with a history of infective endocarditis or prosthetic heart valves should be regarded as a special-risk group and be referred for specialist treatment. Rheumatic fever (particularly when there has been heart damage), insulin-controlled diabetes, anticoagulant therapy and sexually transmitted diseases may affect treatment, and if the practitioner is in any doubt, he or she should consult the patient's medical adviser before commencing treatment. Patients with cardiac abnormalities are usually administered prophylactic antibiotics to prevent infective endocarditis (see **Table 3.2**). The incidence of infective endocarditis in patients with cardiac abnormalities is increased with diabetes mellitus, immunosuppression, alcohol dependence, haemodialysis and intravenous drug abuse.

Table 3.1 Checklist for recording patient information

Rheumatic fever or chorea	Yes/No
Hypertension or cardiac disease	Yes/No
Bleeding disorders	Yes/No
Allergies	Yes/No
Diabetes (or anyone in the family)	
Liver disease (e.g. jaundice or hepatitis) or kidney disease	Yes/No
Pregnant	Yes/No
Taking any prescribed medicine	Yes/No
Under treatment by GP or hospital	Yes/No
Serious illness in last three years	Yes/No
Upper respiratory tract infections	Yes/No

Table 3.2 Prophylactic antibiotic regimens

Procedures under local anaesthesia

Patients not allergic to penicillin who have not been prescribed penicillin more than once in the previous four weeks:

Amoxycillin
— Adults: 3 g single oral dose under supervision one hour before procedure
— Children under 10 years: half adult dose
— Children under 5 years: quarter adult dose

Patients allergic to penicillin or who have had penicillin more than once in the previous four weeks:

Clindamycin
— Adults: 600 mg single oral dose under supervision one hour before procedure
— Children 5–10 years: half adult dose
— Children under 5 years: quarter adult dose

Procedures under general anaesthesia

Patients not allergic to penicillin who have not been prescribed penicillin more than once in the previous four weeks:

Amoxycillin
— Adults: 3 g oral dose four hours before anaesthesia followed by 3 g by mouth as soon as possible after operation
— Children under 10 years: half adult dose
— Children under 5 years: quarter adult dose

Patients allergic to penicillin or who have had more than one dose of penicillin in the previous four weeks:

Teicoplanin and gentamicin
— Adults: intravenous teicoplanin 400 mg and gentamicin 120 mg just before induction of anaesthesia or fifteen minutes before the procedure
— Children under 14 years: intravenous teicoplanin 6 mg/kg plus gentamicin 2 mg/kg

Advice on particular regimens is changing constantly: the operator should check with opinion that is current at the time of operation.

Any patient susceptible to infective endocarditis should use an oral antiseptic chlorhexidine gel (1%) applied to the dry gingival margin, or a chlorhexidine mouthwash (0.2%) 5 min before undergoing dental procedures. This should reduce the severity of any bacteraemia and may be used to supplement the antibiotic prophylaxis.

The initial consultation is most effectively carried out beside a desk with both patient and operator seated; patients find this less stressful than immediately being asked to sit in a dental chair (**3.1**).

The patient's attitudes to dental treatment must be assessed during the first appointment, and the dentist should consider the following questions:

1. Has the patient received much previous dental treatment?
2. Is the patient particularly nervous?
3. Will he or she be able to tolerate endodontics?
4. Should treatment be undertaken in short sessions?
5. Is one particular time of day more suitable than others?
6. Is cost of treatment important?

Chief complaint

Listen carefully to the patient's explanation of his/her condition and use the patient's own words to record it. Obtain a detailed description of any pain: its nature (sharp, dull, throbbing, radiating); any initiating factors; duration; frequency; association with time of day; is relief obtained with analgesics?

CLINICAL EXAMINATION

Extraoral

Extraoral examination is carried out for facial swelling, asymmetry and the presence of lymph nodes. Facial swelling is best viewed from above the patient (**3.2, 3.3**).

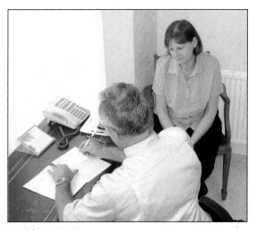

3.1 Consultation

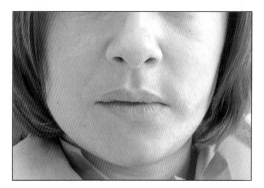

3.2 Any facial swelling should be noted

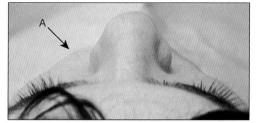

3.3 Facial swelling is best seen from above the patient

Intraoral

The intraoral soft tissues, oral hygiene (**3.4**), general periodontal condition (**3.5**), incidence of caries (**3.6**), missing or unopposed teeth (**3.7**), standard and amount of dental treatment (**3.8**), tooth wear and faceting (**3.9**) should all be assessed.

Ease of access

An assessment should be made of the ease of access, particularly to the posterior part of the mouth. As a general guide, if a patient's mouth will not open wide enough to allow two fingers to pass between the incisors endodontic treatment of the molars is inadvisable (**3.10**). Some patients, with small mouths particularly the elderly, find it difficult to keep their mouth sufficiently wide open for long periods, using a mouth prop, which they may relax upon during treatment, does help (**3.11**)

Radiographic assessment

This is of the utmost importance. Preoperative periapical radiographs should be taken using the paralleling technique (**3.12**). If a patent

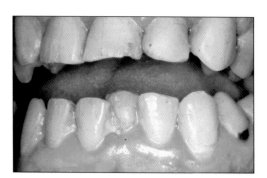

3.4 Poor oral hygiene

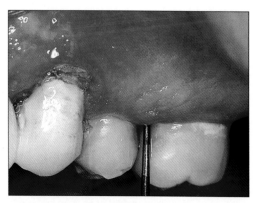

3.5 Periodontal condition

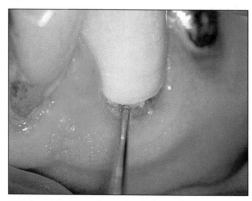

3.6 Loose bridge abutment with caries beneath

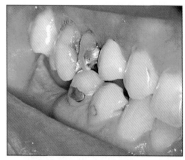

3.7 Missing and unopposed teeth

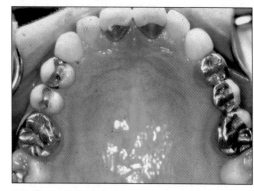

3.8 General dental state

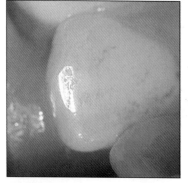

3.9 Facet

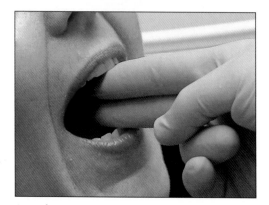

3.10 Access assessed with two fingers

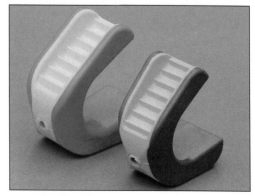

3.11 Mouth props

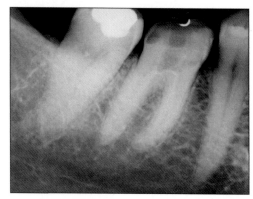

3.12 Radiograph taken with parallel technique

sinus is present preoperatively a radiograph may be taken with a size 20 or 25 gutta-percha point in place. The point should be inserted into the sinus and gently teased by rolling the tip back and forth between the fingers until resistance or discomfort is encountered (**3.13–3.15**).

If endodontic treatment is being considered, the following should be assessed on radiographs: shape, curvature and number of roots; presence and morphology of root canals; size of pulp chamber; type and size of coronal restoration; presence of periradicular disease; periodontal bone loss, internal or external resorption; and root fracture. If the tooth has been treated previously it should be possible to assess the type of root filling material used and the presence of any procedural errors such as perforation, untreated canals or a fractured instrument. The radiograph will often indicate to the operator the cause of the problem and the probable ease of treatment. In **Figure 3.16** the radiograph shows a maxillary first molar with horizontal and furcation bone loss, possible inflammatory resorption of the disto-buccal root and a gutta-percha point passing into the furcation. The tooth should be extracted. **Figure 3.17** shows two maxillary premolars, the first of which has a periapical radiolucency and an inadequate paste root filling, the second showing gross caries in the coronal portion of the root canal.

The first premolar was root filled (**3.18**) and the second extracted and replaced with bridgework.

CLINICAL TESTS

Clinical tests are used for routine assessment or to locate and diagnose the source of pulpal pain. Many clinical tests are available but none is wholly reliable. It is not necessary to use all the tests in each case. The correlation between clinical symptoms and pulpal histology is poor; the operator faced with a case of pulpal pain must use his/her experience to decide whether the pulp is irreversibly damaged and has to be removed or whether removing the cause of the irritation will preserve the pulp. Correct diagnosis depends on tests and the operator's experience and acumen. As a guide, before a pulp cavity is accessed two independent indications for treatment should be established.

Palpation

The soft tissues overlying the apices of the teeth are palpated (**3.19**). The patient will report any tender area. Hard and soft swellings will be apparent: if hard, the site and size should be noted; if soft, the

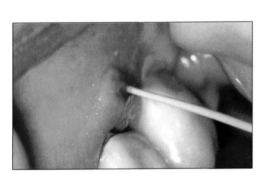

3.13 Gutta-percha in sinus

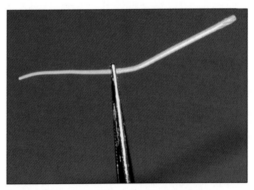

3.14 Depth of insertion of gutta-percha

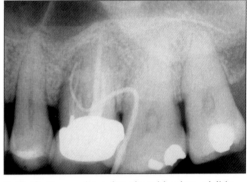

3.15 Gutta-percha point placed in sinus visible on radiograph

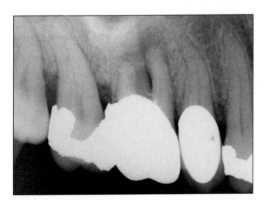

3.16 Maxillary first molar with furcal bone loss, inflammatory resorption, and possible perforation into furcation with gutta-percha. Tooth to be extracted

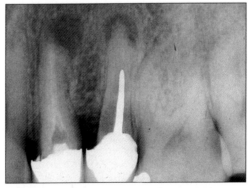

3.17 Inadequate root filling in first premolar and gross caries in second premolar

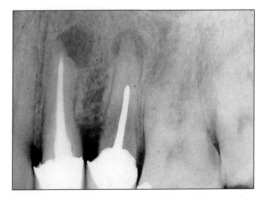

3.18 First premolar root treated. Second premolar due for extraction

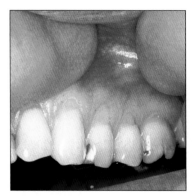

3.19 Palpation

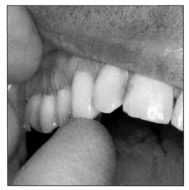

3.20 Percussion

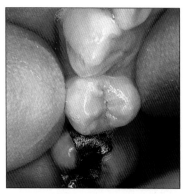

3.21 Mobility

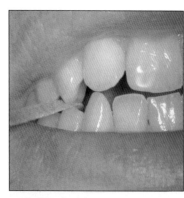

3.22 Wood stick

swelling should be palpated with two fingers to see if it is fluctuant. One finger is placed at either end of the swelling and pressure applied; if the swelling is fluctuant movement of the fluid beneath the oral mucosa will be apparent.

Percussion

Gentle tapping with a finger (both vertically and laterally) will locate a tender tooth (**3.20**). If ankylosis of a tooth is suspected, tapping with a mirror handle in the long axis of the tooth will confirm the diagnosis: an ankylosed tooth has a distinctive high pitched ring.

Mobility

Mobility of a tooth is assessed by placing a finger on each side and pressing with one finger (**3.21**). The amount of movement is judged in relation to a proximal tooth.

Mobility may be graded as *slight* (mobility 1), which is considered normal, *moderate* (mobility 2), or *extensive* (mobility 3) in a lateral or mesiodistal direction, combined with vertical displacement in the alveolus.

Biting

Diagnosis of incompletely fractured teeth is one of the most difficult diagnoses in endodontics. A fracture is seldom visible in its early stages and may lie beneath a restoration. A patient presenting with pain related to chewing but with no evidence of periradicular inflammation may be suspected of having a fracture. Biting on a wooden stick or rubber wheel may elicit pain, usually on release of biting pressure (**3.22**).

Fibreoptic light

Transmission of a powerful light through teeth will show interproximal caries and (of particular interest in endodontics) a fracture. Extraneous light is reduced; the fibreoptic light placed next to the neck of the tooth and moved along its surface. The light will not pass across the fracture line due to reflection, so the part of the tooth

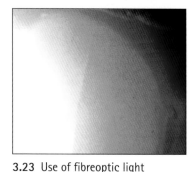

3.23 Use of fibreoptic light showing tooth fracture

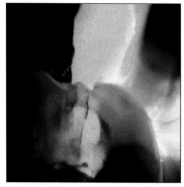

3.24 Mandibular molar with distal fracture

nearest to the light is bright and that beyond the fracture remains dark: **3.23** shows this effect. Figure **3.24** shows a mandibular first molar with a coronal restoration removed – a fracture line is visible in the distal wall.

Pulp testing

This method is used only to decide whether the pulp is responsive; it tests the ability of the nerves within the pulp to conduct impulses but gives no indication of the state of the blood supply. Pulp testing neither quantifies disease nor measures health, and should not be used to judge the degree of pulpal disease. Pulp tests should be used only to assess vitality of the pulp.

Electric pulp tester

The electric pulp tester (EPT) uses gradations of electric current (alternating or direct) to excite a response from the nervous tissues within the pulp. Most modern pulp testers are monopolar.

An example of a pulp tester, the Analytic Technology Endo Analyser, is shown (**3.25**). The instrument has a dual function acting as both a pulp tester and an electronic apex locator (EAL). When used as a pulp tester a pulsating stimulus is produced starting at a low value and automatically increasing. The pulse amplitude of the

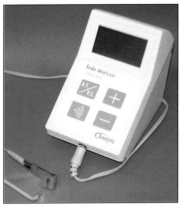

3.25 Unit has a dual function both as a pulp tester and an apex locator

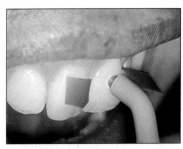

3.26 Pulp tester applied to buccal surface of tooth isolated with strips of rubber dam. Toothpaste used as a conducting medium

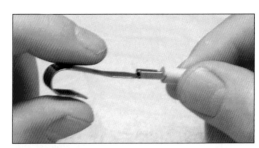

3.27 Patient controls the pulp tester

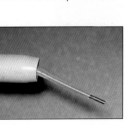

3.28 Special tip for pulp testing beneath crowns

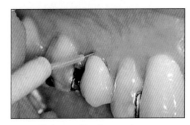

3.29 Pulp testing beneath crown

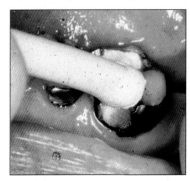

3.30 Hot gutta-percha applied to tooth

stimulus begins at 15 volts and rises to a maximum of 350 volts. When used as an apex locator the apical foramen is located by monitoring the electrical impedance between two electrodes. The first electrode is a metal clip placed over the patient's lip. The second electrode is touched onto a root canal instrument inserted into the canal. The EAL measures the values of impedance in the canal over five signal frequencies.

Pulp testing technique The tooth to be tested should be dried and isolated with cotton wool or rubber dam (**3.26**). Note that the rubber dam is applied as small strips placed between the teeth. A conducting medium must be used – the one most readily available is toothpaste. The pulp tester is applied to the middle third of the tooth, avoiding contact with the soft tissues, and any restorations. A lip electrode is placed over the patients lip. If the pulp is vital the patient feels a tingling sensation. A more user-friendly method is to ask the patient to hold the lip electrode. The plastic cable is held in one hand and the metal electrode between the forefinger and thumb of the other hand as shown in **Figure 3.27**. This method allows the patient to have control by letting go with the fingers holding the metal electrode as soon as they feel any sensation. As a general rule electric pulp testers should not be used on patients who have a cardiac pacemaker because of possible electrical interference. However, modern pacemakers are well shielded, which will reduce the risk of interference.

Pulp testing of crowned teeth is possible, provided that a small area of dentine or enamel can be contacted without touching the gingival tissue. A special tip for the Analytic Technology pulp tester (**3.28**) is being used on the patient shown in **Figure 3.29**.

Disadvantages Electric pulp testing has several disadvantages:
1. It gives no indication of the state of the vascular supply, which would give a more reliable measure of the vitality of the pulp.
2. False-positive readings may be obtained owing to stimulation of nerve fibres in the periodontium.
3. Readings taken from posterior teeth may be misleading because some combination of vital and non-vital root canal pulps may be present.

Thermal pulp testing

Thermal pulp testing involves either applying or removing heat from a tooth. Neither test is completely reliable, both producing false-positive and false-negative readings.

Heat

Dry heat The last 3 mm of the end of a stick of gutta-percha or composition is heated in a flame for two seconds and applied to the suspect tooth (**3.30**). Two precautions are necessary to avoid the patient receiving sudden acute pain: (1) the tooth surface should be lightly coated with petroleum jelly to prevent the composition from sticking and care taken not to overheat the stick as it may stick to the tooth if overheated, despite the application of lubricant; and (2) local anaesthetic should be kept to hand. Another method is to use the heat generated from a rubber wheel in a standard handpiece.

Hot water Some patients report pain with hot drinks, but do not react to heated gutta-percha. This may be due to the presence of porcelain-bonded crowns or large restorations, which insulate the pulp. Hot water should be sipped and held in the mouth, first over the mandibular quadrant on the affected side and then over the maxillary quadrant if this does not elicit a response. An alternative method is to use a rubber dam to isolate each tooth in turn. If a response is noted, local anaesthetic is applied to the suspect tooth and the heat reapplied. No response means that the tooth with pulpitis has been identified.

Cold One method of testing the pulp's reaction to cold is to soak a cotton bud with ethyl chloride and apply it to the tooth (**3.31**, **3.32**). An alternative method is to prepare ice sticks by filling the plastic protective covers for hypodermic needles with water and freezing them. To make them ready for use one end is removed by warming it slightly in the hand (**3.33**). Some operators prefer to use a carbon dioxide probe (**3.34**, **3.35**) because it gives an intense reproducible response, and does not affect the adjacent teeth (which an air blast or ice stick may do).

Local analgesia

When the patient presents with pain or if thermal testing can provoke the pain, an infiltration injection of local analgesic may be used to identify the tooth. An intraligamental injection localizes the effect of the analgesic, although the proximal teeth may still be affected. Note that the bevel of the needle in **Figure 3.36** points away from the tooth to allow easier penetration into the periodontal ligament.

Caries removal and dressing

The first stage of treatment of a carious tooth is to remove the caries and establish whether pulp and/or tooth may be saved.

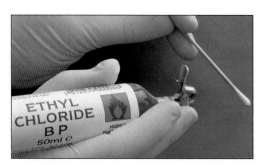

3.31 Ethyl chloride is sprayed onto a cotton bud

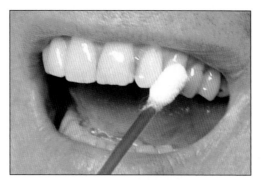

3.32 Cold cotton bud applied to mid third of buccal surface of tooth

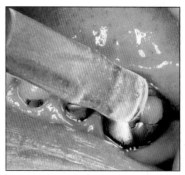

3.33 Ice stick applied to tooth

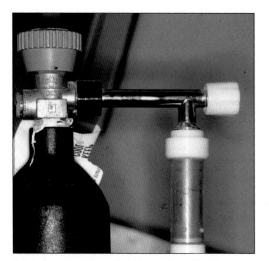

3.34 Apparatus required for carbon dioxide pulp testing

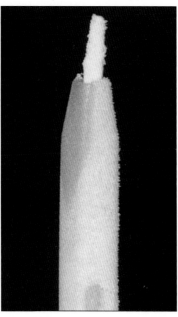

3.35 Carbon dioxide stick

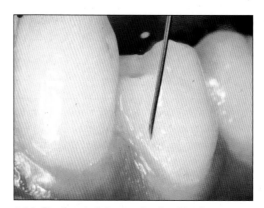

3.36 The bevel of the needle should point away from the tooth

Cutting a test cavity

As a last resort a test cavity may be cut in a tooth, which is believed to be pulpless. In the author's experience this test is not reliable because a positive response may be obtained from a tooth with a necrotic pulp.

Further tests

On occasion it may be necessary to carry out a preliminary procedure before the final treatment plan can be made. For example:

- check crowns and bridge retainers to see if cementation has failed;
- attempt to locate a sclerosed root canal;
- remove a restoration to examine the floor of the cavity for a fracture;
- attempt to remove a post to see if orthograde root canal treatment may be carried out; or
- fit a diagnostic occlusal splint to eliminate muscular pain.

Future possibilities

More precise tests are required to assess the state of the pulp. Research has centred on a device that would assess the quantity of blood flow through the pulp, which would give a better indication of pulp vitality than the present method of testing for nerve response. Research has been carried out on the laser Doppler effect, pulse oximetry, dual-wave length spectrophotometry and infrared non-contact thermometry. To date, there is no commercial unit available for general practice.

DIAGNOSIS

Once the patient has been assessed and the clinical examination and tests completed diagnosis should be possible. The clinician should have a simple classification of pulpal disease and its possible sequelae that complements the rudimentary tests available. It must be emphasized that diseases of the pulp and periradicular tissues do not necessarily cause pain.

Normal pulp

This will be asymptomatic and give only a mild, transitory response to stimulation with thermal or electrical tests. Percussion and palpation do not cause pain. Radiographs show a definite pulp chamber and canal, which will be smaller and narrower in the older patient. The width of the periodontal ligament is normal, with no evidence of resorption.

Dentinal pain may be experienced when the dentine is exposed to the oral cavity, with thermal changes or exposure to sweet food or drink. The pulp is not normally affected.

Concussed pulp

The pulp may be concussed following trauma to the tooth and may not respond to thermal or electrical stimulation for a period of weeks or months. The tooth should be checked at regular intervals until the pulp tests return to normal or, if they do not, root canal treatment should be considered.

Reversible pulpitis

Hot or cold will cause a quick sharp pain, which lingers for seconds after the stimulus is removed. The pain does not radiate and the tooth is otherwise symptomless. The radiograph shows no disease.

Irreversible pulpitis

The pain encountered in this condition may vary – from none to spontaneous intermittent paroxysms or continuous pain – and may radiate from the maxilla to the mandible or vice versa. Pain commonly occurs at night, when it may be worse than during the day because lying down increases the intrapulpal pressure. In the early stages the patient is unable to locate the affected tooth but as pulpal inflammation spreads and toxins pass out through the apical foramen the tooth may become painful to touch. Application of heat or cold will generally start the pain, which gradually increases in intensity then slowly dies away and may last for a few minutes up to several hours. Radiographs will show changes associated with the root apex when pulpitis is well advanced, but occasionally apical rarefaction will occur at an earlier stage with pulpitis. **Figure 3.37** shows a mandibular first molar with coronal caries. The patient was experiencing episodes of pain particularly at night and the tooth was tender. There is a widened periodontal ligament space around both the mesial and distal roots. There is a halo of condensing osteitis around the distal root.

Pulpal necrosis

Necrosis may occur following irreversible pulpitis or as a result of trauma disrupting the blood supply to the pulp. Thermal and electrical pulp testing will produce no response, although in a posterior tooth the pulp tissue in more than one of the canals may be vital, which makes tests inconclusive. In most cases a radiograph will show periradicular changes. In **Figure 3.38** a periapical radiolucent area is evident around the apical portion of the root of the distal molar. When pulpal disease has spread to the periradicular tissue the tooth frequently responds to palpation and percussion.

Acute periapical inflammation

Acute inflammation may be due to an extension of pulpal disease, trauma, a high restoration or endodontic treatment that has inadvertently been extended beyond the apical foremen. If the inflammation is caused by trauma the pulp may remain vital. The tooth is very tender to touch. Radiographic change will be minimal, but may show a little widening of the periodontal ligament. **Figure 3.39** shows the posterior abutment tooth to a bridge, which had become decemented and carious (**3.40**); the pulp is still vital (**3.41**). The pulp was extirpated and root canals prepared (**3.42**).

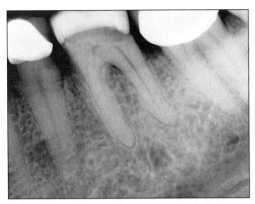

3.37 Irreversible pulpitis of mandibular first molar showing a widened periodontal ligament space around both apices

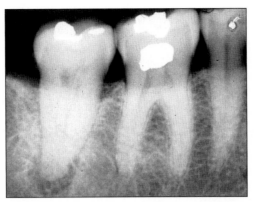

3.38 Mandibular second molar with well defined periradicular area

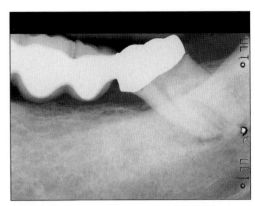

3.39 Posterior abutment to a bridge with early radiographic changes

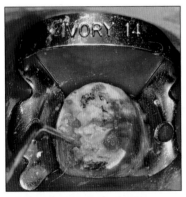

3.40 Bridge removed showing gross caries

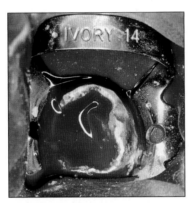

3.41 Carious exposure with hyperaemic pulp

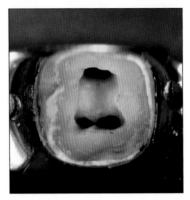

3.42 Pulp extirpated and canals prepared

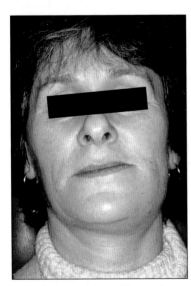

3.43 Patient with swelling and pyrexia

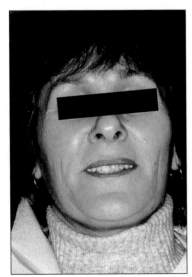

3.44 Patient one week later

Acute apical abscess

An acute apical abscess implies the presence of purulent exudate around the apex. The tooth is extremely tender to touch and palpation of the overlying gingiva painful. Swelling develops in the later stages and the tooth becomes mobile. Pain usually abates when the swelling appears. In severe cases the patient is febrile. The patient in **Figure 3.43** has swelling and pyrexia, which has disappeared a week later following treatment (**3.44**). Radiographically the appearance is similar to acute periapical inflammation. A chronic lesion may flare up into an acute apical abscess – in such cases there will be periradicular rarefaction.

Chronic apical periodontitis

This is a long-standing asymptomatic inflammation around the apex. From time to time the patient may become aware of the tooth. Radiolucency is apparent, although this varies from a widened periodontal ligament to a large area (**3.45**). There may be evidence of a sinus tract. The pulp will be non-vital.

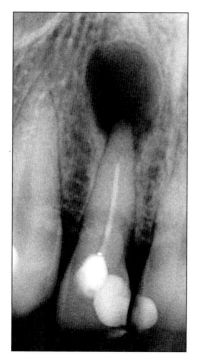

3.45 Lateral incisor with large periapical radiolucency

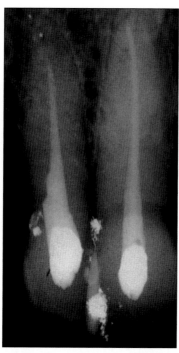

3.46 Atypical facial pain. Patient has had a considerable amount of treatment in the maxillary right quadrant for pain, without effect

Resorption

Internal

Internal resorption occurs as a result of chronic pulpitis. The tooth is usually symptomless. Diagnosis is made by the appearance of a smooth widening of the pulp on the radiograph. Root canal treatment should be carried out without delay (see Chapter 14).

External

External resorption may present in several forms (Chapter 14). It is important to identify the type of resorption so that appropriate treatment may be given. The main difficulty is in differentiating between internal and external resorption. Radiographs are invaluable in the diagnosis.

Fractured teeth

The obvious cause of tooth fracture is trauma but both restored and unrestored teeth with no history of trauma may fracture. Any restoration, which acts as a wedge in the tooth, for example a cast inlay or a mesio-occlusal-distal amalgam, may cause the tooth to fracture. The incidence of tooth fracture is highest in the second

mandibular molar, usually in the saggittal plane. Fractures can be difficult to diagnose and because both the pulp and the periodontium may be affected the range of symptoms is wide.

Fractured crown with vital pulp

This often presents as a non-localized pain associated with eating. There may be a history of trauma but more often the patient cannot remember any traumatic incident. The severity of the symptoms usually depends on the degree of bacterial contamination of the pulp. The patient may or may not be aware of pain during chewing. The fracture is extremely difficult to locate, particularly if it runs obliquely beneath the cusp of a molar. If not treated the pulp will become necrotic.

Fractured crown with non-vital pulp

This may be asymptomatic or may cause mild intermittent pain on chewing.

Fractured crown and root with vital pulp

Symptoms are similar to the crown-only fracture, except that the pain is more likely to occur during chewing – typically on release of the food bolus.

Fractured crown and root with a non-vital pulp

The fracture is usually long-standing and is easier to locate than in the case of vital pulp for two reasons: (1) the fracture line will have become stained and will show up with fibreoptic light; and (2) the pain will be due mainly to stretching of the periodontal ligament as the fractured parts move during mastication. If the fracture has started from the apex of the root and the tooth has been root filled the fracture was probably caused by excessive use of force during treatment.

Atypical facial pain

This condition refers to apparent dental pain, which has no organic cause. The patients are predominantly female and the range of symptoms diverse. The condition is difficult to diagnose and often the patient has been suffering pain for a considerable time. A thorough investigation must be carried out and any pathology treated. If symptoms persist the patient should be referred for specialist treatment. An example of atypical facial pain is given in **Figure 3.46**: a 43-year-old woman complained of pain in the maxillary right incisor region. The central and lateral incisors had been root treated and the canine root treated and apicected without providing the patient with any relief from pain. The patient was referred to a consultant who specialized in atypical facial pain and was successfully treated with antidepressants.

Chapter 4

Radiography

R T Walker and J E Brown

Accurate dental radiographs are an essential requirement for the practice of endodontics. High-quality periapical radiographs improve initial diagnosis and assist greatly in success of treatment. Operators should endeavour to achieve high technical standards in order to ensure accuracy and minimize the number of film exposures needed to complete a clinical procedure. It is important to have a clear understanding of the materials, equipment, techniques and safety standards governing this discipline.

RADIOGRAPHIC EQUIPMENT

The X-ray machine

The machine used (**4.1**) should conform to the requirements of the Ionizing Radiations Regulations 1999. The three *exposure factors* are exposure time, current and voltage. The current and exposure time influence the quantity of X-rays produced, and this is normally controlled by altering the exposure time as current is generally fixed at around 7–10 mA. Voltage influences the penetrating power of the X-ray beam. Tube voltage should be no lower than 50 kV, and preferably 60–70 kV for intraoral radiography.

The tube head

This houses the X-ray tube and transformer (**4.2**) and allows only the X-rays that form the beam to pass out. The tube produces a divergent beam, which is collimated by a diaphragm and/or a metal cylinder. Collimation to give a rectangular beam, similar to a size 2 periapical film, is recommended since this reduces the patient dose by approximately 50% compared with conventional 6 cm circular collimation. Machines employing direct current (DC) are preferred to conventional half-wave rectified units since they result in shorter exposure times and a lower skin dose. The filtration of the beam should be equivalent to no less than 1.5 mm aluminium for voltages up to and including 70 kV. A spacer cone allows accurate alignment of the beam and ensures a minimum focus-to-skin distance of 200 mm for voltages of 50 kV or more. The location of the focal spot should be marked on the tube housing and its diameter identified in the equipment specifications. A smaller focal spot diameter is preferred since this gives rise to less penumbra (a diffusion at the edges of objects) and a sharper image.

Electronic timers (**4.3**) are required for accuracy at very short exposure times. Warning lights must indicate 'mains on' and exposure. Equipment must be surveyed for safety at least once every three years and records kept of all service visits.

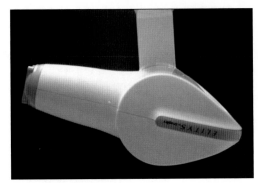

4.1 Modern machine

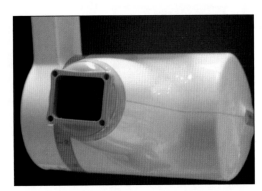

4.2 Modern tube head

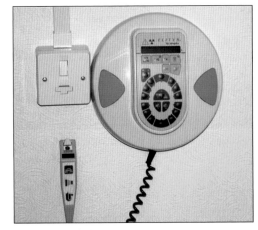

4.3 Electronic timer

Density and contrast

Density is the degree of blackness of a film; *contrast* is the difference in the degrees of blackness of adjacent areas. With a higher voltage, there is better penetration of hard tissues and more shades of grey will be recorded (this is more likely to indicate early pathological changes in bone). At lower kilovoltages there is greater contrast – fewer grey shades are recorded and the image appears more black and white. A 60–70 kV machine suits most dental purposes.

Films

The fastest films available, consistent with satisfactory diagnostic results, should be used. F-speed film is replacing E-speed film as the fastest available, saving a further 20–25% on exposure compared with E-speed film when processed optimally. Size 0 films (34 × 22 mm) are suitable for children and for anterior teeth, size 2 films (40 × 30 mm) for posterior teeth and adults.

Film holders

Film holders are devices designed to hold the film in a stable position within the patient's mouth, avoiding the need to hold the film with a finger. Many incorporate beam-aiming devices to prevent 'cone cutting' and some also include a device for rectangular collimation (**4.4**). Their use improves the diagnostic quality of the image and allows the position of the film and beam to be reproduced during subsequent recall assessment.

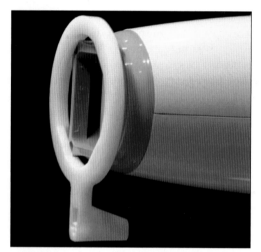

4.4 Circular beam-aiming device with recesses for rectangular collimator

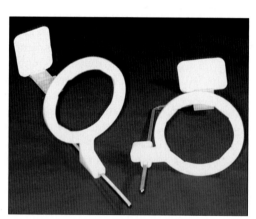

4.5 Rinn XCP film holders

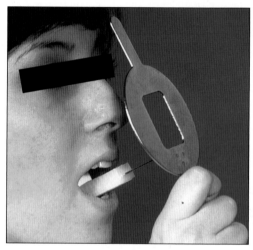

4.6 Masel precision film holder

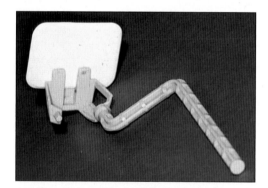

4.7 Rinn Endoray film holder with basket

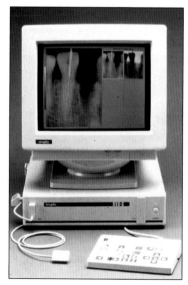

4.8 RVG imaging system

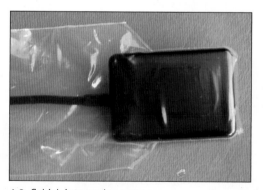

4.9 Schick intraoral sensors

Film holder systems include:

- modified Spencer-Wells forceps;
- Rinn XCP system including anterior and posterior film holders (**4.5**);
- Masel precision film holders (**4.6**);
- Rinn Endoray film holder – a holder designed for taking paralleling technique radiographs in the presence of endodontic hand instruments (**4.7**). The film holder incorporates a 'basket', which fits over the crown of the tooth and endodontic instruments, and on which the patient bites lightly. The X-ray beam may be aligned with the handle and centred through a centring ring.

Digital sensors

Digital radiology (DR) offers many potential advantages in dental and endodontic practice.

DR sensors use miniature TV camera charge-coupled devices (CCD) and phosphorescent screens or photostimulable phosphor plates that are sensitive to X-rays. The CCD is connected to a computer to display the image on a monitor.

The first digital imaging system was radiovisiography (RVG; Trophy Radiologie, Vincennes, France). It eliminated the time spent processing X-ray films and possessed a zoom function, which allowed the magnification of selected areas to try to improve diagnostic performance (**4.8**). Digital image quality has improved with the further development of these intraoral sensors and is now comparable with that of E-speed film (**4.9**).

The sensor unit in digital radiography is the pixel. Image quality is dependent on a number of factors including the number of pixels per unit area contained within the intraoral sensor. Upgrading of the sensor can, therefore, improve image quality. Pixels in the matrix display numerical values dependent on the intensity of X-rays incident on their surface. This data can be manipulated to enhance the information yielded by the radiograph, a significant advantage of digital imaging. The current choice of imaging systems lies between the direct or 'corded' systems such as the Schick CDR® intraoral sensors that simply fit to existing computer equipment (**4.10–4.12**) and the indirect and 'cordless' systems that substitute photostimulable phosphor plates for film. These are used very much like film but must then be laser scanned, introducing a second stage to the technique.

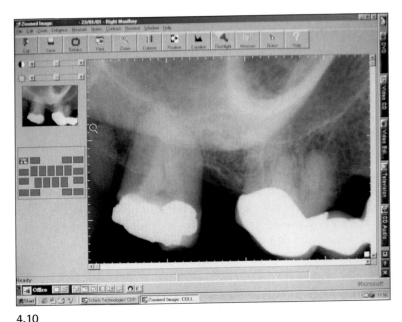

4.10

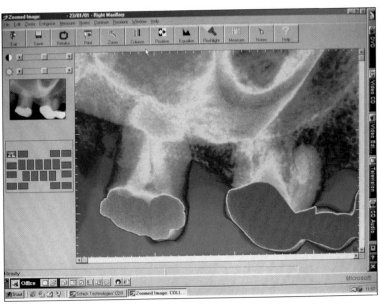

4.11

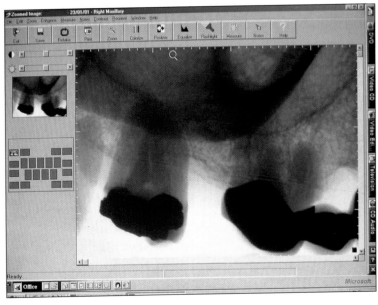

4.12

4.10–4.12 Digital images

Digital radiographic imaging now gives acceptable image quality for potentially lower radiographic exposure to the patient. Images can also be archived and transmitted as necessary.

PROCESSING EQUIPMENT

Processing converts the latent image in the exposed silver halide film emulsion to a permanent image. Correct processing ensures that a proper range of densities is created and that a permanent image of achievable quality is produced. A quick method of chair-side film processing has always been desirable in endodontic radiography. In attempting to achieve a rapid result strict attention should be paid to producing consistently high quality radiographs. Processing may be manual or automatic.

Manual

Manual processing may be undertaken within a darkroom or using a light-proof box within the surgery (**4.13**). Films are passed through four baths: one containing developer; the second water; the third containing fixer; and the fourth containing a final wash. The operator views the processing by the light of a suitable low-intensity film-matched safelight in the darkroom or via a red light-safe viewing panel in the daylight loading box (**4.14**) and may complete the process within 50 seconds using high-speed chemicals. Further fixing and washing is required after examining the radiograph.

Films enclosed within a light-proof container, which also contains developer and fixer, are available. Following exposure the processing fluids are released by pulling two tabs. The Super-X 30 was an example of such a film type and took approximately 80 seconds to process. The disadvantages of using film of this type include absence of a lead foil, rapid deterioration of image quality, and an inability to use it with a paralleling film holder.

Automatic

Automatic machines essentially consist of roller assemblies that transport and immerse films through developing, fixing, washing and drying stations (**4.15**). Processing time is usually 4–6 minutes, a greater speed being achieved by heating the solutions to above room temperature and omitting the first wash. Automatic processors are convenient, provide dry films ready for filing and give good quality results if maintained properly, but are expensive and require regular cleaning.

The Ionizing Radiations Regulations 1999 require all dental practices in the UK to employ a Quality Assurance programme to ensure that the exposure and processing of radiographs results in consistently good quality films. A protocol for recording an assessment of the quality of each radiograph and monitoring processing solutions is central to this programme.

VIEWING AND STORAGE EQUIPMENT

Viewers

The greatest amount of diagnostic information is gained when a radiograph is viewed under magnification on a clean viewing box and masked to exclude extraneous light. A simple viewer that magnifies the image and cuts out glare is illustrated (**4.16**).

Mounts

Radiographs should be named, dated and filed systematically. They may be stored in the patient's clinical records but should ideally be mounted to protect the film during examination, storage or referral. It is usual to place radiographs in labelled pouches or to laminate them between two sheets of acetate (**4.17**), either by stapling the sheets together, using adhesive transparent 'sticky-back plastic' or by using a heat-sealing laminating machine.

SAFETY AND REGULATIONS

The Ionizing Radiations Regulations 1999 and the Ionizing Radiation (Medical Exposure) Regulations 2000 (IRMER) lay down requirements for the safe use of radiation in the workplace and for the protection of patients, staff and the general public. It is the responsibility of all staff to be familiar with legislation relevant to them. The dangers of excessive radiation are minimal, provided simple precautions are observed. Four categories of personnel are identified under the IRMER 2000 regulations:

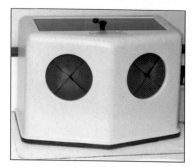

4.13 Light-proof processing box

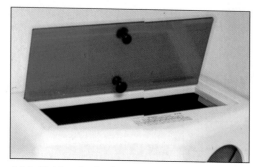

4.14 Light-safe viewing panel

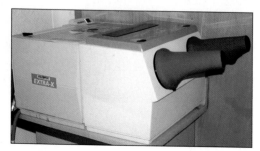

4.15 Velopex automatic processing unit

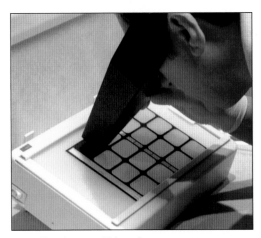

4.16 Simple magnifying viewer

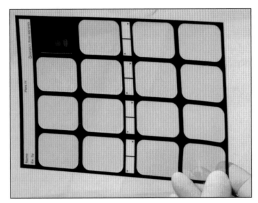

4.17 Mount for radiographs

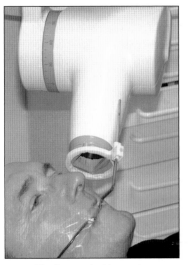

4.18 Film/sensor holder and beam-aiming device in use

1. The *referrer* who requests the radiograph.
2. The *practitioner* whose responsibility is to decide if the radiograph can be justified.
3. The *operator* who carries out any aspect of the exposure procedure.
4. *The employer (legal person)* who takes responsibility for the radiation instillation and staff working within it.

In dental practice the dental surgeon may fulfil several or all of these roles. The most important decision any practitioner should make is whether the use of X-rays is clinically necessary. Safety considerations of radiological techniques fall into three areas:

1. The patient.
2. The operator.
3. The equipment.

Patients

To justify any radiograph, the risk to the patient from an X-ray exposure must be outweighed by the benefit of the diagnostic information given by the radiograph. The risk must be minimized by reducing the dose as far as possible. Techniques should be used which avoid exposures passing towards the patient's body and gonads. Paralleling technique for periapicals is preferred for this reason. Lead aprons are no longer recommended for routine dental radiography since the use of such techniques with modern, high kilovolt equipment, rectangular collimation and fast films produce less scatter towards the body and are more effective at reducing dose.

Exposures need to be set to the minimum exposure time possible. Patients should not hold the film packet in position with their fingers; film holders or forceps should be used (**4.18**) and no one other than the patient should be within the *controlled area* during the exposure. The *controlled area* is an exclusion zone around the X-ray tube head when it is in operation. It extends for a distance of 2 m around the tube head and patient (for tubes operating at up to and including 70 kV) and for a distance along the primary beam until it is attenuated by a radiopaque wall or shield of suitable thickness.

Operators and other staff

All staff involved in dental radiography should understand the dangers of radiation and be conversant with the precautions necessary for proper handling of equipment and patients. Every practice should appoint a Radiation Protection Supervisor (RPS) from within the dental staff to oversee day-to-day radiation safety, and a Radiation Protection Advisor (RPA) – a qualified medical physicist – to advise the practice on radiation protection measures and to carry out equipment checks. Local rules relating to radiation protection in the practice should be conveniently displayed. Only people adequately trained for their role should take part in dental radiography and no one under 16 years should be allowed to work with ionizing radiation.

Several units are used for measuring radiation:

1. The *exposure* is a measure of the energy of the X-ray beam emitted by the X-ray tube. It measures ionization per unit mass of air and is expressed in units of coulombs per kilogram (C kg^{-1}).
2. *Radiation Absorbed Dose (D)* is the amount of energy absorbed from the X-ray beam per unit mass of tissue. It gives the absorbed energy in joules/kg and is expressed in Grays (Gy) and milliGrays (mGy).
3. The *Effective Dose (E)* is a measure that considers the relative harm of the radiation emitted and the relative sensitivity of the tissues exposed. This then allows doses from different investigations of different parts of the body to be compared, by converting all doses to an equivalent whole body dose. It is expressed in Sieverts (Sv) and milliSieverts (mSv).

Staff exposure to radiation should be closely monitored, using film badges or thermoluminescent dosimeters (**4.19**) if an individual's workload exceeds 150 radiographs per week or if an X-ray tube is relocated. Radiation dosage is reduced if the following precautions are observed:

- the operator must stand outside the controlled area;
- the operator should never hold the film, tube housing or patient during the exposure;
- when not in use the X-ray machine should be disconnected from the mains to prevent inadvertent exposure;
- an exposure warning display should light up outside a door, during exposure, if the door may be opened directly into the controlled area during radiography;
- in the case of an accidental overexposure, the incident should be reported to the Health & Safety Executive and records kept for 50 years.

Equipment

Equipment for dental radiography must be installed in accordance with national standards and manufacturer's instructions and checked for safety by an independent radiation physicist before use. It should be sited, e.g. against an outside wall, so that the beam is unlikely to pass towards any frequently occupied area or that area should be sufficiently shielded. Equipment must be checked at least once every three years and records of all maintenance and repairs should be kept. If any fault develops (e.g. faulty warning lights, timers or other electrical problems) the equipment should be disconnected from the mains supply and not used until it has been checked and repaired.

RADIOGRAPHIC TECHNIQUES

Paralleling periapical projections

The ideal imaging geometry for a radiograph would place the object and film close together, with their long axes parallel. The X-ray beam would then be directed at 90° to the long axes of these two structures. It is rarely possible to achieve this ideal positioning in the mouth, except in the lower molar area, but it is usually possible to align the tooth parallel with the film with a small separating distance. A separation of object and film creates magnification of the object, but this is overcome in the paralleling technique by the use of a longer focal spot to object distance (ffd), creating a more parallel beam.

A film holder with a beam-aiming device is necessary to support the film upright in the mouth and to ensure accurate alignment of the collimated beam. **Figure 4.20** shows a paralleling periapical radiograph of the central incisors being taken using a Rinn film/sensor holder and localizing ring. The resultant digital radiographic image is also shown (**4.21**).

The advantages of paralleling technique are:

- greater geometric accuracy (e.g. **4.22**);
- reproducibility;
- fewer retakes (films held securely & technique less prone to errors);
- lower radiation dose (beam not directed towards the body trunk, finger not holding film & therefore not irradiated, use of high kilovolt modern machines);
- superior images of upper molar roots (zygomatic butress projected above the molar apices (**4.23**);
- superior image of bone margins;
- superior images of interproximal regions (the positioning is closer to that of bitewings therefore interproximal caries may be assessed).

Inevitably, this technique has some limitations, being more difficult to achieve ideal positioning in patients with shallow palates, with a pronounced gag reflex or with rubber dam in place. Compromises involve the use of cotton wool rolls (**4.24**), tongue spatulas and forceps (**4.25**).

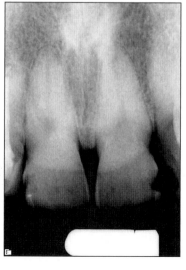

4.21 Digital image of maxillary central incisors using paralleling technique

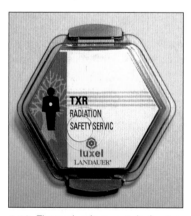

4.19 Thermoluminescent dosimeter

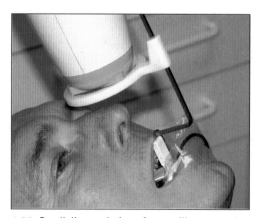

4.20 Paralleling technique for maxillary central incisors

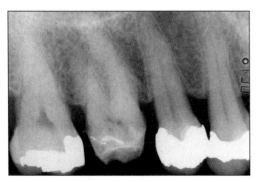

4.22 Parallel image of maxillary posterior teeth

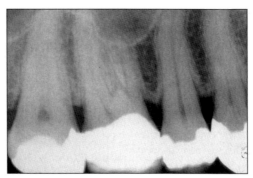

4.23 Parallel image of maxillary molar roots (see **4.29** for bisecting angle view)

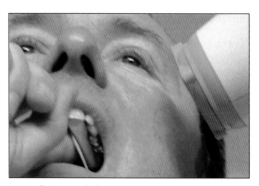

4.24 Cotton rolls in use

Bisecting angle periapical projections

In this technique the film is placed against the tooth and the angle between the long axis of tooth and film is visualized and bisected. The X-ray beam is centred on the apex of the tooth, transecting the bisecting line at 90° (**4.26**). In the lower molar region the film and tooth may be almost parallel but in the upper anterior regions a considerable angle may result between the tooth and the film causing a pronounced angulation of the beam downwards towards the body (**4.27**).

The bisecting angle technique may be performed without film/sensor holders (although the patient must then hold the film with their finger or forceps), is quick and easy to use with rubber dam in place and is relatively comfortable for all patients, even those with small mouths. It is, however, difficult to avoid distortion and an accurate image can never be guaranteed. Other faults such as displaced or bent films and 'cone cutting' are more likely than with film/sensor holders (**4.28**). Anatomical structures such as the zygomatic

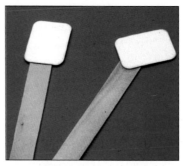

4.25 Use of tongue spatulas to support intraoral films

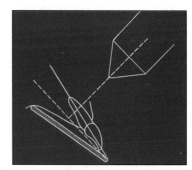

4.26 Principle of the bisecting angle periapical projection

arch are frequently superimposed over the apices of the upper posterior teeth and the relationship between roots, other anatomical structures and alveolar bone may be distorted (**4.29**). It is also difficult to reproduce a periapical view for review and recall purposes.

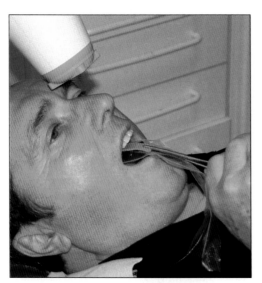

4.27 Bisecting angle periapical projection of maxillary central incisors

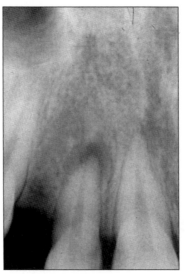

4.28 Image produced by misplaced film in bisecting angle technique

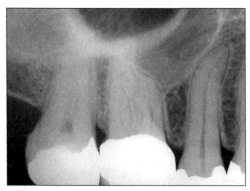

4.29 Superimposition of the zygomatic arch in bisecting angle technique (see **4.23** for parallel view)

Parallax techniques

Horizontal and vertical parallax techniques are most useful in endodontics in the diagnostic and treatment phases. Identifying the shift of the X-ray beam between two radiographs of the same area and the resultant shift in the positions of the two objects in the images can identify positions of neighbouring objects. A useful acronym is the *SLOB* rule – this stands for *Same Lingual, Opposite Buccal*. To apply this rule you must first know the position of the X-ray tube for each of two radiographs taken of the tooth or area of interest. Next, study the resultant radiographs and compare the position of the object of interest with a neighbouring reference tooth. If the X-ray tube *and* object under investigation have moved in the *same* direction in relation to a reference object then the object of interest lies *lingual* to it. If the X-ray tube and the object of interest move in *opposite* directions then the object lies *buccal* to the reference object.

Horizontal parallax can be used to indicate the position of intradental structures in relation to the external surface of the tooth. This is very useful in the identification of perforations (**4.30–4.35**). Both horizontal and vertical parallax can be used to good effect to selectively image individual roots of a multirooted tooth (**4.36, 4.37**).

QUALITY ASSURANCE

Good quality radiographs are required for accurate diagnosis. If high standards of image quality are to be maintained and radiation dose to the patient minimized, a quality assurance programme for radiography is essential and is mandatory under UK legislation. Such a programme is composed of:

- written procedures for the acquisition and processing of radiographs;
- a system of quality-control measures which are carried out at regular, predetermined intervals;
- systems for the monitoring and audit of image quality in order to identify errors and enable their correction.

This requirement is applicable to both conventional and digital radiography. An important aspect of quality assurance is the identification of film faults – these must be recognized and understood in order to correct the error.

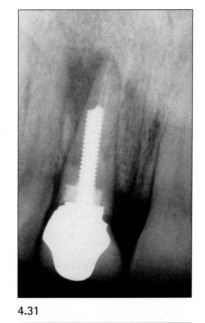

4.30

4.31

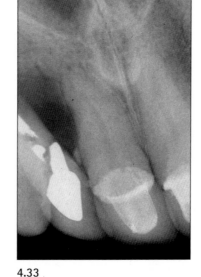

4.32

4.33

4.30–4.33 Horizontal parallax used to identify perforated post

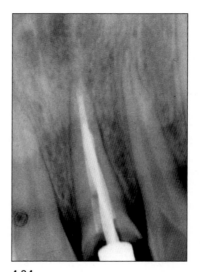

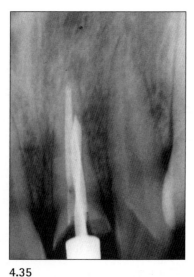

4.34

4.35

4.34–4.35 Horizontal parallax used to identify perforated post preparation

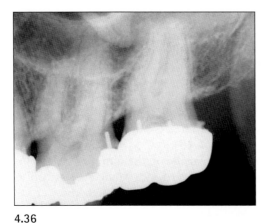

4.36

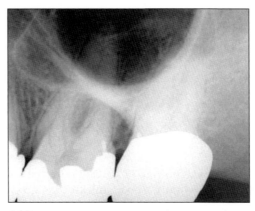

4.37

4.36–4.37 Vertical parallax used to improve imaging of palatal root of maxillary molar

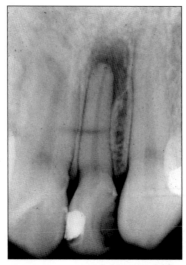

4.38 Dark line produced on bent film

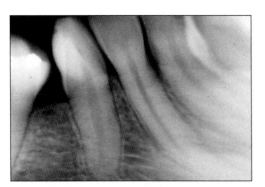

4.39 Distorted image produced by bent film

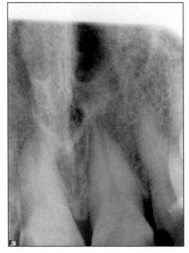

4.40 Coning off of digital image

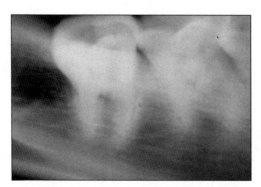

4.41 Blurred image produced by patient movement

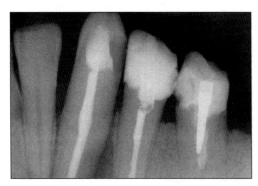

4.42 Incomplete image produced by poor film/sensor placement

Errors in technique

Certain errors may occur as a result of faulty radiographic technique and should be prevented (many of these are equally applicable to digital intraoral radiography):

- bent film gives rise to dark lines (**4.38**);
- distortion occurs when the film is curved under pressure, particularly when finger pressure is used to hold the film in place (**4.39**) or when the film is allowed to bend in the film holder;
- a partial image ('coning off') results from failure to aim the main beam at the centre of the film. This error leaves a white unexposed portion of the radiograph. This is more likely with the smaller beam created by rectangular collimation, and therefore film holders are recommended to ensure accurate alignment (**4.40**);
- if the patient, film or tube moves during exposure the image will appear blurred (**4.41**);
- an incomplete image is formed when the film or sensor is not placed sufficiently far into the mouth – a particular problem with bulky digital sensors but helped by the use of film holders tailored for sensor support (**4.42**);

- extraneous radio-opaque objects such as saliva ejectors (**4.43**), rubber dam clamps, frames and spectacles may become superimposed on the area to be radiographed;
- if the film is placed back-to-front in the mouth with the back of the film facing the tube, the radiograph appears light and carries a pattern derived from the lead foil in the film packet (**4.44**).

Errors in processing

Other errors may occur during film processing:

- prolonged exposure or developing times, high processing temperatures or a high concentration of developer will produce dark films (**4.45**);

- fogging (**4.46**) represents a gradual increase in background density and also makes the film appear dark. This may occur if the film has been stored incorrectly or for too long, if there is additional exposure to light or radiation or if a faulty safe light is used;
- insufficient exposure or development time, exhausted developer, low processing temperatures or use of excessively diluted developer are likely to produce light films (**4.47**);
- when the film is still wet the emulsion is soft and easily scratched by fingernails or film hangers (**4.48**);
- streaks, spots and marks may be made on the film, especially by dirty rollers in automatic processors (**4.49**). Meticulous attention must be paid to careful wet processing and thorough and regular cleaning of automatic processor tank and roller systems.

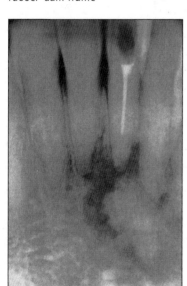

4.43 Image obscured by metal rubber-dam frame

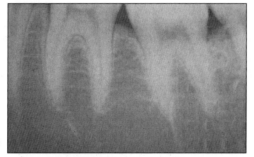

4.44 Image produced when film is placed with tube side away from tube

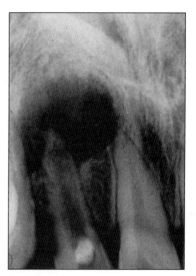

4.45 Dark image

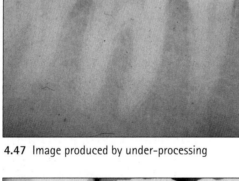

4.47 Image produced by under-processing

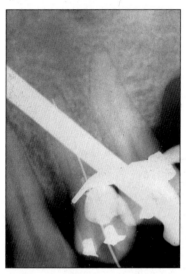

4.46 Fogged image

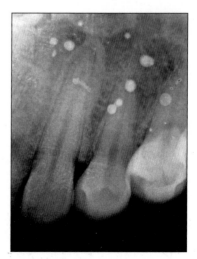

4.48 Damaged film emulsion

4.49 Marks introduced during wet film processing (fixer splashes)

Old or spare films should be passed through automatic processors as 'cleaning films' at the beginning of each day to remove dried concretions that have formed on the rollers overnight.

INTERPRETATION OF RADIOGRAPHS

The interpretation of radiographs should be approached in a logical fashion in order to avoid mistaking an artefact or area of normal anatomy for an abnormality. The operator should be familiar with the radiographic appearances of normal anatomical structures before attempting to identify abnormalities.

Normal radiographic landmarks

Enamel, dentine and cementum

Enamel is the most radio-opaque structure in the mouth. Dentine is darker and has a uniform density. Cementum cannot be distinguished from dentine. Radiographic 'burn out' occurs in the cervical region, between the cement–enamel junction and the alveolar crest, and may be confused with root caries or secondary caries beneath a mesial or distal box (**4.50**).

Cancellous bone

The trabeculae have a coarser pattern in the mandible than in the maxilla, where they are slightly denser, finer and more lace-like.

Periodontal ligament

This appears as a narrow, even radiolucent line around the root surface. It is also referred to as the periodontal ligament space. Genuine widening of this space is indicative of pathological change.

Lamina dura

This is the name given to the white line forming the lining of the tooth socket seen on radiographs and represents the margin of the socket.

Pulp space

The pulp chamber and larger root canals are usually readily visible on the radiograph, but finer canals are more difficult to see. Root canals that appear to be completely sclerosed rarely are. Stones are common in the pulp and present as a problem only when they block root canals.

Maxillary antrum

This may extend from the premolar region in the maxilla to the tuberosity. The floor of the antrum may be closely associated with the roots of the premolars and molars and may dip between the roots (**4.51**). The floor of the antrum appears as a white cortical line and should be carefully traced to check continuity when possible periapical change is suspected.

The anterior maxillary region

Figure 4.52 identifies common landmarks in this region.

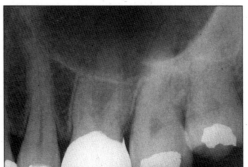

4.51 Appearance of large maxillary antrum

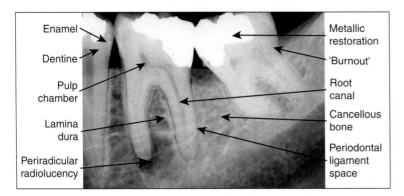

4.50 Radiographic appearance of posterior teeth

Enamel · Dentine · Pulp chamber · Lamina dura · Periradicular radiolucency · Metallic restoration · 'Burnout' · Root canal · Cancellous bone · Periodontal ligament space

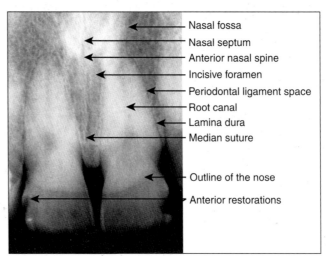

4.52 Radiographic appearance of maxillary anterior region

Nasal fossa · Nasal septum · Anterior nasal spine · Incisive foramen · Periodontal ligament space · Root canal · Lamina dura · Median suture · Outline of the nose · Anterior restorations

Common errors in interpretation

False widening of the periodontal ligament space

The dark appearance of the periodontal ligament space may become more pronounced when an air space (such as the maxillary antrum) or other radiolucency is superimposed on it, giving the erroneous impression of widening of this space (**4.53**). Similarly the white line of the lamina dura may appear less opaque when an air space or other radiolucency is superimposed on it (**4.54**) making it less visible and increasing the impression of breakdown of normal anatomical features at the apex. Thus apical pathology may be suggested when a radiolucent area is superimposed over a normal apex.

The maxillary antrum

The margin of the maxillary antrum may appear loculated and take on the appearance of a cyst (**4.55**).

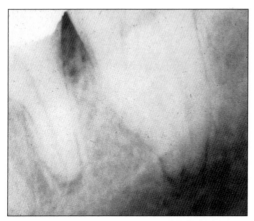

4.53 False widening of the PDL space in mandibular second molar – evidence of presence of periradicular lesion on distal root of the first molar

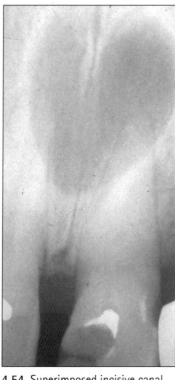

4.54 Superimposed incisive canal cyst giving impression of loss of lamina dura around the apex of a maxillary incisor

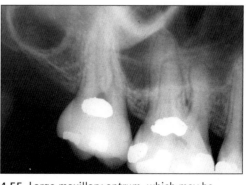

4.55 Large maxillary antrum, which may be confused with a cyst

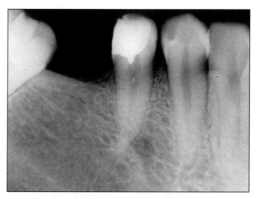

4.58 Radiographic appearance of a mental foramen

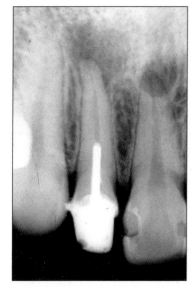

4.56 Maxillary lateral incisor with a periradicular lesion – maxillary central incisor with superimposed incisive canal

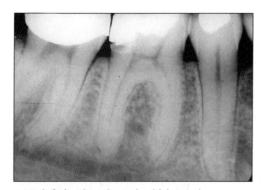

4.57 Inferior dental canal, which may be confused with periradicular lesion

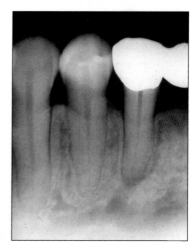

4.59 Inferior dental canal and mental foramen, which might be confused with periradicular lesion

Incisive foramen

This circular or oval radiolucent shadow of the incisive foramen may be superimposed over the apex of a central incisor and be mistaken for a periapical lesion (**4.56**).

Inferior dental canal

The mandibular or inferior dental canal runs from the mandibular foramen on the medial aspect of the ascending ramus of the mandible to the mental foramen in the premolar region. It is seen as a radiolucent band that may be close to or coincident with the roots of the lower molar and premolar teeth. Here it may be mistaken for a lesion (**4.57**).

Mental foramen

The mental foramen is situated below and distal to the apex of the mandibular first premolar (**4.58**). Occasionally the angulation of a periapical radiograph may result in superimposition of the structure on the apex of one of the premolars. The foramen may then be confused with a periradicular lesion (**4.59**).

Lesions involving the periodontal ligament space

Periradicular lesions

These are the most common apical radiolucencies. Long-standing lesions and those from a chronic inflammatory process are usually well defined (**4.60**) and may even develop a radio-opaque margin of reactive bone (**4.61**). Early lesions are identified by thickening of the periodontal ligament space (**4.62**) – these can progress to discrete areas of radiolucency (**4.43**) and may, at a later stage, become larger and more diffuse in appearance (**4.63**).

Lateral periradicular lesions

Widening of the periodontal ligament space and formation of radiolucencies unrelated to the apex (**4.64**) are associated with infection within the lateral canals. These canals may become visible only after canal obturation (**4.65**).

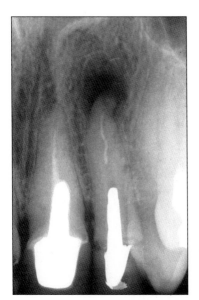

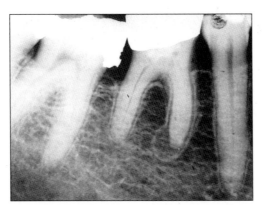

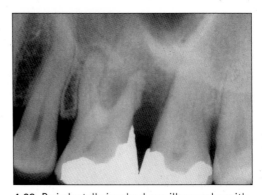

4.60 Maxillary lateral incisor with well-defined periradicular lesion

4.61 Mandibular molar with periradicular lesion with radiopaque margin

4.62 Periodontally involved maxillary molar with widening of the periodontal ligament space of the mesiobuccal root

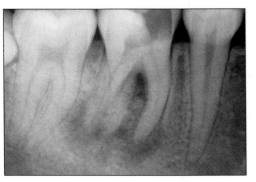

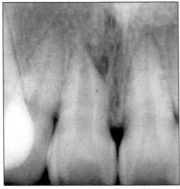

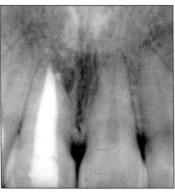

4.63 Mandibular molar with large diffuse periradicular radiolucency

4.64 Central incisor with lateral periradicular radiolucency

4.65 Central incisor with obturated lateral canal

Fractured root lesions

Radiolucencies associated with the pathology of fractured roots are often widespread along the involved root (**4.66**). The ability to determine the presence of a fracture will depend upon the plane of the fracture in relation to the main X-ray beam (**4.67**). If the beam does not pass through the fracture it may well remain undetected.

Perforation lesions

Perforations (**4.68**) can lead to rapid bone loss, the diffuse appearance of the radiolucency reflecting the more acute inflammatory process initiated. The presence of a post-retained restoration in a tooth with a large diffuse lesion involving more than just the apical region should arouse suspicion of a perforation or fracture (**4.69**).

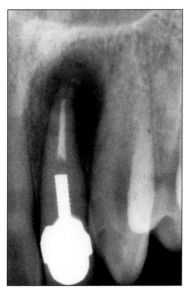

4.66 Diffuse radiolucency related to fractured maxillary incisor

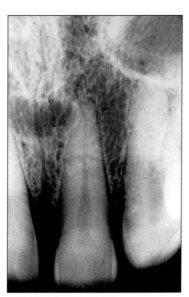

4.67 Maxillary central incisor with horizontal root fracture

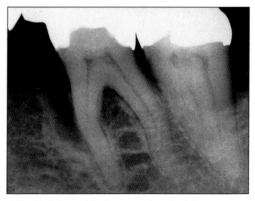

4.68 Maxillary second premolar with root perforation

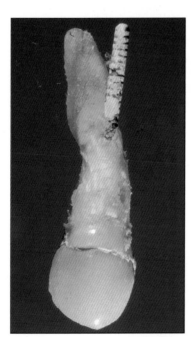

4.69 Extracted perforated second premolar

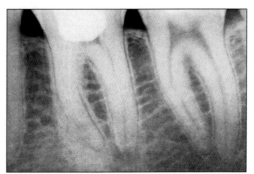

4.70 Sclerosing osteitis related to the mesial root of a mandibular first molar

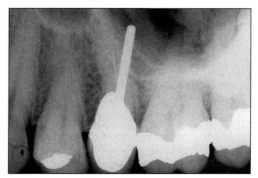

4.71 Periodontal lesion associated with mandibular molar

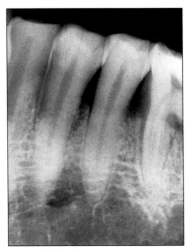

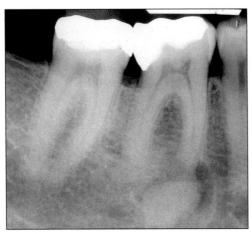

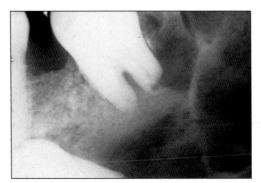

4.72 Dense bony trabecular pattern around the roots of vital teeth

4.73 Fibro-cemento-osseous-dysplasia related to a mandibular molar

4.74 Extensive radiolucency produced by a lesion of non-endodontic origin

Sclerosing osteitis

This appears as a zone of peripheral radio-opacity (**4.70**) and is indicative of a long-standing, low-grade apical infection, which gives rise to a circumscribed proliferation of the periapical bone. It is usually related to a non-vital pulp or one that is in the process of degeneration. The condition is often symptomless.

Lesions not of intrapulpal origin

It is important to be able to distinguish lesions of endodontic origin from those arising from other disease processes.

Periodontal lesions

Periodontal lesions within bone can give rise to radiographic changes, which can be confused with periradicular areas (**4.71**). The teeth involved usually remain vital despite the bone loss.

Idiopathic osteosclerosis

Areas of dense bone may frequently be encountered within the trabecular spaces and may represent a developmental anomaly or occasionally a compensatory response to abnormal stress. The radiographic appearance may closely resemble that of sclerosing osteitis. However, the tooth reacts normally to vitality testing (**4.72**).

Fibro-cemento-osseous dysplasia

Fibro-cemento-osseous lesions present in their early stages as radiolucent areas, commonly in relation to the apices of the mandibular incisors known here as periapical fibro-cemento-osseous dysplasia (**4.73**). These lesions mature over a 5 to 10-year period with gradual infill of dense cemento-osseous material to create radio-opacities. The teeth remain vital and endodontic treatment is not required.

Other local and systemic pathology

Many inflammatory, cystic and neoplastic lesions may arise in the jaws which are not of endodontic origin (**4.74**). These are capable of destroying or remodelling neighbouring bone and of displacing or resorbing teeth. In many cases the teeth remain vital if the lesion originates outside the periodontium. The operator should always be alert to the possibility of non-dental causes of bone destruction.

The origin of such lesions may be divided into:

- infections (localized and spreading);
- trauma;
- cysts (odontogenic and non-odontogenic);
- tumours (benign and malignant);
- giant cell lesions;
- fibro-cemento-osseous lesions;
- metabolic and endocrine lesions;
- idiopathic lesions.

Chapter 5

Treatment options

K Gulabivala and R T Walker

GOALS OF OVERALL PATIENT CARE AND ROLE OF ENDODONTICS

The health and well-being of an individual is influenced by factors as diverse as their genetic make-up, environment, nutrition and interaction with society. These factors all play a part in the physical, psychological, social, cultural and spiritual aspects of the well-being of the individual. Health-care workers in general should have an awareness of the complex interplay between such factors and their potential influence on the outcome of any health-improving measure. Those involved in the direct delivery of any intervention that may impinge on these factors should understand the nature of the broadest effect of that intervention. Oral health care is perceived by many in the general health care profession to play only a small part in the overall well-being of the individual. The truth, however, is that oral and dental problems may influence and in turn be influenced by the overall well being of the individual. Management of oral and dental health is therefore no less important than management of the overall health of people. It requires a broad-based appreciation of life (including, social, cultural, individual, psychological and spiritual contexts) in parallel with the biological and clinical knowledge and skills necessary to deal with diseases of the pulp and periradicular tissues. The dentist must, therefore, be both a physician and surgeon.

Dentistry is no more than a specialty of medicine but the management of complex oral problems requires broad as well as specific advanced training and this has resulted in the development of sub-specialties. This means dentists are able to develop their skills in a given subspecialty and practice within that sphere to the exclusion of other aspects. Restriction to such a narrow sphere of practice (such as endodontics) enables the development of highly skilled and knowledgeable individuals able to deal with especially difficult problems. This does, however, mean that the onus of ensuring the coordinated and appropriate delivery of whole mouth and patient care must rest with the referring general dental practitioner, in conjunction with other specialists and the medical practitioner where necessary.

The knowledge and skills of endodontics have to be deployed judiciously to ensure that the patient receives appropriate care. In order to do this, the dentist should be equally well versed in all aspects of dentistry and understand the role of each in overall management, as well as potential overlaps and interactions between the subdisciplines. In the context of a health care profession, the 'endodontist' must be a human being first, dentist second and endodontist last.

TREATMENT OPTION SELECTION AND TREATMENT PLANNING

Treatment planning, as the term implies, is the planning of the management of a patient's dental problems in a systematic and ordered way that assumes a complete knowledge of the patient's needs, the precise nature of the problems and the prognoses of possible options under consideration. It is rare in dentistry, however, for both patient and dentist to have such a complete picture of the problems and outcomes of options. The phase of assessment or establishment of a more complete picture of the problem(s), therefore, often overlaps with the phases of decision-making, planning and delivery of treatment. Anticipation of a particular outcome while desirable is not always a certainty. The term 'provisional treatment plan' is used to describe the overlapping phases of diagnosis and treatment when further information is sought to garner a clearer picture. A 'definitive treatment plan' will emerge as the information becomes more complete and the wishes of the patient and dentist crystallize into a more concrete proposal. Unfortunately, even under the best set of circumstances, the most complete and definitive picture of the problems is seldom reached and together with the variations inherent in each dentist's knowledge, experience, skills and judgement, this gives rise to the differences evident in treatment planning between operators. Conscientious dentists, therefore, strive to reach this goal throughout their professional lives in what has now become formally recognized as continuing professional development (CPD). Unfortunately, some practitioners take the receipt of their practicing licence as the end of professional development. Their frame of reference extends no further than the teachings given at undergraduate level. Decision-making for them is a matter of following the simple decision-tree given as expedient teaching. Their knowledge is written in black and white, is clear and simple but unfortunately never approaches the truth. Their intellect and skills consequently never flower into their full potential. The true difficulty in treatment planning is only realized by the conscious and conscientious endeavour to improve the service delivered to patients.

The aim of this chapter is to highlight the factors important in planning the endodontic management of pulpal and periradicular diseases and how to prioritize them in the context of the patient's overall and dental needs. Treatment planning encompasses the phases of:

- establishing the nature of the problem;
- mutual interrogation and negotiation (between patient and dentist) that precedes the decision-making inherent in selecting the best course of action;
- planning required to deliver the selected treatment in an effective and efficient sequence.

THE IDEAL TREATMENT PLANNING SCENARIO

The textbook depiction of treatment planning commences *at the first encounter with the patient*, when a full assessment is made of the patient's overall dental and oral problems. In this diagnostic phase, a detailed systematic appraisal is made in the classical manner described in Chapter 3. The end-point of this is a series of conclusions about the general health of the patient and their current oral and dental problems. This will include the state of their dentition, including that of the periodontium, the teeth (presence of caries or tooth surface loss and their pulpal and periapical status) and any restorations. A number of different solutions will be possible for management of the patient's problems but the specific treatment options selected will be dictated by a number of other factors such as technical feasibility, cost and time involved, dentist's preferences based on their skills, and the patient's age, wishes and compliance in oral care. In the ideal scenario, each option should be evaluated in an objective way taking the above factors into account, weighing the effectiveness and projected long-term prognosis (based on outcome data) with compliance, cost and time commitment. As the number of dental problems to be addressed increases (5.1), so does the interaction between options for individual problems. This may have the overall effect of either complicating management or simplifying it because more radical solutions (such as extraction) become more appropriate. In any case, the options will be discussed with the patient and after appropriate negotiation and clarification a mutually agreed choice of treatment or '*treatment plan*' will be made (**Box 5.1**).

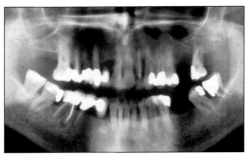

5.1 Orthopantomogram (OPG) of difficult problems

A plan is then made of the sequence in which treatment will be executed, called the '*plan of treatment*' (**Box 5.2**). Once the treatment is completed, the patient will be recruited to a recall system to evaluate and maintain the work. At these recall reviews note will be taken of any changes and dealt with according to a preplanned scheme for dealing with failure (planning for failure should be considered as part of the overall long-term treatment plan).

Box 5.1 Treatment plan

Scenario – a patient presents in pain with a poorly maintained mouth, several carious and periapical lesions and gingival inflammation. Following history and examination, the treatment plan is as follows but beyond pain management is conditional on compliance. It includes:

1. Diet investigation.
2. Scale and polish and oral hygiene instruction.
3. Treatment of carious lesions.
4. Extractions of unrestorable teeth.
5. Root canal treatment of teeth with periapical lesions.
6. Root canal retreatment of root-filled teeth with periapical lesions.
7. Periapical surgery if required.
8. Provision of crowns.
9. Provision of denture.

Box 5.2 Plan of treatment

The 'plan of treatment' to deliver the 'treatment plan' will consist of checks to gauge compliance and success in pain management. It may progress as follows:

1. Treatment of acute problems including incision and drainage, first stage root canal treatment, extractions.
2. Immediate denture if necessary, oral hygiene instruction, diet instruction and fluoride mouthwash.
3. Stabilize carious lesions in conjunction with scale and polish and reinforcement of oral hygiene instructions.
4. Gauge compliance in home-care and gingival health with further oral hygiene instruction as necessary.
5. Provide definitive plastic restorations for carious teeth in order of priority dependent on presence of sensitivity and integrity of temporaries.
6. Complete all root canal treatments where teeth restorable.
7. Carry out periapical surgery where necessary.
8. Review prognosis of treated teeth, design definitive denture or fixed prosthesis and decide teeth requiring cast restorations (compliance should be absolute at this stage).
9. Provide crowns.
10. Provide definitive denture.

THE REALITY IN PRACTICE

In general practice, however, where a patient has often been under long-term care by a particular practice or dentist, the majority of interactions with the patient are part of continuing care. A plan of management will have been established at some point in the past and in the simplest cases, requires no more than a review (recall) to evaluate a change in overall status. Under these circumstances, the sudden precipitation of a pulpal or periapical problem may be managed in isolation as long as there are no complex restorative implications (**5.2**). Where there are such complex restorative implications, the desire or lack of desire (on the part of the dentist) to tackle them may influence management of the endodontic problem (**5.3**). It is therefore important that a rational analysis of the situation is carried out and difficult restorative decisions taken as necessary rather than deferred to another time when the situation is likely to be worse.

In many patients on long-term recall, the dentist may place individual teeth on probation and review their status at a subsequent time because of uncertainty about a diagnosis or the progression of a lesion (**5.4**). A number of potential problems, not causing current difficulties will therefore have been identified but a mutually agreed decision made to leave alone and review. Such a plan of action is not uncommon in mouths which are heavily restored and where changes can precipitate a radical review of the overall dental strategy for the patient plan, with major implications of time and cost. Small changes to the situation may be managed by minimal intervention and a 'patchwork' approach. The situation, however, must be understood between the patient and dentist in the so-called *informed consent* approach. The tooth in **Figure 5.4** has been retreated (**5.5**) and placed on continuing review until a mutually agreed decision can be reached with regard to the restorative options.

Under some circumstances, with the passage of time, the mutually agreed plan may be forgotten or fade from memory, particularly where detailed records are not maintained. Under these circumstances, the precipitation of a pulpal or periapical problem and even worse multiple problems that occur in rapid succession may cause the need for a radical review of the options. The sudden accumulation of such unfavourable events may prompt the patient to seek a second opinion. The nature of this next encounter, in all likelihood with somebody with a different perspective, may raise different opinions about the previous management. The precise nature of the previous mutually agreed treatment plan might not be fully appreciated in the absence of accurate and detailed records. The vagaries and subtleties that lead to differences in management approach may cause patient dissatisfaction, which sometimes (and in contemporary society increasingly frequently) leads to legal action. It is therefore best to keep detailed records of initial findings, option appraisals, rationale for decisions and informed consent for treatment.

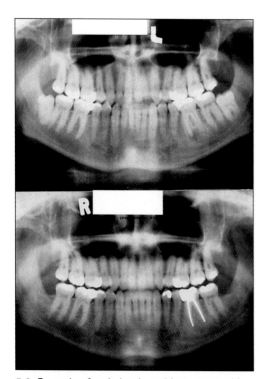

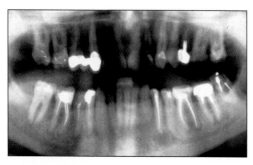

5.3 Example of endodontic problems that have complex restorative implications

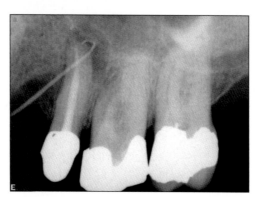

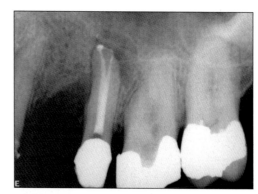

5.2 Example of endodontic problem managed in isolation

5.4 Symptomless 25 has been reviewed for some time and now has a sinus

5.5 The same 25 has been retreated and is now under review to assess healing before making a decision about restorative options

FACTORS INFLUENCING TREATMENT PLANNING

Treatment planning is a challenging and complex decision-making process by both the operator and patient that involves a two-way interrogation and negotiation between them, leading preferably to short-, medium-, and long-term goals for the management of the patient's dentition. Difficulties are often caused by the contradictory requirements and perceptions of dentist and patient. The ways in which these may be resolved are numerous, even forming the basis for practice-marketing strategies. The factors influencing the decision-making process are many. Factors that may confound the process include differences in perception and goals between the dentist and patient. Some examples are listed in **Table 5.1**. The dentist must be

Table 5.1 Patient and dentist perceptions

Patient's complaint	Dentist's perception and goals	Patient's perception and goals
Pain and swelling	Requires emergency scheduling but also planning for definitive solution	Priority is to eliminate immediate problem, definitive solution not always a priority
Eating and chewing compromised	Aim to define sources of useful support for prostheses, balancing feasibility with learning curve for patient and side-effects	Has expectations of establishing normal uncompromised function
Aesthetics compromised	Aim to define source of problem(s) and technical feasibility of correction	Expectation of ideal aesthetics (that may not match that of the dentist or that achievable)
Previous history of dental treatment	Aim to establish the residual problems of extensive previous dental work	May harbour feelings of mistrust because of past experience and may now be seeking correction
Medical history	Aim to identify factors that may compromise dental treatment Identify if the dental condition may be responsible for any systemic illness?	Coping with added burden of their systemic problems may lessen patient's priority of dental care Will wish to know if the teeth are causing the systemic problems?
Extraoral examination	Exclude other causes of pain and establish TMJ and mandibular function for restorative evaluation	Liable to harbour doubts about relation between dental problems and extraoral factors
Intraoral examination	Aim to gauge general oral condition first before focusing on the specific sites of complaint so as not to miss clues	May question the need to evaluate 'peripheral factors' Will wish dentist to investigate the problem, as they perceive it
Oral hygiene	Aim to identify deficiencies to improve overall dental condition	Will always be crestfallen and disbelieving, 'but I spend hours cleaning my teeth!'
Soft tissues	Aim to confirm evidence for and location of infection and inflammation by visual and tactile examination	May perceive that elicitation of pain is not confirmation for diagnostic reasons but aggravation of pain Will expect dentist to believe them
Teeth and restorative status	Aim to identify missing units and need for replacement, state of residual dentition and restorations, confirming sources of discomfort and pain	Probing and percussion of teeth is often perceived as aggravation of pain Its purpose should always be explained
Periodontal status	Aim to establish the state of periodontal foundation for long-term stability and to identify and correct any problems	Will usually find the probing uncomfortable, viewing any bleeding caused by inflamed sites as trauma induced by the dentist and source of further problems
Occlusal status	Aim to establish functional relationship between opposing teeth, accounting for occlusal wear, habits and potential future loading of proposed restorations	Almost universally will deny that they parafunction or that their mandible reaches extreme excursions proven by tell-tale faceting and contact relationships
Special tests	Aim to reveal the status of unseen or invisible tissues, namely pulp and periapical tissues	May find pulp tests painful and aggravating and will be cautious of X-radiation
Diagnoses	Aim to report the series of conclusions	May be daunted by unexpected findings and reports, sometimes causing emotional responses
Treatment option appraisal	Aim to objectively evaluate the treatment options to determine the most suitable choice for the patient's long-term benefit	Priority usually placed on aesthetics and short-term benefits Importance of function and long-term considerations should be stressed

aware of the potential for such problems and be prepared to take appropriate action to circumvent them.

This hypothetical but familiar illustration of operator and patient's perspectives, which many will identify with, illustrates some sources of problematic communication. Effective communication is the key to arriving at a mutually satisfactory treatment plan.

The complexities of decision-making are further explored by examining different case scenarios based on a simple situation.

INFLUENCE OF VARIOUS FACTORS ON TREATMENT PLANNING IN A SIMPLE SITUATION

In any given situation the options available to treat pulpal or peri-apical disease may be to carry out pulp therapy, root canal treatment, root canal retreatment, periapical surgery, root resection or extraction. The last option also requires a consideration of the alternative restorative options. Apart from feasibility, the cost and long-term priorities of the patient have to be weighed.

A cost–benefit analysis should be performed to aid the decision-making process as illustrated below in **Table 5.2**. The outcome of such an analysis, though, is likely to be different depending upon the exact details of the situation.

As an example, consider the various presentations of an endodontic problem associated with a maxillary central incisor in an otherwise intact dental arch.

Scenario 1

Consider the not uncommon scenario of the pulp in a maxillary incisor of an otherwise intact dentition becoming compromised by a severe traumatic injury in a young, mature adult (**5.6**). The options of pulp therapy or root canal treatment may be considered. The choice will centre on the prognosis of each treatment (based on

biological factors) and the long-term benefit to the patient. If the tooth is not restoratively compromised and the root is mature, the high prevalence of pulp necrosis in such cases may lean the decision towards root canal treatment and the appropriate restoration as having a high chance of success (**5.7, 5.8**). Other restorative factors may not come into the equation at this stage but will be discussed with the patient.

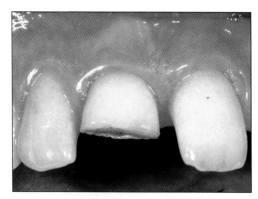

5.6 Traumatized maxillary incisor

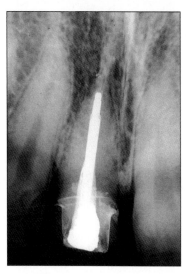

5.7 Maxillary incisor following endodontic treatment

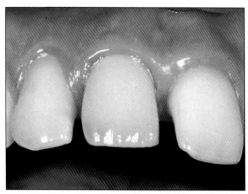

5.8 Maxillary incisor restored

Table 5.2 Weighing of prognosis and relative cost of endodontic and restorative options (based on average figures)

Treatment option	Relative cost	Prognosis (% survival/years)
Root canal treatment	1.0	Difficult to determine as
Conventional retreatment and new post retained restoration	2.3	dependent on individual prognostic factors
		Each case has to be
Surgical endodontics	1.5	weighed independently
Extraction/leave unrestored	0.2	
Extraction/denture	1.4	
Extraction/bridge	3.8	
Extraction/implant	4.3	

NB the relative cost may change depending on contemporary and local trends.

Scenario 2

If, under the same circumstances, the patient was younger with an incompletely formed root, the decision may now lean towards, the more conservative pulp therapy (**5.9**) in order to aid completion of root formation and improve the long-term restorative prognosis (**5.10**). In the event that the traumatic injury in such circumstances is accompanied by severe coronal tooth fracture, the restorative prognosis may be further jeopardized (**5.11a–c**). Consideration of early replacement may have to be tempered by the psychological need to avoid loss of the tooth as well as to delay permanent replacement during the growth phase of the individual, especially if an implant-retained crown is a possible alternative. The compromised tooth may therefore be retained as a suitable space maintainer until a more definitive solution can be executed.

Scenario 3

Consider an identical scenario but where a traumatized, intact, mature, maxillary central incisor has been left untreated for years as the pulp slowly succumbs and the patient seeks attention either because of an acute infection or the discolouration caused by secondary dentine formation and/or pulp necrosis (**5.12**). On radiographic examination, it is found that the canal is sclerosed (**5.13**) and only evident in the apical third of the root associated with a periapical lesion. Now other considerations come into play including the potential for successful outcome by conventional or surgical means, as well as the desire for correcting the discolouration. In the matter of the former problem, it has to be established, whether the operator is confident of locating the canal using a conventional coronal approach (**5.14**), which would improve the chances of success (**5.15**). If not, injudicious dentine removal may result in compromised restorability of the tooth. A surgical approach may stand a better chance of finding the canal but may not help eradicate the major part of the infection in the root canal system, compromising the chances of successful healing (**5.16a–c**). In addition, the absence of access to the pulp chamber also compromises the chances of internal bleaching of the tooth to help correct the discolouration. In this scenario, there are an increasing number of uncertainties as outcomes are less certain. The decision-making now has to be aided by weighing the relative chances of success of the different endodontic options and finally also the restorative/aesthetic outcome.

Scenario 4

Consider that the same scenario presents many years later but this time without having caused the patient any symptoms, the sole concern being tooth discolouration. The intact tooth will in all probability give negative pulp test responses and may or may not be associated with a periapical radiolucency. In the case of a periapical lesion the decision is easier as it would be reasonable to recommend root canal treatment, bleaching (**5.17**, **5.18**) and if necessary a

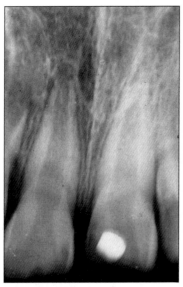

5.9 Traumatized maxillary incisor with an open apex, receiving pulp therapy

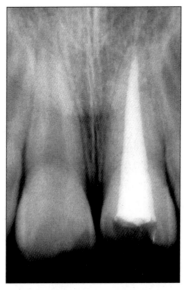

5.10 Traumatized maxillary incisor root filled following root closure

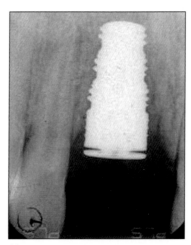

5.11 (a) UR1 under calcium hydroxide therapy to induce root end closure following traumatic injury; (b) same tooth following cervical level fracture; (c) replacement with an implant, still in the process of integrating

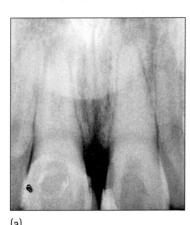

(a)

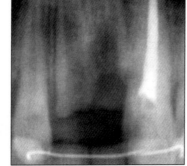

(b)

(c)

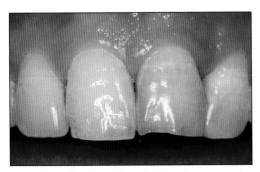

5.12 Discolouration of tooth following trauma

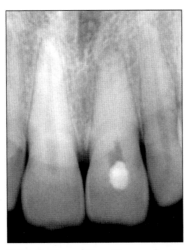

5.13 Radiographic evidence of pulp calcification and dentine sclerosis

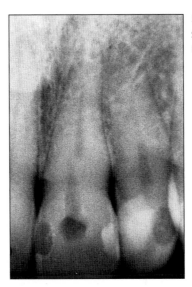

5.14 Example of sclerosed canal in maxillary incisor

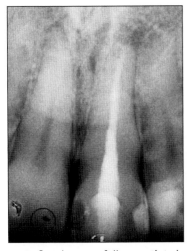

5.15 Canal successfully negotiated and obturated

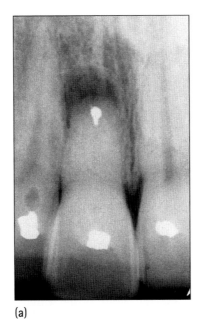

(a)

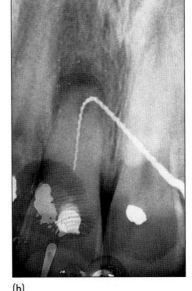

(b)

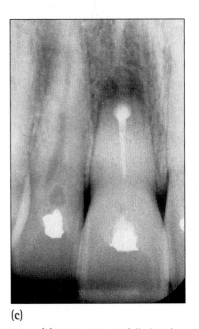

(c)

5.16 (a) Sclerosed canal in central incisor managed by apicectomy and root-end filling; (b) the treatment failed and required a further procedure when retrograde root canal treatment was performed; (c) final retrograde root filling

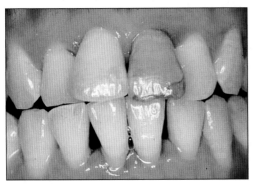

5.17 Central incisor requiring endodontic treatment and bleaching

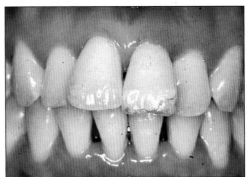

5.18 Bleached central incisor

porcelain veneer to mask residual discolouration caused by increased thickness of sclerosed dentine. The morbidity of treatment, that is, the potential of an acute flare-up, should also be considered since about 10–15% of asymptomatic periapical lesions, without sinus tracts, become acute on commencement of root canal treatment. The decision is even more difficult in the absence of a periapical lesion because of the potential to infect a necrotic pulp and precipitate further problems.

Scenario 5

Consider another variation on the above scenario, where the tooth has already been root treated and restored with a post-crown. The patient now presents years later with a periapical lesion (**5.19**). This confronts the dentist with additional endodontic and restorative dimensions that must be considered. The endodontic question to address is the reason for treatment failure. The causes of failure include persistent intraradicular infection, new intraradicular infection, extraradicular infection, cyst, foreign body reaction, healing by scar tissue and radicular fracture. It is virtually impossible to predict which of these factors may be the prime causative factor in the absence of other clinical clues. The presence of acute infection may narrow down the options. The presence of uninstrumented apical canal space may suggest persistent infection, whereas, a recently decemented and recemented post crown may suggest a newly established infection or root fracture. If intraradicular infection is implicated, then conventional retreatment may be the treatment of choice. In this case, the restorability of the tooth, the retrievability of the post-core and root filling should be weighed up, as should the potential for root fracture during post removal. The natural consequence of this will also be the need for redoing the root canal treatment and placing a new post crown. The chances of success using this approach should be weighed against a surgical option where the existing crown is preserved (assuming good pre-existing

margins, contours and aesthetics) and retrograde apical treatment considered (**5.20**). This has the advantage of correcting causes of failure other than intraradicular infection. It must be remembered that if a conventional approach is selected and the cause of the problem turns out to be extraradicular infection or a cyst, surgical correction may still be required in addition. Under these circumstances, the decision-making process is therefore more complicated. If it is found that the root length is short or that the restorative management is compromised by the existing canal shape, size and length, extraction and prosthetic replacement should also be considered.

Under these circumstances, further assessments have to be made for alternative replacements. The options include, leaving alone, a denture, bridge or implant. A number of factors now need to be considered, including the size and shape of the vault of the palate (for a denture), the restorative status of the adjacent teeth, including their size for the purposes of adhesive bonding, the quality and quantity of bone in the site at present as a possible indicator of bone after extraction for an implant and finally the occlusal relationship with opposing teeth. The prognoses of each of these options, as well as their cost, should be considered.

Scenario 6

The superimposition of a medical condition such as rheumatic fever that renders the patient susceptible to infective endocarditis may sway the balance of the decision depending upon the predictability of the outcome. The type of endodontic treatment planned for a particular patient should take into account the patient's general health and dental state.

SUMMARY OF FACTORS AFFECTING TREATMENT PLANNING

This illustration shows how the balance of the decision may be swayed by the interaction of a number variables including the age, desire and means of the patient, endodontic status of the tooth, the restorative status of the tooth and that of adjacent teeth, the overall and specific periodontal condition of involved teeth, the overall and specific occlusal relationship of involved teeth and the prognoses and cost of the different options of treatment.

Similar considerations apply to posterior multirooted teeth. However, the root canal anatomy and its influence on management prospects have also to be considered (**5.21**). The situation becomes further complicated in teeth that have been previously treated and may have iatrogenic problems such as broken instruments (**5.22**) and canal transportation (**5.23**).

FACTORS INFLUENCING TREATMENT PLANNING IN A COMPLEX CASE

The complexity of interacting factors increases further when more than one tooth is involved, whether they are adjacent or separated by

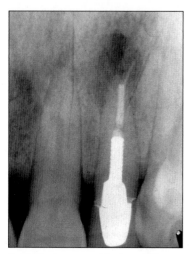

5.19 Post-crowned incisor with periapical lesion

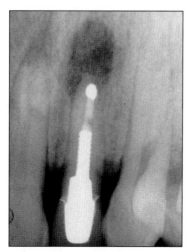

5.20 Retrograde apical treatment of post-crowned incisor

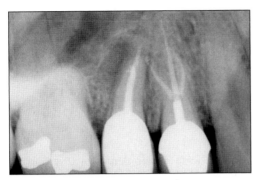

5.21 Multirooted maxillary premolar

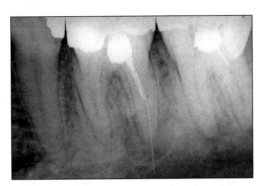

5.22 Mandibular molar with iatrogenic problems

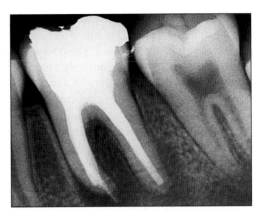

5.23 Radiograph of root-treated molar with evidence of canal transportation

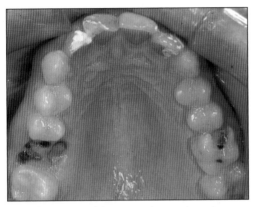

5.24 Patient requiring extensive treatment

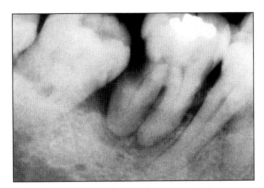

5.25 Very carious, periodontally involved mandibular molar

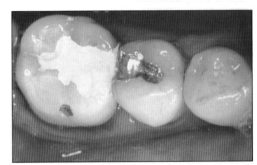

5.26 Provisional sedative restoration in a molar

other teeth or in different arches. Where multiple teeth are involved each should be independently evaluated initially and then the interacting aspects considered. It will often be intuitively obvious when the simple solution should take precedence over overly complicated efforts to preserve all teeth at all costs.

Once the treatment options have been selected, the next phase involves the planning of the sequence of delivery of the treatment. In the case of single teeth, this is straightforward, but becomes increasingly complicated with involvement of multiple teeth, of which some may be symptomatic and others may require temporization.

THE SEQUENCE OF TREATMENT DELIVERY

Figure 5.24 shows the case of a patient with multiple restorative and endodontic problems.

There are three stages in the planning process. These are:

- planned initial treatment;
- planned definitive treatment;
- planned review.

Planned initial treatment

Immediate relief of symptoms

The immediate relief of pain is a valuable service and should precede other forms of treatment. The provision of emergency endodontic care for patients in pain of pulpal or periradicular origin need not be anxiety ridden or time consuming, and can assist in building the reputation of a practitioner.

The treatment required for the immediate relief of pain may be obvious – for example a very carious, periodontally involved, unrestorable tooth may be extracted (**5.25**).

Where a tooth has recurrent caries, treatment of the provoked pain may only require the removal of caries, placement of an indirect pulp capping with calcium hydroxide, and the placement of a provisional sedative restoration (**5.26**).

Where the appropriate treatment is not quite so obvious, as in some cases of post-restorative pain, interim relief may be achieved by correction of occlusal interferences and inadequate or excessive approximal contacts, to allow the stressed pulp to recover from the restorative episode.

Cracked teeth with symptoms of irreversible pulpitis may require endodontic treatment for the relief of symptoms before making a definitive decision about the restorative future of the tooth. For example, endodontic treatment may be commenced in a painful tooth with a suspected fracture before undertaking further investigations to establish the true prognosis (**5.27**).

Teeth with established intraradicular infection may present with severe pain and/or localized or diffuse swelling (**5.28**). Treatment in these situations is based on the need for the establishment of drainage (**5.29**), thorough disinfection of the tooth and, where necessary, the prescription of analgesics and antibiotics. The use of antibiotics alone in the relief of acute symptoms is considered inappropriate.

Stabilization

Stabilization involves halting the progress of primary dental disease in the dentition. Both caries and periodontal disease fall into this category.

When disease is at an advanced stage and threatens the survival of a tooth or teeth, its progression may be controlled without the delivery of full effective, definitive treatment. The most easily understood example of this is the dressing of carious teeth to arrest caries progression and protect the pulp. The primary phase in periodontal therapy may involve oral-hygiene instruction and debridement.

The same principle may be applied to pulpally involved teeth. Endodontic treatment may be instituted and the canals in the teeth provisionally dressed to control the development of periradicular disease without completing the definitive therapy (**5.30**). Endodontically speaking, the teeth are placed 'on hold' while other aspects of the patient's total care are being managed.

Prevention

A patient's understanding and belief about dental disease and its treatment may affect his/her motivation, attitude to attendance and compliance to treatment. Initial planned treatment should always incorporate an element of behavioural conditioning to address the patient's beliefs and attitudes.

This approach is crucial for the long-term prevention of dental caries and periodontal disease.

Effective planning should always incorporate prevention. In addition to the identification of the aetiology of the dental disease present, patient education becomes the basis of any preventative regime. This may include dietary advice, home oral-health measures, and the use of fluoride supplements.

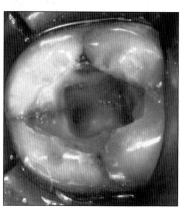

5.27 Endodontic treatment commenced in painful fractured molar

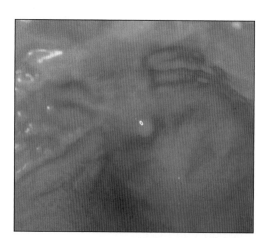

5.28 Swelling of the palate related to endodontic intraradicular infection

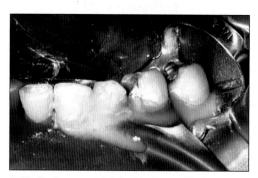

5.29 Drainage established in a mandibular canine

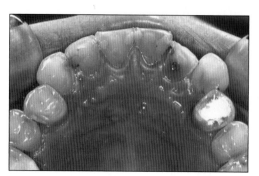

5.30 Endodontic stabilization of maxillary first premolar

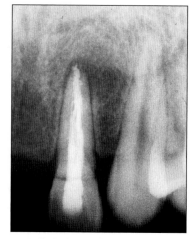

5.31 Endodontically unsound incisor

Planned definitive treatment

Definitive treatment options may involve pulp therapy, root canal treatment, root canal retreatment, surgical treatment, review or extraction. Where the loss of teeth becomes a factor then replacement options should be considered. These involve the construction of fixed and removable prostheses or the provision of implants. The choice of treatment may be influenced by specific factors.

Overall treatment

The general state of a patient's dentition is an indicator of dental disease experience. The age, condition and maintenance of restorations and the presence of recurrent disease are all factors that may influence the decision-making.

It should be remembered that not all teeth with pulpal and periradicular disease are candidates for endodontic treatment, and on occasions the retention of a pulpally compromised tooth should be questioned if it unnecessarily complicates the restorative plan. One such example is an endodontically compromised remaining incisor, where the restorative option is a removable prosthesis (5.31). Sometimes teeth with perfectly normal pulps are judged to require endodontic treatment for restorative reasons, as in the case of the restorative realignment of teeth or overdenture construction (5.32, 5.33).

Endodontic treatment of teeth with low-grade symptoms may also be considered when there is the likelihood of them receiving extensive restorations or they are required as abutments for fixed prostheses (5.34, 5.35). The difficulty and expense of treating teeth with large cast or ceramometal restorations should always be borne in mind.

Decisions made in both simple and more complex treatment plans should follow the knowledge gained from research and evidence-based practice.

Access and the final restoration

When planning the endodontic treatment of a tooth the physical demands of the final restoration should be considered. The way in which the access and root canal preparation will influence the amount of remaining coronal tooth substance and canal space for post construction should be borne in mind. Good access leads to success in endodontics, but access produced without thought may make the restoration of the tooth more difficult (5.36).

Restorability of teeth

Following endodontic treatment it should be possible to restore a tooth to function and health. Particular attention needs to be given to the support that can be provided for a coronal restoration and the position of finishing margins. Finishing margins benefit from being above the alveolar crest, and preferably supragingival. If the prospects of providing an adequate restoration seem remote, extraction should be considered as an alternative treatment.

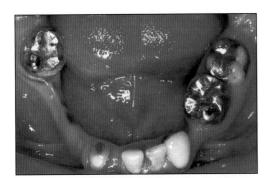

5.32 Elective root canal treatment for mandibular canine

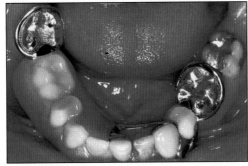

5.33 Overdenture in place

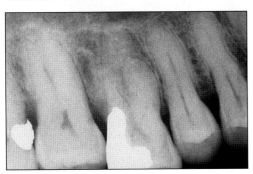

5.34 Molar requiring restoration with questionable vitality

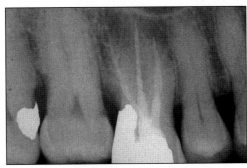

5.35 Molar endodontics completed prior to restoration

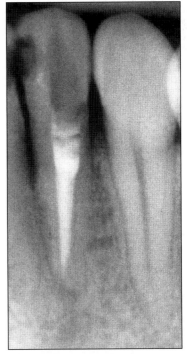

5.36 Overzealous access in mandibular incisor leads to unnecessary loss of dentine

Well-treated teeth may require elaborate and innovative restorations and possible surgery to satisfy the physical and marginal requirements of the final restoration. Further details are given in Chapter 16.

Good treatment strategies should also take into account possible failure. By planning for failure operators and patients are in a much better position to cope with outcomes that are not as originally hoped for.

Periodontal support

Loss of periodontal attachment on its own is not a contraindication for endodontic treatment. Provided a tooth has, or can be made to have, a healthy periodontal apparatus, endodontic treatment may be carried out (**5.37**).

Strategic importance of teeth

Before deciding whether to retain or extract a tooth, the importance of a particular tooth in the dental arch should be considered before embarking upon endodontic treatment. Clearly, unopposed and functionless teeth (**5.38**) are strategically less important than single standing teeth, which often prevent the need for a free-end saddle denture (**5.39**).

Canal anatomy

Bizarre root forms and root canal anatomy, congenital grooves and dilacerations may all present difficulties if endodontic treatment is attempted (**5.40–5.42**). These unusual forms may affect the outcome of treatment.

Root resorption

The loss of tooth tissue structure may lead to fracture (**5.43, 5.44**). The prognosis for teeth affected by internal resorption is good. The process may be arrested by pulp removal and, provided the remaining tooth substance is strong enough, the tooth can be retained (**5.45, 5.46**). Treatment of resorption arising on the external surface of the root is less predictable (**5.47**). External inflammatory resorption is treatable and responds to root canal treatment. The treatment of other types of external resorption is unpredictable. Defects can be repaired surgically (**5.48**) and also made supragingival. There is, however, a tendency for this type of external resorption to continue.

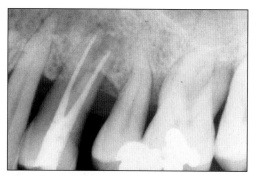

5.37 Root-filled tooth with loss of periodontal support

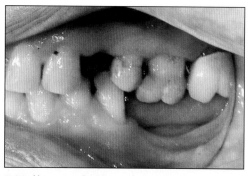

5.38 Unopposed molar

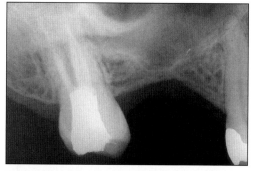

5.39 Tooth defending the need for a free-end saddle

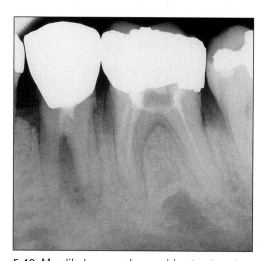

5.40 Mandibular premolar requiring treatment

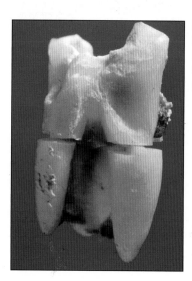

5.41 Irregular root form of the premolar

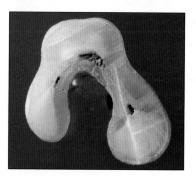

5.42 Complex canal anatomy of the premolar

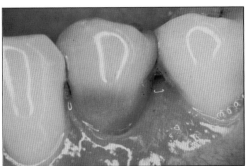

5.43 Mandibular premolar with internal resorption

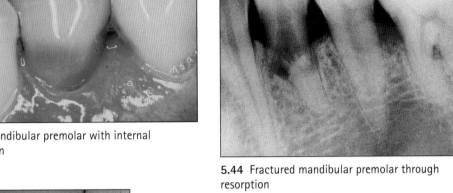

5.44 Fractured mandibular premolar through resorption

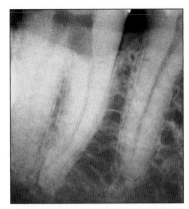

5.45 Radiographic evidence of internal resorption in a mandibular molar

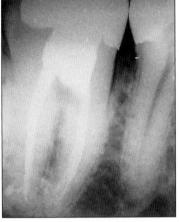

5.46 Root treatment performed to arrest the resorption

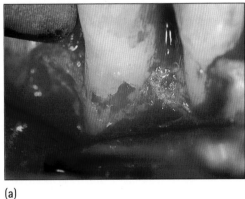

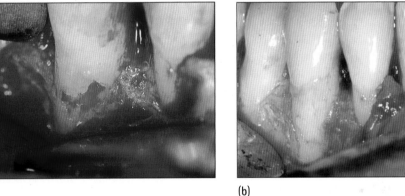

(a)   (b)

5.48 (a) External root resorption at surgery; (b) surgical repair of the resorptive defect with glass ionomer cement

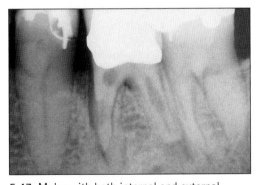

5.47 Molar with both internal and external resorption

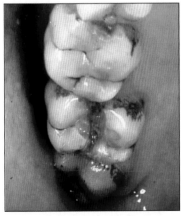

5.49 Vertical fracture of a maxillary molar

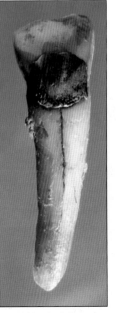

5.50 Vertical fracture in an anterior tooth

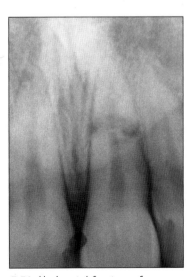

5.51 Horizontal fracture of a maxillary incisor

Root fractures

Fractures that communicate with the oral environment provide a route for infection. Vertically fractured teeth (**5.49, 5.50**) have a worse prognosis than those with horizontal fractures (**5.51**), which are also easier to detect radiographically.

Crown-root fractures passing through the attachment apparatus and involving alveolar bone require careful assessment to establish accurately the endodontic and restorative needs of the remaining tooth substance. Posterior teeth with fractures involving the floor of the pulp chamber have poor long-term prospects.

Sclerosed canals

Root canals that are not visible radiographically may be very difficult to locate and negotiate if endodontic treatment is necessary (**5.52–5.59**). However, in many cases they are possible to find and treat. It is impossible to predict the outcome of treatment until an

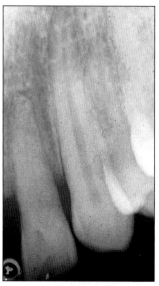

5.52 Sclerosed root canal in maxillary incisor

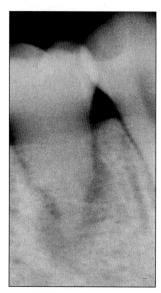

5.53 Sclerosed root canal in mandibular premolar

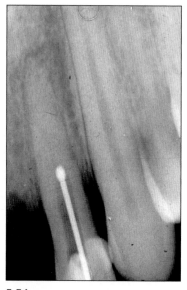

5.54
5.54–5.55 Drilling to locate canals

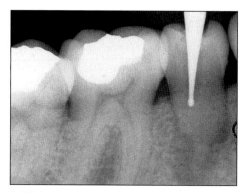

5.55

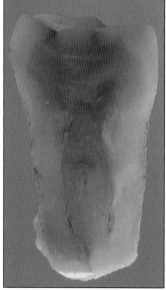

5.56

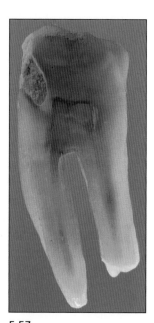

5.57
5.56–5.57 Sclerosed pulp chamber and canals in multirooted teeth

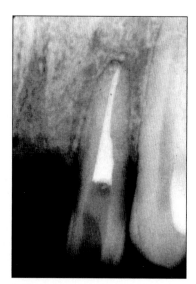

5.58 Canal in maxillary incisor located and treated

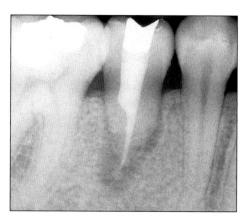

5.59 Canal in mandibular premolar located and treated

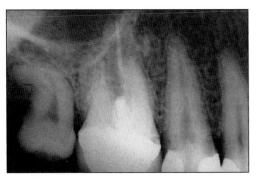

5.60 Maxillary molar requiring retreatment

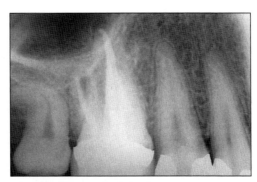

5.61 Maxillary molar following retreatment

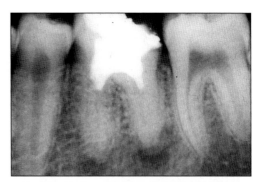

5.62 Mandibular molar requiring retreatment

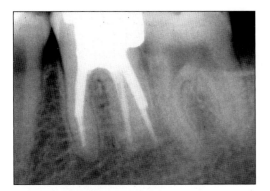

5.63 Mandibular molar six months after retreatment and restoration

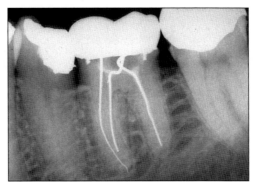

5.64 Mandibular molar with silver points requiring retreatment

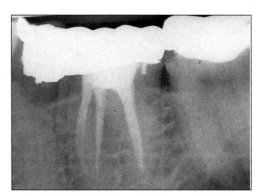

5.65 Mandibular molar following retreatment

attempt has been made to locate them. Teeth with a history of trauma experience progressive narrowing of the pulp space. Such teeth should be reviewed radiographically and if there is evidence of sclerotic change endodontic treatment should not be contemplated until there are radiographic periradicular indications of necrotic change occurring within the canal.

Previous root treatment

The decision to retreat a previously root-filled tooth (**5.60, 5.61**) should be based on clear criteria. If the treatment appears to be failing (**5.62–5.63**) because it shows symptoms, sinus tracts, persistent or developing radiolucencies, separated instruments and iatrogenic perforations, retreatment may be considered (**5.64, 5.65**).

The management of symptom-free periradicular lesions in previously root-treated teeth seems to give rise to considerable management variations. The inclination of a dentist to propose endodontic retreatment would seem to be variable. There does not appear to be a definite retreatment criterion for stable symptomless periradicular lesions.

The replacement of coronal restorations in endodontically treated teeth can occasionally give rise to symptoms, but why this should be so is not fully understood. It has been suggested that altered occlusal loading, the effects of post-space preparation and restoration cementation hydrostatic pressures may account for the problems. Such problems are possibly related to coronal reinfection of the canal system.

Previously treated teeth requiring new restorations should be examined with care, and if the adequacy of the sealing of the pulp space is in doubt retreatment should be considered.

Where post-retained restorations exist in teeth requiring endodontic treatment a choice has to be made regarding the approach to treatment. Conservative treatment is likely to damage the restoration, and post removal might precipitate a root fracture. Conservative treatment gives a better opportunity to clean the canal system and eliminate coronal leakage as a possible cause for failure but does not treat extraradicular infection. A surgical retrograde approach to retreatment preserves existing restorations but does not eliminate coronal leakage as a cause of failure. It is difficult to clean the canal system thoroughly. However, a surgical approach offers an opportunity to eradicate extraradicular infection (**5.66–5.68**).

In cases involving retreatment of teeth with large and irregular-looking lesions the use of decompression (**5.69–5.73**) and biopsy techniques should be considered to establish a clear diagnosis.

Finally, the practitioner should always assess his or her ability to improve on the existing situation. If this ability is in doubt, referral to a colleague specializing in this area should be considered.

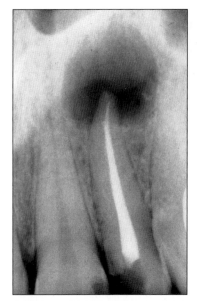

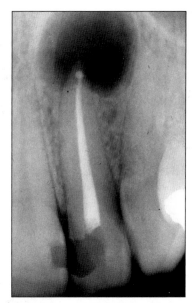

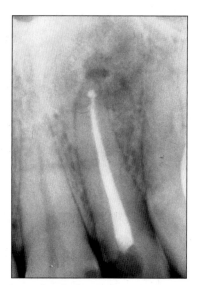

5.66 Lateral incisor fails to respond to conventional root canal treatment

5.67 Surgery performed to eradicate possible extraradicular infection

5.68 Resolution of the periradicular lesion

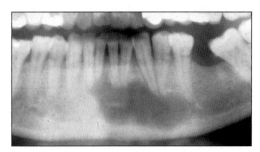

5.69 Large lesion in mandible

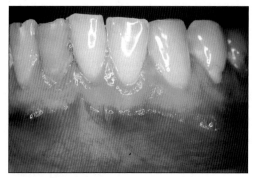

5.70 Lesion situated between left mandibular lateral incisor and canine

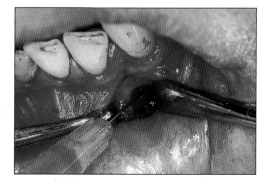

5.71 Penetration of lesion

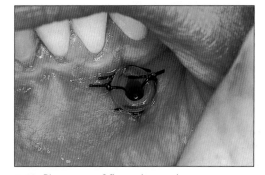

5.72 Placement of flanged cannula

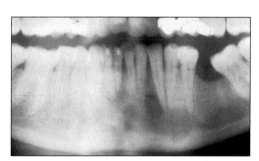

5.73 Radiographic evidence of decompression

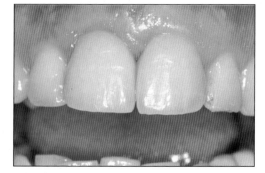

5.74 Clinical image of implant-retained crowns

Implants

The apparent success of single-tooth implants has prompted extravagant claims in some quarters to the effect that the treatment modality may spell the end of endodontics. Implants are just one of several tooth replacement options and nothing more. They have good success rates but are judged by a different set of criteria that are better described as survival rates rather than success (**5.74, 5.75**). Most patients will wish to retain their own natural teeth and extraction must be a considered decision based on exhaustion of all possibilities to save them within a reasonable time and cost frame.

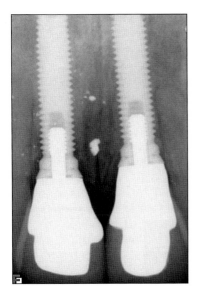

5.75 Radiograph of single tooth implant

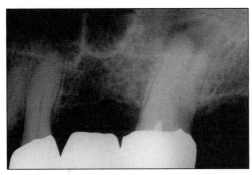

5.76 Periradicular lesion related to bridge abutment

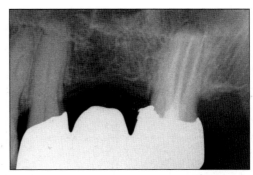

5.77 Healing following root canal treatment (one year later)

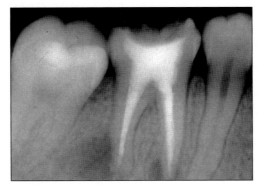

5.78 Postoperative radiograph of lesion

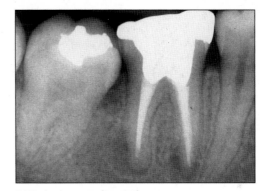

5.79 Lesion remains static

A cost–benefit analysis of the options showed retention of the tooth to be a better option (Moiseiwitsch & Caplan 2001) but this will be a changing comparison as the cost of the treatment changes.

Single or multiple visit treatment

It is becoming popular for members of the dental profession to favour the completion of endodontic treatment in one visit.

Currently accepted criteria for the completion of endodontic treatment include lack of symptoms and a prepared pulp space free of microorganisms.

When considering whether to complete treatment in one visit or more it is worth thinking about the possible advantages and disadvantages of both the single- and multiple-visit approach.

Where endodontic treatment is being performed on a vital tooth, the bacterial content of the tooth is minimal and a single visit approach is favoured, thus reducing the possibility of bacterial entry into the tooth through coronal leakage of the provisional restoration. The single visit also allows for immediate and intimate knowledge of the canal anatomy of the tooth and all important reference points. Patients also favour single visits because there is less time spent in the dental office with less anxiety and local anaesthetic. Patients with medical histories that require the administration of antibiotics for treatment also benefit from receiving care in a single visit.

When dealing with a long-standing infection in a tooth, it may be wise to consider the disinfection of the tooth over more than one visit. This approach allows greater time and the use of a medicament to supplement the chair-side irrigation and disinfection procedures. This approach seems to favour the treatment and retreatment of teeth with periradicular lesions with swelling and draining sinuses.

Retreatment cases lend themselves to a multi-visit approach because of the time required to remove restorations and root fillings, and the presence of resistant bacterial strains.

Planned review

Reassessment and re-evaluation of the status of dental health of patients is an integral part of the planning process. It involves examining the patient again; often taking elements of the history again, re-establishing a diagnosis, and formulating a new treatment plan for whatever new or residual problems are encountered.

Clinical and radiographic follow-up, at regular intervals for an indefinite period, are essential for the assessment of endodontic treatment. Observation periods of at least four years are desirable (**5.76, 5.77**). Endodontic treatment should be assessed annually.

Indications of success are absence of pain, swelling and other symptoms, no sinus tract, no loss of function, and radiographic evidence of a normal periodontal ligament space around the root.

The outcome of treatment is considered uncertain if radiographs reveal that a lesion has remained the same size or has diminished in size, but total repair has not occurred (**5.78, 5.79**).

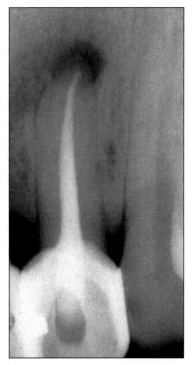

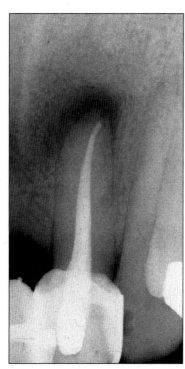

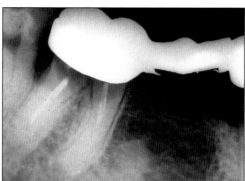

5.82 Caries leading to failure of restoration

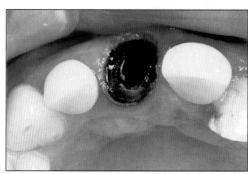

5.83 Caries in a root canal

5.80 Pre-existing lesion

5.81 Lesion increasing in size

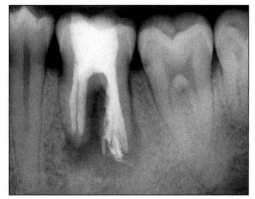

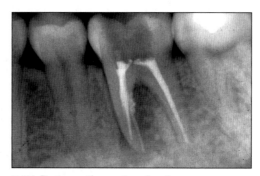

5.84 Postoperative root fracture

5.85 Postoperative root perforation

Treatment is considered to have failed if radiographs reveal that a lesion has appeared following endodontic treatment or a pre-existing lesion has increased in size (**5.80, 5.81**) or there is conflicting evidence with respect to symptoms and radiographic evaluation. For example, a tooth may have persistent low-grade symptoms and yet appear healthy on radiography.

Factors that may lead to secondary failure of a previously successful endodontic treatment include recurrent caries and coronal leakage (**5.82**), caries extending into the root canal (**5.83**) or furcation, root fracture (**5.84**) or perforation (**5.85**).

In conclusion, all dental treatment should be undertaken applying the principle of continuous review. Endodontic treatment provides definite indications for scheduling review appointments and should be looked upon as an integral part of treatment planning.

Reference

Moisiewitsch JRD, Caplan D (2001) A cost–benefit comparison between single tooth implant and endodontics. *J Endod* **27**, 235.

Chapter 6

Pre-endodontic management

C J R Stock and K Gulabivala

Endodontics can be one of the most satisfying aspects of dental practice, provided it is performed in a well-managed working environment. Consideration should be given to specific organizational requirements, which affect the operator, the staff, the patient and ultimately the tooth to be treated.

THE CLINICAL AREA

The clinical area, or 'operatory', benefits from having a fresh, bright, warm and welcoming atmosphere. The design, layout and décor help contribute a great deal to enhance its image. An environment that has been constructed to allow staff to work efficiently, with comfort and ease, will decrease stress, encourage smooth, relaxed working days, and increase job satisfaction. The operatory should be designed in an uncluttered fashion to facilitate movement to and from the working area.

Equipment location

The organization of endodontic equipment requires some thought and should be planned carefully to satisfy the needs of the operator's working methods.

Cabinetry and cupboards in an L- or U-shaped configuration should be placed within the working area of both operator and assistant. Work can often be simplified by considering the most useful positions to place the more commonly used instruments.

The distance that the hand instruments have to travel during procedures should be minimized – use of a mobile cabinet or cervical tray (**6.1**) may achieve this. A mobile cabinet provides flexibility with a worktop area and drawers, which may be sited close to the patient. Simple cervical trays without handpiece and 3-in-1 cord fittings will also allow instruments to be approximated to the tooth being treated.

Ultrasonic units are used regularly in endodontics; these units should be as easily accessible as conventional hand-pieces and not be seen as an addition to the usual dental equipment. Ultrasonic units may be mounted as a permanent fixture on the dental unit, or stored in an accessible position. Sliding shelves or drawers are most useful in this respect (**6.2**).

Radiographic viewers should also be sited within easy reach. The viewer may be placed on a nearby work surface or in a sliding drawer.

Work surface organization

The work surfaces of dental units and cupboards readily collect infected material and surfaces should be chosen that are easy to keep clean. The junction between the work surface and the wall should cove to aid cleaning. Any joints on the work surface should be sealed to prevent accumulation of contaminated matter and allow cleaning.

Between clinical sessions all work surfaces, including those that are apparently uncontaminated, should be cleaned with a detergent or a microbicidal disinfectant.

Contamination zones

Work surfaces should be defined as zones of high or low contamination.

Surfaces liable to become contaminated with body fluids or infected matter should be identified and designated high contamination zones. These areas benefit from impervious disposable coverings that can be changed and the surface beneath cleaned between patients. All disposable and sterilizable instruments and trays fall within this area.

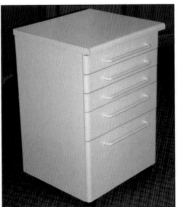

6.1 Mobile cabinet

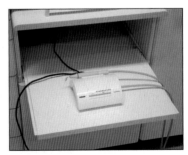

6.2 Ultrasonic unit in sliding drawer

Low contamination zones include all other areas that, during normal clinical procedures, are not expected to become impregnated with infected material. In these areas procedures should be adopted to limit the number of surfaces touched each time a patient is treated.

Water supplies

All waterlines and airlines should be fitted with antiretraction valves to help prevent contamination of the lines. Water retraction valves may aspirate infective material back into the tubing. Handpieces with water sprays should be allowed to discharge water into the sink for 20–30 seconds after each patient. Overnight microbial accumulation can be reduced if the handpiece is run for two minutes at the beginning of each day. Many units now have a bottled water system, disinfectants advised by the manufacturer may be run through the system at the end of each day to reduce the microbial load and prevent the build up of biofilm. Specific agents are now available to eradicate biofilms in dental-unit water lines.

Instrumentation and storage

A very wide range of instruments designed specifically for endodontic treatment is available. Some of these instruments have been used for many years; others are new and, in some cases, highly technical. The instruments described in this book are readily available and commonly used.

Generally used instruments and materials include:

- basic instruments packs;
- rotary instruments,
  friction grip burs,
  conventional burs,
  safe-ended burs,
  Gates–Glidden burs;
- hand instruments,
  barbed broaches,
  files,
  other root canal instruments;

- rubber dam and accessories;
- power-assisted instruments,
  nickel titanium rotaries,
  ultrasonic;
- measuring devices,
  electronic,
  rules, gauges, stops;
- instrument and post-retrieval kits;
- irrigating syringes and needles;
- paper points;
- gutta-percha points both ISO and larger tapers;
- instruments for lateral and vertical condensation of gutta-percha;
- instruments for thermomechanical compaction of gutta-percha;
- equipment for thermoplastic injection of gutta-percha;
- equipment for solid core gutta-percha techniques.

Consideration must be given to storing, cleaning and sterilizing all these items.

The basic instrument pack

A presterilized basic pack (**6.3**, **6.4**) is required for all routine root canal procedures. The pack contains:

- front surface mirror;
- two endodontic locking tweezers;
- canal probe;
- briault probe;
- long-shanked excavator;
- flat plastic;
- ruler;
- mixing spatula;
- Mitchell's trimmer.

Use of the *front surface mirror* overcomes the problems associated with double images, which are produced when the reflecting surface is beneath a layer of glass. The *endodontic locking tweezers* allow small items to be gripped safely and transferred between assistant and operator (**6.5**). They are particularly useful when handling gutta-percha points, paper points and cotton-wool pledgets. The

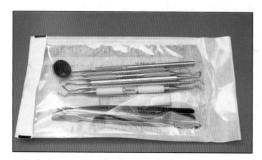

6.3 Endo pack in sterile pouch

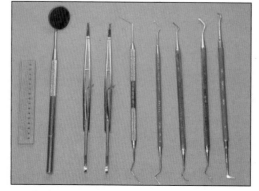

6.4 Endo pack

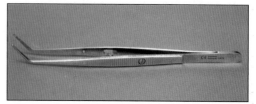

6.5 Endo-locking tweezers

tips of the beaks should be blunt and grooved. A *Mitchell's trimmer* may be used to remove cement and either temporary or permanent crowns. The *canal probe* should be long, fine, sharp and strong. It is used to feel the floor of the pulp chamber when locating canal orifices. A *Briault probe* is used to feel for overhangs when removing the roof of the pulp chamber. Two other probes, although not included in the basic kit, are useful in periodontal assessment and are worth mentioning here: the *explorer EXD3CH* (**6.6**) (used to examine restorations such as bridges), *furcation probe* with markings (for measuring the extent of periodontal furcation involvement in posterior teeth); and a *pocket measuring probe* with a fine shank, blunt end, and millimetre markings (as illustrated in Chapter 11). *Long-shanked excavators* (**6.7**) come in a range of designs to allow access to the pulp chamber. These are used for scooping out the remains of the pulp and excess gutta-percha; also for flicking away pulp stones. The *flat plastic* assists in placement of interappointment provisional restorations. The *ruler* is used to measure instrument lengths for calculating root canal length.

CLEANING AND STERILIZATION

All instruments contaminated with oral and other body fluids should be cleaned and sterilized after use. There are three stages to the sterilization process: presterilization cleaning, sterilization and storage. Dentists should note the manufacturers' instructions and ensure these are followed. There is a progressive move towards using instruments once only. Many nickel titanium rotary files have a sign on the packet showing a number 2 with a diagonal line running though it, which means for one use only (**6.8**). It should be noted that a new packet of files should be sterilized before use unless it arrives in a presterilized pack. Many dental instruments are now available for one use only and are presented in presterilized packs (**6.9**).

Presterilization cleaning

Used instruments may be heavily contaminated with body matter, which harbours and protects microorganisms. The instruments should be cleaned thoroughly before being sterilized. Cleaning can be done by hand using long-handled kitchen type brush, warm water and a detergent, an ultrasonic bath, enzyme cleaners or an instrument washing machine. Gross debris is removed from small files by stabbing them into sponges impregnated with detergent. The person cleaning instruments should always wear protective gloves to avoid inoculation with debris. Ultrasonic baths (**6.10**) are the most reliable way of eliminating gross debris. A detergent should be used in the bath not a disinfectant.

Sterilization

Chemical methods

Chemical solutions only disinfect and should be used only for those items that may not be sterilized by conventional methods. Chemicals have variable effects on different microorganisms, a reduced efficiency in the presence of organic matter, a tendency to deteriorate with storage and may be toxic. Of the solutions available, those containing

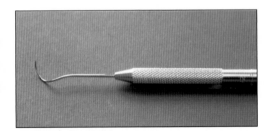

6.6 Explorer EXD3CH

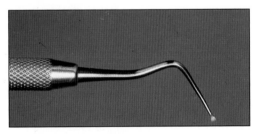

6.7 Long-shanked excavator

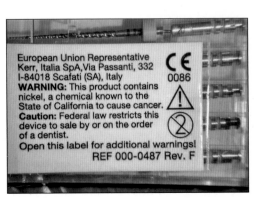

6.8 Symbol indicating single use only

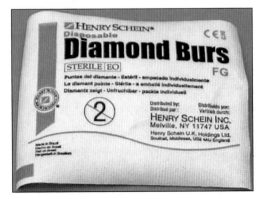

6.9 Single use only diamond burs

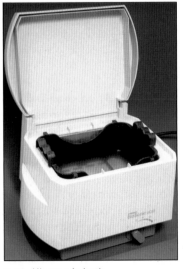

6.10 Ultrasonic bath

glutaraldehyde seem to be the most effective against hepatitis B and HIV. Sterilizing solutions should be stored in a closed container at all times. Certain patients may become sensitized to the chemicals used in sterilizing instruments, and other methods are preferred.

Hot-air ovens

Dry heat is widely used in sterilization, a temperature of 160°C is recommended with a holding time of 120 minutes. Hot-air ovens tend to use a long cycle and the high temperatures reached may damage some instruments. This form of sterilization is most useful for paper points, cotton wool, oils and powders.

Pressure steam (autoclave)

This method of sterilization is effective and has a reasonably short cycle (3 min at 134°C). The effectiveness of autoclaving wrapped instruments in sterilizing chambers that are not evacuated has been called into question and steam-sterilizers with a vacuum phase are generally recommended (**6.11**). However, this type of sterilization has the disadvantage of causing corrosion and dulling of sharp instruments and is unsuitable for sterilizing cotton wool and paper products.

Checking successful sterilization

Successful sterilization depends upon the consistent reproducibility of sterilization conditions. Autoclaves should therefore be validated before use and their performance monitored routinely. Correct operation of the autoclave must be checked every day that the autoclave is used. This can be achieved by recording the readings given as printouts or readings on the instrument panels. The readings should be compared with the recommended values.

Storage

The most convenient storage systems for endodontic instruments involve the use of trays, boxes and test tubes.

Metal containers

(**Figures 6.12** and **6.13**) are available in a variety of styles. Most boxes have lids and magazines for instruments; some are designed for autoclaves and others for sterilization in a hot-air oven. A recent improvement for the smaller autoclavable boxes has been to add a simple device to show how many times the instruments have been sterilized. With the larger boxes sterile instruments are taken from one box and, after use, are placed in a second box. At the end of the working day the box is replenished and sterilized for use the next day. Using this process many instruments are sterilized several times without being used, which may reduce the cutting efficiency of the hand instruments. The move towards single use for root canal files would suggest these metal boxes are obsolescent.

Disposable trays are now used in many practices (**6.14**) and fit in with the emerging concept of single use.

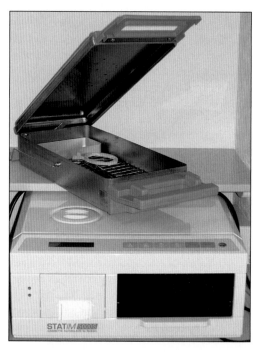

6.11 Vacuum autoclave for use in the dental operatory

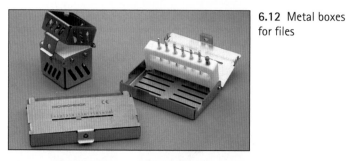

6.12 Metal boxes for files

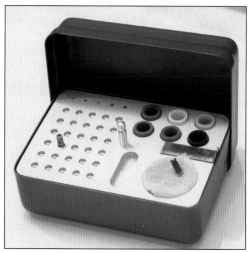

6.13 Large metal box

File holders

There are several file holders on the market; they carry enough instruments for one treatment or part of the treatment (**6.15, 6.16**). This simple stand for files closes flat to prevent the instruments falling out in the autoclave.

Files may be placed in a foam insert held by an Endoring (**6.17**). This finger-held device allows the operator or nurse to have both hands free. A ruler lies in front and small cups may be placed at the side for example EDTA paste. The foam insert has been specially developed so that files placed in it may be sterilized in an autoclave

(**6.18**). The foam inserts are one use only and provide a convenient way of disposing of the instruments into a sharps container after use. Using the insert in this way reduces the chance of a needle stick injury.

Standard 11 mm wide Pyrex test tubes with colour-coded caps are convenient receptacles for sets of six hand instruments (**6.19**). The instruments are sterilized in an autoclave within the test tube. The test tubes may be stored in racks (**6.20**) or compartments within a drawer. Different-coloured caps are available for easy identification. Selected instruments are removed from the test tube and placed in either a stand or sterile sponge.

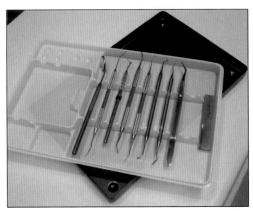

6.14 Disposable tray

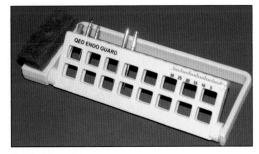

6.15 File holder

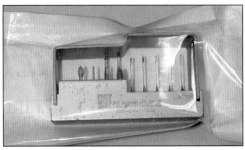

6.16 Sterilizable file holder (courtesy of Peter Endo)

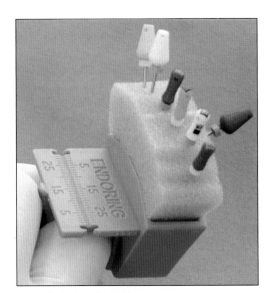

6.17 Endoring file holder

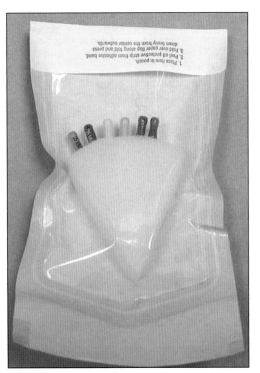

6.18 Sterilizable foam inserts (courtesy of Peter Endo)

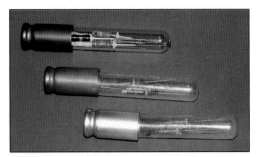

6.19 Pyrex test tubes

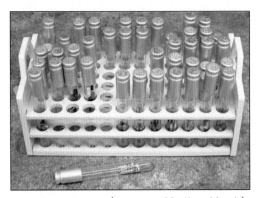

6.20 Test-tube rack (courtesy of Dr Koos Marais)

Pastes and medicaments

A wide variety of pastes and medicaments are available for endodontic treatment, many of them housed in syringes. A suitable rack for these is shown (**6.21**). Sleeves are available for cross-infection control. After each use the sleeve and tip are discarded. **Figure 6.22** shows calcium hydroxide being placed into the canal system with a capillary tip.

Infection control

Each practice must have an infection-control policy. This describes the practice policy for all aspects of infection control and provides a useful guide to the training necessary for each member of staff. Clinical staff should be vaccinated against the common illnesses shown in the list below. The immune status of staff must be checked for rubella and hepatitis B.

Recommended vaccinations for dental staff:

- diphtheria;
- hepatitis B;
- pertussis;
- poliomyelitis;
- rubella;
- tetanus;
- tuberculosis.

During the history taking, patients might disclose that they are HIV or HBV carriers. HBV carriers and patients with HIV who are otherwise well may be treated routinely in dental practice, but patients with HIV who are in ill health or who have oral manifestations of the disease should be referred for expert advice. Confidentiality should always be preserved and the obligation to provide care realized. Refusal to treat these patients is illogical – undiagnosed carriers of infectious disease pass undetected through practices every day. Operators who are HBV- or HIV-positive should seek appropriate advice.

Dental interest in Creutzfeld–Jacob disease (CJD) and the related conditions centres on the risk of their transmission from human to human during dental treatment. There is no known case of this happening. However, those patients suspected of being infected require special infection-control procedures. 'Prions', the infectious agents that cause CJD and related conditions, are much more difficult to destroy than conventional microorganisms. Suspected cases should be referred to hospital for dental treatment.

All staff should understand the modes of transmission of infections, sterilization and infection-control requirements, the proper use of protective clothing and equipment, the remedial actions to be taken in the event of accidents, the importance of general hygiene and of keeping immunizations up to date.

Inoculation injuries are the most common route for transmission of blood-borne viral and other infections in dentistry. Great care

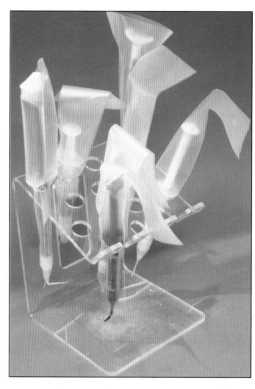

6.21 Rack for endodontic syringes

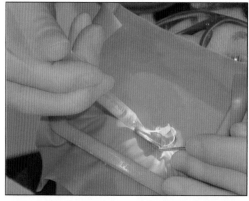

6.22 Calcium hydroxide syringe in use

should be taken when handling all sharps and specially designated bins should be used in their disposal. Needle-protection devices are available and should be used for resheathing.

THE DENTAL NURSE

The dental nurse should be well trained and hold a relevant qualification. In a specialized field such as endodontics in-house training is also necessary to ensure that the nurse understands fully the various techniques employed. Emergency and resuscitation training requirements should also be met.

Anticipation

One of the greatest assets a dental nurse can have is the ability to anticipate the needs of patient and operator. The nurse should be aware of the aspects of care that optimize a patient's comfort, safety and protection. Dental nurses should be encouraged not to adjust the patient's chair until the medical history has been established – and certainly not before explaining what is about to happen – because sudden chair movements may frighten patients unnecessarily. Particular attention should be paid to the angulation of the chair and the head position. It is wise to ask the patient if they are comfortable.

The patient must wear spectacles, to protect their eyes, and a disposable waterproof bib (**6.23**). These items protect against splashes, dropped instruments and spillage of sodium hypochlorite.

With the patient supine, the assistant should sit slightly higher than the operator to allow adequate visibility (**6.24**). Adjustment of the light is the nurse's responsibility.

If patients spend long periods lying supine, the chair should be returned to the upright position slowly on completion of treatment, and the patient asked to sit for a moment or two before leaving the chair – this will prevent problems arising from postural hypotension.

In order to provide effective operator support the nurse must anticipate the actions of the operator. Clinical procedures should be understood and learned thoroughly and a rationalized work sequence developed between the operator and nurse. Use of arranged spoken and unspoken signals improve the efficiency and flow of working movements.

Close support

The specific operations involved in endodontics are generally delicate and require a high level of concentration on the part of the operator. Control of the operating field is one of the main aims of close support. The operator and nurse control visibility, soft tissues, moisture and saliva, instruments, water coolants and contaminants.

In endodontics the greatest aid in achieving this degree of control is a rubber dam. Isolation using a rubber dam can greatly improve efficiency by gaining time normally lost by patients rinsing, dentists continually changing wet cotton rolls and assistants struggling with saliva ejectors.

Instrument transfer

This should be smooth, safe, and unobtrusive and require a minimum amount of movement on the part of the operator. Transfer of instruments should take place in the so-called transfer zone which lies over the patient's neck at chin level. Instrument exchange becomes important during the obturation phase of root canal treatment, when the system of parallel transfer can be employed to advantage as it allows the alternate exchange of spreading instrument and accessory cones to be accomplished speedily.

A dental nurse can be of considerable help during rubber dam placement (**6.25**), instrument transfer, canal irrigation, and suction procedures. **Figure 6.26** shows the nurse holding the aspirator tip close to the tooth without hindering the operator's access. Similarly, a small surgical tip is placed close to the tooth (**6.27**) so that sodium hypochlorite may be removed efficiently without obstructing the operators view. Paper points and gutta-percha points are exchanged between operator and nurse efficiently using endo-locking tweezers with the parallel technique. **Figure 6.28** shows the nurse removing a paper point and placing a new paper point in the operator's hand (**6.29**). Notice that the instruments lie parallel to each other during transfer.

The nurse should also be able to judge the length of hand instruments required and set working lengths when instructed (**6.30**). A quick and efficient method of transferring an instrument after use to the nurse is shown in **Figure 6.31**, the operator holds the instrument towards the nurse who spears the instrument into the sponge. This simple movement reduces the chance of needle stick injury.

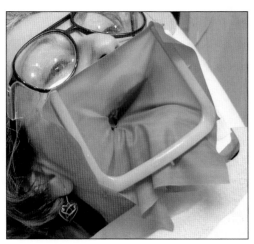

6.23 Rubber dam, eye protection and waterproof bib

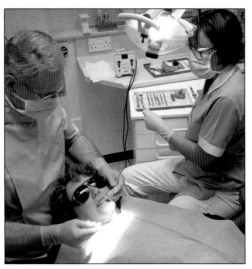

6.24 Nurse seated slightly higher than operator

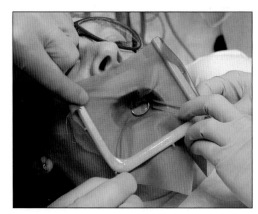

6.25 Rubber dam placement

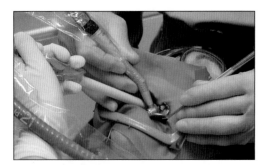

6.26 Close support aspiration

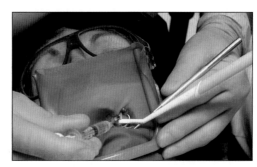

6.27 Surgical tip used for the aspiration of sodium hypochlorite

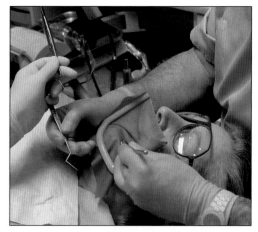

6.28 Exchange of paper points

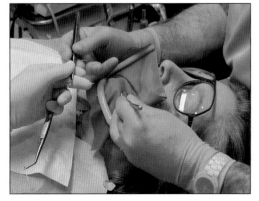

6.29 Transferring new paper point to the operator

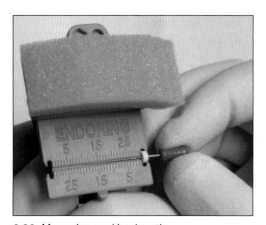

6.30 Measuring working length

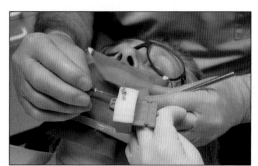

6.31 Instrument transfer to foam insert

THE PATIENT

Education and information

All treatment should be fully explained to the patient before any is carried out. Patients who understand the treatment that they are about to undergo will be less anxious, easier to handle and more appreciative. Information may be made available in the waiting room – patients are most receptive in the few minutes before their appointment – in the form of leaflets produced by the practice or commercially available (**6.32**). In the clinical area the dentist should use models (**6.33**), which make the procedures easier to explain: a patient will understand the radiographs better if he or she is given a basic knowledge of anatomy. Digital radiography, which shows an enlarged image of the patients' tooth on a monitor, is helpful in providing an explanation of the treatment.

Most (if not all) patients attending the dental practice for the first time will be nervous. A calm, pleasant manner, showing that you are concerned about the patient's welfare, will make treatment easier for both patient and operator.

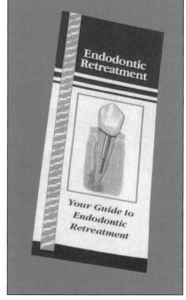

6.32 Patient information

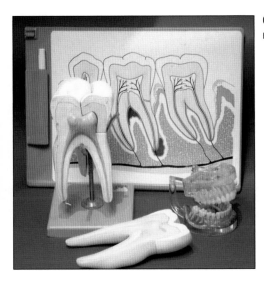

6.33 Education models

Anaesthesia and analgesia

Pain control is a most important aspect of endodontic procedures: the patient's confidence will be gained if they undergo a painless procedure. *Analgesia* removes pain sensation without loss of tactile sense. Anaesthesia results in complete loss of all sensation, and may be induced locally or generally (when the patient will lose consciousness). In dentistry analgesia is usually all that is required because we wish merely to remove pain; occasionally, with an injection, we may achieve anaesthesia but this is surplus to requirements. Local anaesthesia is more accurately described as local analgesia.

Before treatment begins the type of analgesia or anaesthesia must be chosen. Guidelines for this decision are given below.

Routine root canal treatment

Regional or infiltration local analgesia is all that is necessary.

Acute hyperaemic pulp

Regional or infiltration analgesia is usually adopted, followed by additional local analgesic (for details see Chapter 13).

Anxious patient

Gag reflex In mild cases once the rubber dam is applied treatment may be carried out routinely with local analgesia as the patient has an effective barrier and is unaware of instruments or fingers in his or her mouth. In the more severe cases intravenous sedation or relative analgesia will control the reflex.

General anaesthesia in the dental chair is governed by strict regulations (Department of Health 1990), which have restricted its use in general dental practice. However, one or more of the following methods may manage the vast majority of anxious patients satisfactorily.

Relative analgesia This is a safe, easy technique using varying quantities of a mixture of nitrous oxide (N_2O) and oxygen (O_2) administered via a nasal mask. However, difficulties may arise in that the nosepiece may hinder the operator in root treatment and endodontic surgery in the maxillary incisal region. Other disadvantages include the set-up costs and the possible hazards of air 'pollution' within the surgery environment.

Oral sedation A suitable benzodiazepine may be prescribed for the night before and/or one hour preoperatively. Many drugs are available for this purpose and the operator is advised to consult the relevant literature for correct dosage, contraindications, precautions and other important data. In common with oral, nasal, and intravenous sedation, consent for the procedure and pre- and postoperative instructions must be in writing and be obtained before the sedative is taken. For all types of sedation, the operator must be chaperoned, and a responsible adult must accompany all patients home.

Nasal sedation Concentrated forms of midazolam are being produced which can be sprayed into the nasal cavity resulting in a rapid onset (about ten minutes) of action. This technique is especially suited for patients with physical or learning difficulties, and for children.

Intravenous sedation Intravenous sedation may be used for any endodontic procedure. It has a quicker recovery time and is considered safer than general anaesthesia, making it more suitable for the ambulatory patient. In the UK there is no place for general anaesthesia except in the hospital setting. Indeed, only 'conscious sedation' is permitted, a state in which the patient is calm, relaxed, and in verbal contact with the operator. In other parts of the world, notably the USA, 'deep sedation' is also utilized but requires substantial skill and experience on the part of the sedationist.

Intravenous sedation is ideally administered by an anaesthetist or dedicated sedationist. The technique involves using various drugs, most commonly the benzodiazepines such as diazepam and midazolam. Analgesics are occasionally given in addition to a benzodiazepine to produce a finer quality of sedation and to raise the pain threshold; this is particularly useful for those who find local anaesthetic injections disproportionately painful, and in patients in whom inferior dental blocks do not 'take' very well. Patients with medical conditions such as Parkinson's disease or epilepsy, as well as those with strong gag reflexes, can be controlled well with this technique. Antisialogogues such as atropine may be added to the sedation to produce a dry field.

Careful titration of these drugs by an appropriately trained and skilled sedationist allows long and/or difficult procedures to be carried out with relative ease, particularly for anxious patients, most of whom welcome the side effect of profound amnesia!

Endodontic surgery

If more than two teeth are to be apicected intravenous sedation may be necessary.

Medication

Following treatment, the patient should be advised to take a suitable analgesic for any postoperative pain. There is some evidence to show that taking a non-steroidal anti-inflammatory drug one hour before treatment can reduce postoperative pain.

Patients who are already on medication must be advised of any change during the endodontic treatment. The patient's medical advisor should be contacted if it is thought necessary to alter the dosage or to stop a drug that has been prescribed (for example warfarin or steroid therapy).

Patients requiring antibiotic cover

Patients at risk from infective endocarditis (**Table 6.1**) should be given antibiotic cover (see also Chapter 3). Some patients (those who have already suffered an attack of infective endocarditis or require a general anaesthetic and are either allergic to penicillin or have already had more than one course of penicillin in the previous month) are at special risk and must be referred to hospital for endodontic treatment.

All patients at risk should be encouraged to maintain a high degree of oral health to reduce the severity of possible bacteraemias. Patients who require endodontic surgery should be advised to take a chlorhexidine mouthwash, starting 24 hours before surgery and continuing for 4–5 days afterwards.

Patients with HIV/HBV

Every patient must be considered a possible source of infection from herpes simplex 1 and 2, HBV and HIV. The operator should always wear barrier protection: gloves; mask; and protective spectacles during treatment, and gloves should be changed after each patient. The risks of transmission of HBV during dental treatment are well known, but HIV is less easily transmitted. By providing a physical barrier between the operating site and the patient's saliva, a rubber dam reduces the contaminated aerosol effect and therefore the risk of infection. All health workers should receive regular vaccination against hepatitis B. HIV-positive patients in good health may be treated in general dental practice, but if they show evidence of ill health or oral manifestations of disease then they should be referred to special units for advice or treatment.

THE TOOTH

Removal of calculus and plaque from teeth

Prior to careful examination of the involved tooth and its isolation, it is important to remove any calculus and debris. This will facilitate examination as well as prevent impaction of debris and calculus into the periodontium during rubber dam application. It may also be convenient at this point to floss through the contacts where rubber dam is to be applied to ensure freedom of contact. It is sometimes necessary to trim overhanging amalgams or to remove them prior to satisfactory isolation.

Table 6.1   Patients at risk from infective endocarditis

History of infective endocarditis	Rheumatic heart disease
Ventricular septal defect	Degenerative valve disease
Patient ductus arteriosus	Persistent heart murmur
Coarctation of the aorta	Atrial septal defect repaired
Prosthetic heart valve	with a patch

Removal of caries/restorations

Any carious, leaking or suspect restorations must be removed. The amalgam illustrated (**6.34**) is obviously carious and should be removed see (**6.35, 6.36**). Both radiographic and clinical signs of caries should prompt entire removal of the restoration prior to consideration for endodontic treatment.

When a bridge abutment or crown requires root canal treatment they should always be checked to see if they have been decemented by hooking a Briault or American Pattern probe under the pontic, near the retainer, and applying pressure to remove them: bubbles around the retainer margins of bridges and in extreme cases a slight sucking noise indicate decementation. Even solitary crowns may sometimes be sufficiently devoid of luting cement without actually coming off and it is worth applying controlled axial force with a pair of towel clips to ensure absence of looseness. In the case illustrated (**6.37**) the bridge must be removed. More subtle signs of leakage should be sought, including marginal discolouration of the tooth or staining of the restoration, both from the external aspect as well as

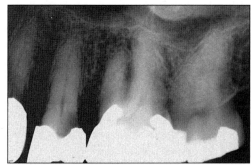

6.34 Carious maxillary premolar

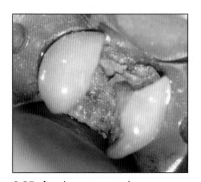

6.35 Amalgam removed

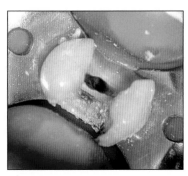

6.36 Caries removed and access gained

from within the access cavity when it is judged that the existing restoration is sound enough to keep and work through. Even at the second visit of root canal treatment, the cotton wool placed in the access cavity (to prevent the temporary restoration from blocking the canals) should be examined for signs of staining caused by possible leakage around residual restorative material.

Assessment of restorability of teeth

Large plastic restorations (amalgams and composites) and crown or bridge retainers make it difficult to assess the long-term restorative prognosis of teeth without their removal. Such restorations should usually be removed and an assessment made of the residual tooth tissue in the context of the future restoration so as to avoid the embarrassing situation of satisfactorily root treating an un-restorable tooth (6.38). It is difficult to give clear guidelines for restorability but an attempt is made in Chapter 16.

Provisional restoration of broken-down teeth

The most important reason for placing provisional restorations in/on broken down teeth is to protect and retain the occlusal and proximal space that will be occupied by any future restoration. A common problem is that neglect of such space preservation allows occlusal and/or mesial tooth drifting with consequent loss of space rendering the tooth unrestorable without complicated orthodontic intervention.

Broken-down teeth should be restored to meet space protection criteria as well as to allow the placement of a rubber dam. More definitive restoration of the tooth before root treatment is unnecessary, time-consuming, and may jeopardize the final restoration. The best possible view of the floor of the pulp chamber is seen in severely broken-down teeth (6.39), although such rampant access cavity preparation is not recommended!

It is usually possible to place a clamp on a broken-down tooth but on rare occasions some build-up or a crown lengthening procedure is required to remove excess gingival tissue and expose the margins of the tooth.

If a clamp cannot be placed because of significant loss of tooth substance the tooth may be built up with a restorative material such as a light-cured composite to allow clamp placement and temporary filling (see below, 6.54). Another option is to fit and cement a copper band or steel orthodontic band around the tooth with glass ionomer cement. The band must fit accurately otherwise the attachment apparatus will be damaged and at subsequent visits confuse the judgement of progress of treatment, as the patient may report the tooth to be tender on pressure. Where possible, the band must be left clear of the gingival margin. The case illustrated (6.40), shows a first mandibular molar with a fracture line in both the distal and buccal walls of the crown. A copper band was selected, cut (6.41) and trimmed with a stone to fit (6.42), cotton wool placed in the pulp chamber with softened stick gutta-percha over the top, and the band cemented.

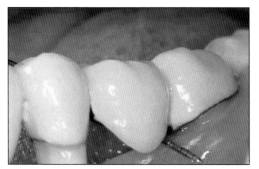
6.37 Decemented distal abutment of posterior bridge

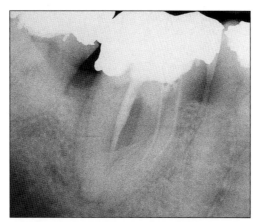
6.38 Unrestorable tooth

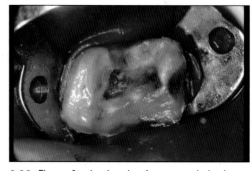
6.39 Floor of pulp chamber in a severely broken-down tooth

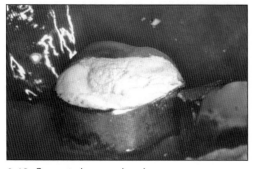
6.40 Cemented copper band

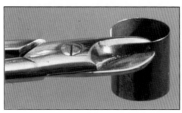
6.41 Cutting a copper band

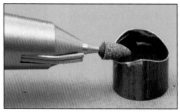
6.42 Trimming a copper band using a stone

Where the tooth tissue loss is great enough to prevent easy placement of a rubber dam clamp, the predictable restorability of the tooth must be questioned. Alternative options should be carefully considered before progressing further.

Periodontal tissue management

There are several reasons why the periodontal tissues should receive attention before root treatment, including removal of excess tissue to allow the placement of a rubber dam. The periodontal health around the tooth margin is examined, any inflammation pointed out to the patient and oral hygiene instruction given. Inflammation-free gingival tissues make for easier and cleaner tooth isolation. Furthermore, any discomfort caused by local gingival inflammation will be eradicated before commencing root canal treatment and enable confusion-free evaluation of the tooth as treatment progresses. If a surgical procedure is planned, gingival tissues free of inflammation provide the best tissue texture for surgical manipulation and provide a predictable outcome in replacement of the tissues. Root canal treatment will be often followed by a permanent restoration, often a crown whose accurate margin placement is reliant upon good gingival health. When the proximal contact between a restoration in the tooth under treatment and its neighbour is poor, consideration should be given to its replacement with one that has a better contact relationship in order to protect the periodontal tissues. This is especially important in periodontally susceptible patients.

Periodontal probing defects around teeth scheduled for endodontic treatment should be measured in detail using continuous point charting (as shown in Chapter 11) and recorded; in molars exposed furca should also be properly characterized. These provide a baseline for assessment of the effect of endodontic treatment.

Isolation using rubber dam and other devices

Rubber dam isolation is the single most useful procedure for making dentistry and in particular endodontics easier. It has many advantages, which can be listed as follows:

- **Safety** Rubber dam undoubtedly provides the best protection for the oropharynx and should be used during root canal treatment (**6.43**). They further protect the soft tissues of the mouth and lips from the potentially caustic effects of any root canal irrigants or medicaments.
- **Prevention of cross-infection** Rubber dam acts as a barrier and prevents aerosol formation from the mouth when air-driven or ultrasonically activated instruments are used in the mouth. Not only is the risk of cross-infection from such aerosol eliminated but the patient is also protected from the surgical environment. Perhaps most importantly, the barrier prevents salivary microorganisms from entering the root canal environment.
- **Comfort** Contrary to popular belief rubber dam confers a comfortable working environment for the patient, dentist and nurse. It is very rare that a patient may find a rubber dam to be uncomfortable. The reasons are usually feelings of claustrophobia, breathing difficulties, activation of gagging reflex or latex allergy. Each of these may be appropriately addressed and it is rare that a patient cannot be convinced of the benefits of a rubber dam. In fact, once used to it, most will demand its use for treatment. Latex allergies appear to be on the increase and non-latex rubber dam is available as an alternative.
- **Simplifies procedures** Rubber dam provides retraction of the lips and facial tissues and also helps keep the tongue out of the field, although the extent of retraction is determined by the manner in which the rubber dam is framed. A number of options are available and discussed later. It also improves visual and manual access and provides a clean operating field. It reduces the need for the patient to rinse, although they should still be able to swallow and communicate reasonably well. All of this contributes to an improvement in overall efficiency of treatment.

Rubber dam kits

Rubber dam is manufactured in different coloured squares of two sizes: 130 and 150 mm. The larger square is the most convenient for endodontics. A variety of thicknesses are available; heavy (0.25 mm) or extra heavy (0.3 mm) are the least likely to tear. The rubber dam

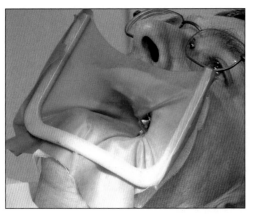

6.43 Rubber dam protecting a patient's oropharynx

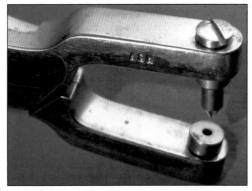

6.44 Rubber dam punch

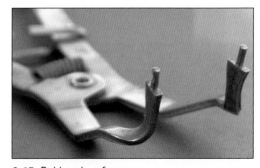

6.45 Rubber dam forceps

has one shiny and one mat surface, these are important in the context of the orientation used during application (explained later).

The *punch* (**6.44**) may be used to make several different-sized holes in the dam but only one medium-sized hole is usually necessary. If several teeth need to be isolated a rubber stamp can be used to locate the holes precisely. The stamp becomes unnecessary when rubber dam is used routinely and for single tooth isolation only.

Forceps (**6.45**) allow clamps to be placed and removed from teeth. The beaks should be deep enough to allow the clamp to be fitted around the gingival margin in a small mouth.

Frames (**6.46**) should be wide enough to provide good access with good retaining spikes for the dam. Retracting frames that provide better cheek retraction using a band that passes around the neck are also available though rarely used nowadays.

Clamps are manufactured in a wide variety of shapes and sizes to suit different teeth and situations. The choice of which one to select depends largely on personal preference, though the main criterion for selection is that the jaws provide a four-point contact for best stability. Root canal treatment requires only a small number of clamps

that will be used routinely. The four clamps shown in **Figure 6.47** are sufficient to cover most situations.

Applying the dam

Root canal treatment usually requires isolation of a single tooth. Two commonly used methods for placing the dam are described. The first of these is to fit the clamp so that all four jaws are in contact with the tooth (**6.48, 6.49**). Having ensured that the clamp is stable on the tooth a single hole is punched in the dam if the clamp is wingless and if winged a larger hole is made (by punching a second hole beside the first one or selecting a larger punch), the dam is then stretched over the clamp bow and the tooth (**6.50**). The second method is to insert the wings of the clamp into a hole punched in the dam, then carry the dam and clamp to the mouth and place them over the tooth (**6.51**); the dam is then slipped off the wings so that it lies around the neck of the tooth.

In both these situations, the rubber dam may not have sufficient opportunity to slip through the contact points to a stable position at

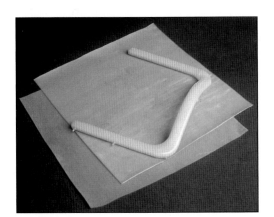

6.46 Rubber dam and plastic frame

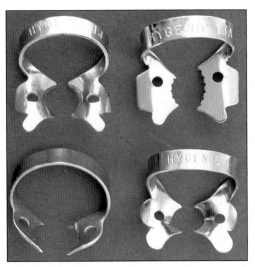

6.47 Clamps from left to right – 14, 13a, W8a, 1

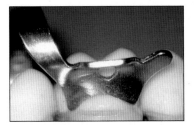

6.48 All four jaws should be in contact with the tooth

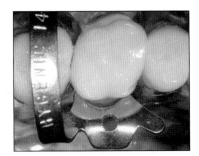

6.49 Jaws in contact with tooth – viewed from above

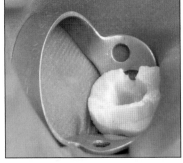

6.50 Rubber is stretched over clamp bow and tooth

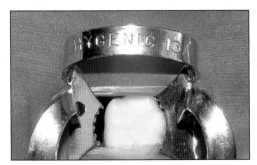

6.51 Clamp and dam carried to the tooth together

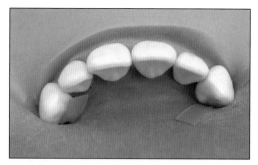

6.52 Dam fitted to anterior teeth without clamps

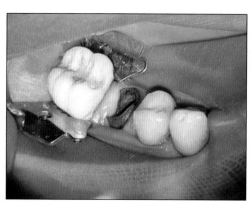

6.53 Split-dam technique

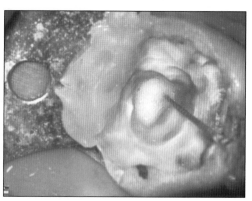

6.54 Clamp retained with etched composite

the gingival margin around the entire circumference of the tooth. As a consequence, the dam may allow some seepage of saliva around its margins. This may be conveniently stemmed with a commercially available gasket such as Oral Seal. This is a paste that is applied to the margin of the dam in small quantities. It absorbs moisture and stems the passage of saliva.

A less commonly used method of rubber dam application but one that gives a better seal is that used in operative dentistry when several teeth are isolated together. In this method the clamp(s) is/are pre-selected as described. The rubber dam is prepared by punching holes designed to match the size and distribution of the teeth so that the sheet is positioned centrally over the operative site, to cover the mouth completely without unequal tension on any side when the frame is applied. The rubber dam is applied by stretching the rubber at selected holes to thin it down. The edges are then 'knifed' into contact between the teeth. This ensures that the rubber dam lies at about the same level around the circumference of the tooth. The dam is inverted, after drying the teeth with a triple syringe, by employing a flat plastic to insert the edge of the dam into the gingival crevice. When the mat surface faces away from the patient's face, the inverted dam surface facing the tooth is also mat and this facilitates the stability of the dam as it is held in position by friction. Although application in this way is a little more time-consuming, it is worth the

time spent because of the moisture-free isolation it provides. The rubber dam clamps are then applied to hold the sheet in place.

In the anterior part of the mouth the dam may be fitted without clamps (**6.52**) using rubber or wooden wedges. In those cases where the tooth is severely broken down there are two options either use the split-dam method (**6.53**) or build a retaining wall on the tooth being treated (**6.54**).

The rubber dam frame may be applied to the front of the dam or to the back depending on preference. When applied to the front, an additional tip is to create little pockets at the bottom corners to collect waste irrigant from the tooth and to prevent it from spilling onto the patient. This is particularly useful for single operators working without continuous nursing support.

Other devices

Many other devices are used to protect the oropharynx but none of them are as effective as rubber dam.

Reference

Department of Health (1990) *Principle recommendations of the report of an expert working party on general anaesthesia, sedation, and resuscitation in dentistry.* London: HMSO.

Chapter 7

Root canal morphology

R T Walker

PULP SPACE ANATOMY

Pulp space

In describing the internal anatomy of teeth it is probably more appropriate to refer to the morphology of the pulp space rather than root canal systems. The pulp space is that part of the pulp–dentine complex which, in a healthy tooth, is occupied by the pulpal tissue, that is the space within the hard tissue of teeth in which, in health, the pulp resides. Due to the structure of the pulp–dentine complex, this also includes over 20% of the dentine. In disease, the space becomes the province of microorganisms.

The pulp space is complex and bears little resemblance to the stylized diagrams that are often used to explain the traditional terms used in describing the anatomy of the pulp. It has to be appreciated that the outlines, shapes, and positions of pulp chambers, root canals and pulpal–periradicular foramina are highly variable. Canals may branch, divide, rejoin and present forms that are considerably more involved than many textbooks of anatomy would lead us to believe. The complex nature of the pulp space is typified by the appearance of a cleared molar specimen (**7.1**).

An understanding of the pulp-space anatomy of teeth is a pre-requisite to the delivery of high-quality root canal treatment. Many of the problems attributable to failure in endodontic treatment relate to an inadequate understanding of the three-dimensional nature of the pulp space. In treatment, it is important to develop a visual picture of the likely location and number of root canals in a particular tooth. It may be necessary to take more than one preoperative radiographic view to gain as much information as possible about the nature of the pulp space before proceeding with the therapy.

A number of comments, which have a significant bearing on the practice of endodontics, can be made about the pulp canals that exist within teeth. Roots and root canals are rarely straight even when they appear so in a normal clinical radiographic projection (**7.2**). The buccal view of this single-rooted tooth does not indicate the curvature evident when the tooth is viewed in a proximal direction. Cleared specimens further re-enforce the complex anatomy (**7.3, 7.4**).

In cross-section root canals tend to take on the shapes of the roots. Where roots are wide in a bucco-lingual direction, the pulp space tends to take on similar proportions to the outline of the root or there may be more than one root canal (**7.5**).

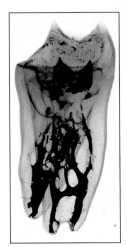

7.1 Cleared mandibular molar

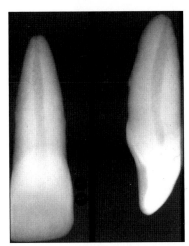

7.2 Buccal and approximal views of a central incisor

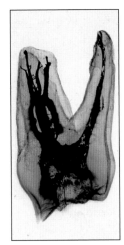

7.3 Cleared maxillary molar

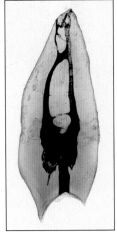

7.4 Cleared maxillary premolar

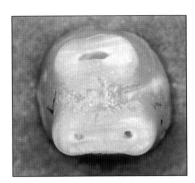

7.5 Sectioned roots of a mandibular molar

The volume of the pulp space is also greater than the normal buccal view might suggest. The mean volumes of teeth of each tooth type have been studied and it would appear that molar pulp spaces occupy large volumes **Table 7.1**.

Single roots do not necessarily have single root canals. Even when clinically there appears to be a single opening into a root canal, separation can lead to two distinct canals (**7.6, 7.7**). Characteristics in the form of fins (**7.8**) and bulges (**7.9**) may also be apparent.

Generally, the diameters of root canals decrease towards the apex of the root of the tooth where they tend to be narrowest, 0–1.5 mm from the foramina. The term used to describe the narrowest point is the *apical constriction*, which may be oval, round or serrated. From this point the canal widens into the foramen, which may open onto the root surface anywhere between 0 and 3 mm from the root apex. There may of course be more than one apical foramen (**7.10–7.12**).

Lateral and accessory canals

These occur anywhere along the length of any root and vary in size from a few microns in width to the size of a main canal. These canals are demonstrated in histological sections (**7.13**), cleared teeth (**7.14**) and clinical radiographs (**7.15**). The blood vessels passing through these canals contribute to the blood supply of the pulp and allow interchange of inflammatory breakdown products between the pulp and the periodontal tissues, which may influence the outcome of endodontic treatment and periodontal health.

Pulp space changes

With the passage of time and the laying down of both secondary and tertiary dentine, pulp space volume tends to decrease. The dental pulp has the ability to react to chronic irritation, usually of microbial origin, by laying down reactive (irritational) dentine, which leads to this decrease in pulp space volume (**7.16**). This process can occur at different rates in different teeth. Interestingly, no canal becomes completely occluded or sclerosed during this process. Often the coronal portions of teeth become obliterated leaving a patent apical portion. Such canals can be difficult to locate and treat when the remaining pulp becomes necrotic or infected (**7.17**).

Table 7.1 Mean volume and standard deviation (SD) of dental pulp cavities

Tooth type	Maxillary		Mandibular	
	Mean volume (mm³)	SD	Mean volume (mm³)	SD
Central incisor	12.4	3.3	6.1	2.5
Lateral incisor	11.4	4.6	7.1	2.1
Canine	14.7	4.8	14.2	5.4
First premolar	18.2	5.1	14.9	5.7
Second premolar	16.5	4.2	14.9	6.3
First molar	68.2	21.4	52.5	8.5
Second molar	44.3	29.7	32.9	8.4
Third molar	22.6	3.3	31.1	11.2

Source: Fanibunda, 1986.

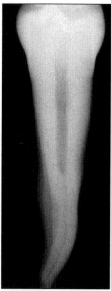

7.6 Buccal radiograph of mandibular first premolar

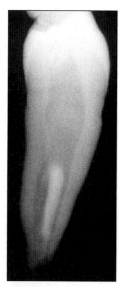

7.7 Approximal radiograph of the mandibular first premolar

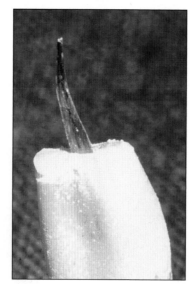

7.8 Pulpal fin in central incisor

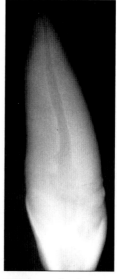

7.9 Approximal radiograph of maxillary canine with pulpal cervical bulge

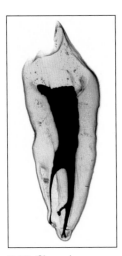

7.10 Cleared mandibular first premolar

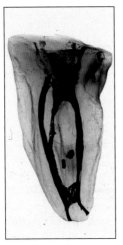

7.11 Cleared mandibular second molar

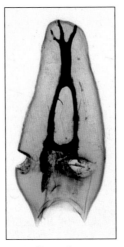

7.12 Cleared maxillary premolar

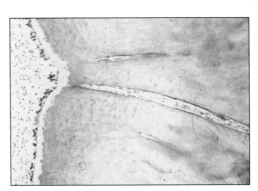

7.13 Lateral canal evident on histological section

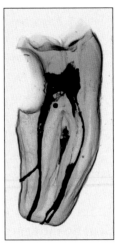

7.14 Cleared mandibular second molar with lateral canal

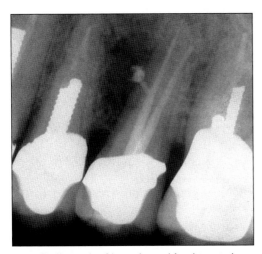

7.15 Radiograph of lateral canal in obturated maxillary premolar

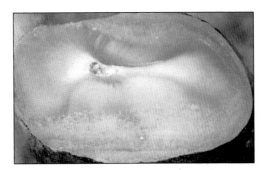

7.16 Partial obliteration of the pulp space

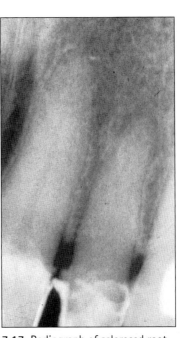

7.17 Radiograph of sclerosed root canal in maxillary lateral incisor

CANAL CONFIGURATIONS

Failure to understand the root form and root canal anatomy of the teeth that we treat is rather like setting out on a long journey without a road map.

Basic biological knowledge

An understanding of the processes that lead to a fully formed tooth helps in differentiating the various patterns or configurations that occur in the anatomy of roots and pulps. Calcification times, eruption and apical root closure dates provide important information in this regard. If eruption dates can be remembered (**Table 7.2**), as a general rule, the calcification of the tooth crown is complete three years before eruption and root end closure three years after eruption.

Table 7.2 Eruption times of adult teeth

Year	Tooth	
6–7	16/26/36/46	31/41
7–8	11/21	32/42
8–9	12/22	
9–10	13/23	33/43
10–11	14/24	34/44
11–12	15/25	35/45
12–13	17/27	37/47
17–22	18/28	38/48

Table 7.3 Average lengths of teeth (mm)

Tooth	Maxillary	Mandibular
Central incisor	22.5	20.7
Lateral incisor	22.0	21.1
Canine	26.5	25.6
First premolar	20.6	21.6
Second premolar	21.5	22.3
First molar	20.8	21.0
Second molar	20.0	19.8

Genetic influences

The proliferation of the dental tissues during development is a genetically-driven activity. The growth and migration of the internal and external enamel epithelium in defining the crown and root forms of teeth is particularly heritable. Familial and racial traits affecting the pulp-space configurations of teeth should be borne in mind.

Congenital malformations, aberrations and complexities

Malformed teeth may display bizarre pulp-space configurations. Most commonly this occurs in invagination, evagination, talon cusps, dilacerations and gemination (**7.18**).

Average values

A knowledge of the average lengths of teeth will help determine the likely depth of insertion of working length instruments (**Table 7.3**). A working understanding of the percentage of teeth that might contain two canals in one root also helps to establish the possible configurations of teeth requiring treatment (**Table 7.4**).

However, the information currently available may not be wholly applicable to teeth in patients of non-Caucasoid origin. Practitioners

Table 7.4 Roots of teeth with two canals (%)

Tooth	Maxillary	Mandibular
Incisor	Rare	41
Canine	Rare	14
First premolar	84 (62 with 2 roots)	30
Second premolar	40	11
First molar	71 (MB root)	87 (M root)
		38 (D root)
Second molar	3 roots/3 canals	2 roots/3 canals
	Root fusion common	Root fusion common

that treat Negroid or Mongoloid populations are aware that these values do not coincide with their own clinical experiences.

Clinical evidence

It is possible to glean additional information with regard to the pulp-space configurations of teeth by using a degree of clinical intuition. Clues may be gained from radiographs by developing a sense of the three-dimensional characteristics of teeth when viewing normal projections.

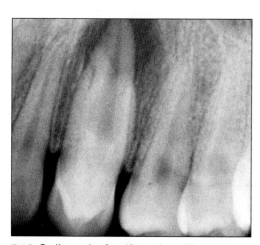

7.18 Radiograph of malformed maxillary canine

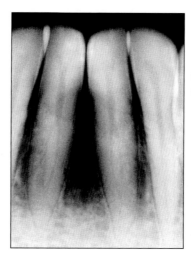

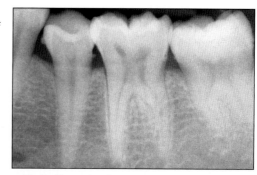

7.19 Radiograph of mandibular incisors with root canal division

7.20 Radiograph of mandibular molar with an extra distal root

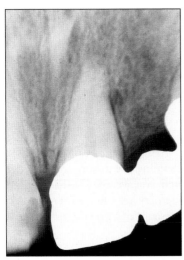

7.21 Periradicular radiolucencies in a maxillary incisor

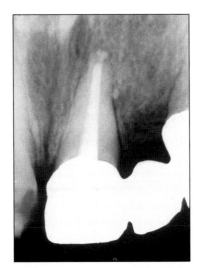

7.22 Obturated incisor with apical and lateral canals

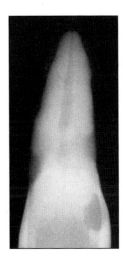

7.23 Buccal radiograph of central incisor

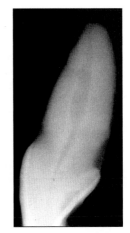

7.24 Approximal radiograph of central incisor with lateral canal

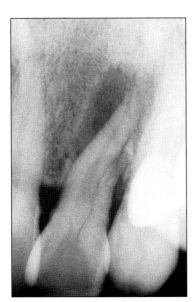

7.25 Radiograph of lateral incisor with two roots

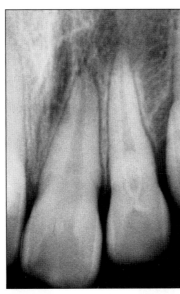

7.26 Radiograph of lateral incisor with an invagination

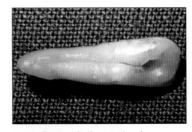

7.27 Congenital grooving in a maxillary lateral incisor

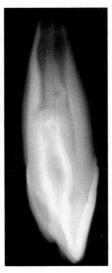

7.28 Radiograph of malformed maxillary lateral incisor

Root canals that disappear radiographically are an indication of canal division (**7.19**).

It is always wise to trace the periodontal ligament space. This is a most useful exercise when searching for extra roots (**7.20**). Thickening of the space in periradicular areas other than the apical region may indicate the presence of lateral and accessory canals (**7.21, 7.22**).

Knob-like appearance of roots may indicate curvatures and the unusual presence of vertical lines suggest gross concavities of the root surface. Further information can be obtained from tactile perception and the angulation of instruments within root canals.

CHARACTERISTICS OF INDIVIDUAL TEETH

Maxillary incisors

The canal is tapering in shape, with an irregular triangular or oval cross-section cervically, which gradually becomes round towards the apex. Generally there is very little apical curvature in central incisors, and where it is present it is either distal or labial. It is extremely rare for these teeth to have more than one root or root canal. It has been suggested that up to 60% of central incisors have accessory canals (**7.23, 7.24**).

The apex of lateral incisors is often curved, generally in a disto-palatal direction. Extra roots and second canals are more likely to be found in lateral incisors (**7.25**), as are developmental grooves and invaginations (**7.26–7.28**).

Maxillary canines

These teeth tend to be the longest of all. The root is wide labio-palatally and the canal does not begin to become round in cross-section until the apical third, where there may be a distal curve. The canal in the coronal third often has a bulge (**7.29, 7.30**).

Maxillary first premolars

This tooth is generally considered to have two roots and two canals (**7.31**). The frequency of two roots is more than 55% in Caucasoids and less than 20% in Mongoloids. Irrespective of race these teeth tend to have two canals (**7.32**). Up to 6% of these teeth have been reported to have three roots and three canals.

Maxillary second premolars

These tend to be single-rooted with a single canal, which is wide in a bucco-lingual direction (**7.33**). Where there are two canals they tend to converge apically.

Maxillary first molars

These teeth are usually three-rooted with four root canals, the additional canal being located in the mesiobuccal root (**7.34**). The minor mesiobuccal canal lies on a line joining the major canal and the palatal canal orifice, 1.82 mm to the lingual on average (**7.35**). As both the canals lie on the buccopalatal plane they are often superimposed on the preoperative radiograph. The presence of a groove on the floor

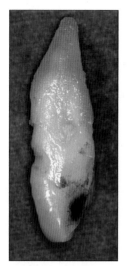

7.29 Specimen maxillary canine

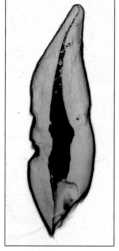

7.30 Specimen maxillary canine cleared

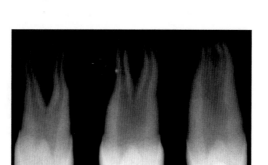

7.31 Radiograph of extracted maxillary first premolars

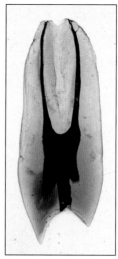

7.32 Cleared Mongoloid maxillary first premolar

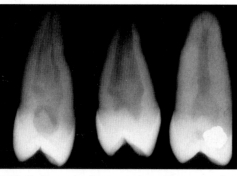

7.33 Radiograph of extracted maxillary second premolars

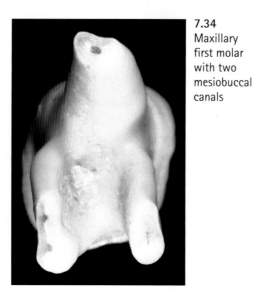

7.34 Maxillary first molar with two mesiobuccal canals

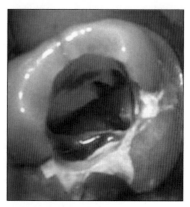

7.35 Four canal orifices in maxillary first molar

of the pulp chamber may be an indication of the likelihood of a second mesiobuccal canal orifice (**7.36**), Which may be only fully exposed after the removal of dentine in the area (**7.37**). The mesiobuccal root often curves distopalatally in the apical third of the root (**7.38**). The distobuccal canal is the shortest of the three canals and leaves the pulp chamber in a distal direction but may curve mesially in the apical half of the root. The palatal canal is the largest and longest of the canals and tends to curve buccally in the apical 4–5 mm (**7.39**). This curvature is not apparent on the radiograph. The variable anatomy of the tooth extends to extra roots and canals (**7.40**).

Maxillary second molars

This tooth is a smaller replica of the first molar. The roots are less divergent and root fusion is much more frequent than in the maxillary first molar (**7.41**, **7.42**), which might give rise to a reduction in the number of canals. The buccal canal orifices tend to be closer together. Teeth with three roots and three canals are prevalent.

Maxillary third molars

The root form and canal anatomy is highly variable. It may possess three roots (**7.43**, **7.44**) but more often fusion occurs and only one or two canals are evident (**7.45**, **7.46**).

Mandibular incisors

Over 40% of these teeth have two canals, which usually join in the apical third (**7.47**). The highest recorded figure for two separate apical foramina is 5.5%.

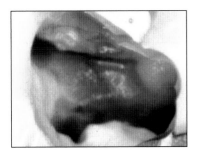

7.36 Groove in the floor of a maxillary first molar

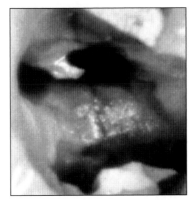

7.37 Mesiobuccal canals evident following removal of the groove

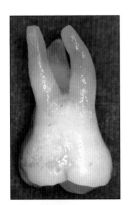

7.38 Right maxillary first molar

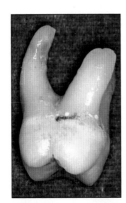

7.39 Buccal curvature of a palatal root of a maxillary first molar

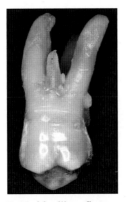

7.40 Maxillary first molar with an extra root

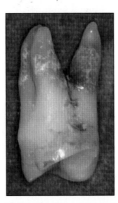

7.41 Maxillary second molar with buccal root fusion

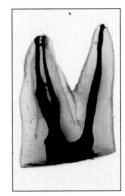

7.42 Maxillary second molar cleared

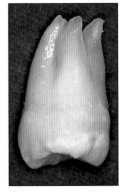

7.43 Maxillary third molar

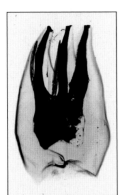

7.44 Maxillary third molar cleared

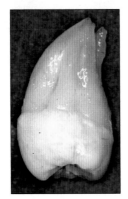

7.45 Maxillary third molar

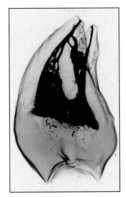

7.46 Maxillary third molar cleared

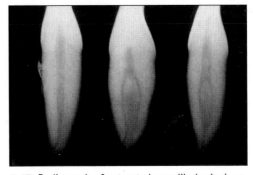

7.47 Radiograph of extracted mandibular incisors

In teeth with a single root canal the canal is normally straight but may curve to the distal (and less often to the labial) side. The grooving found on the mesial and distal surfaces of the roots of these teeth (**7.48**) makes them susceptible to perforation if over-instrumented.

Mandibular canines

The mandibular canine resembles the maxillary canine although its dimensions are smaller (**7.49**). It rarely has two roots but up to 20% may have two root canals (**7.50, 7.51**)

Mandibular first premolars

These teeth occasionally present with a division of roots in the apical half (**7.52**). Up to one-third of these teeth demonstrate division of canals in the apical half of the root, where the canals tend to remain separate and produce separate foramina (**7.53, 7.54**). Three canals appear in less that 2% of the teeth. The existence of 'c'-shaped canals has been reported in these teeth.

Mandibular second premolars

These tend to be single-rooted with a single canal, which is wide in a buccolingual direction (**7.55**). Two canals occur in 25% of cases, when the floor of the pulp chamber extends well below the cervical level.

Mandibular first molars

These teeth usually have two roots (**7.56**). In a Mongoloid variation (which may occur in over 40% of such teeth) a supernumerary disto-lingual root is present (**7.57, 7.58**). The two-rooted molar usually

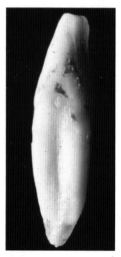

7.48 Approximal groove on mandibular incisor root

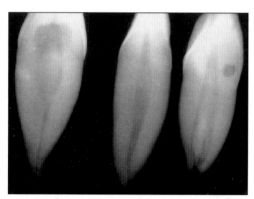

7.49 Radiograph of extracted mandibular canines

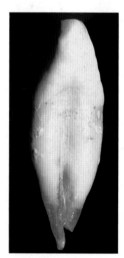

7.50 Mandibular canine with two roots

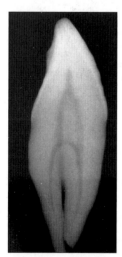

7.51 Radiograph of mandibular canine with two roots

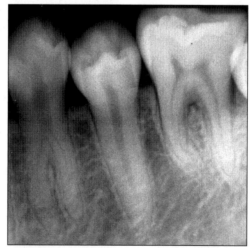

7.52 Radiograph of mandibular first premolar with two roots

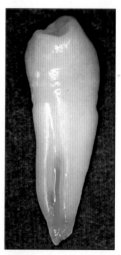

7.53 Extracted specimen of mandibular first premolar

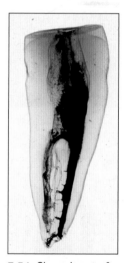

7.54 Cleared root of mandibular first premolar

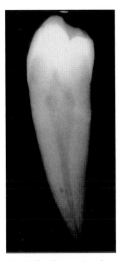

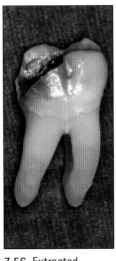

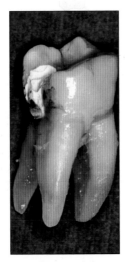

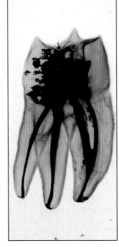

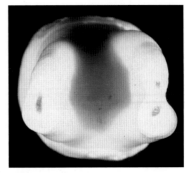

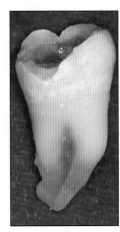

7.55 Radiograph of extracted mandibular second premolar

7.56 Extracted mandibular first molar

7.57 Extracted three-rooted mandibular first molar

7.58 Cleared three-rooted mandibular first molar

7.59 Mandibular first molar with three canals

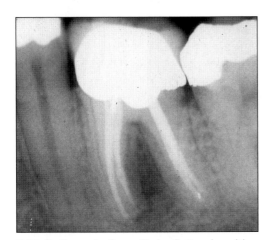

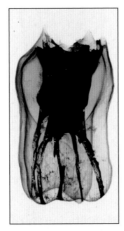

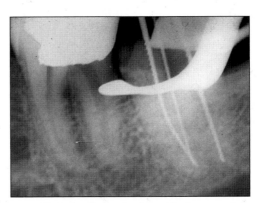

7.60 Radiograph of mandibular first molar with four canals

7.61 Cleared mandibular first molar with five canals

7.62 Clinical radiograph of mandibular second molar

7.63 Mandibular second molar with fused roots

has a canal configuration of three canals; two canals in the mesial root and one in the distal root (**7.59**). There is only one apical foramen in the mesial root in 45% of cases. The single distal canal is usually larger and more oval in cross-section and has a tendency to emerge on the distal side of the root surface short of the anatomical apex. More than 25% of the distal roots have two canals, half of which have separate apical foramina (**7.60**). The frequency of second distal canals appears to be higher in Mongoloid teeth, and specimens with five canals have been observed (**7.61**). The mesiobuccal canal is the most difficult canal to treat because of its tortuous path. It leaves the pulp chamber in a mesial direction,

which alters to a distal direction in the middle of the root. When a second distolingual canal is present it tends to curve towards the buccal. There have been case reports of five and six canals and the presence of a third mesial canal.

Mandibular second molars

In Caucasoid teeth the mesial root has two (occasionally one) canals and the distal root usually has only one canal (**7.62**). The roots tend to be closer together and may fuse (**7.63**). Rarely only one canal is present when both roots are fused (**7.64–7.68**). In Mongoloid

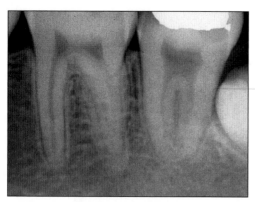

7.64 Clinical radiograph of mandibular second molar

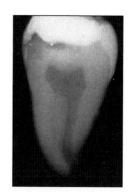

7.65 Buccal radiograph of extracted second molar

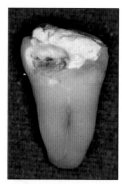

7.66 Approximal radiograph of the extracted second molar

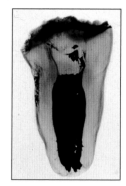

7.67 Lingual view of extracted specimen

7.68 Cleared specimen

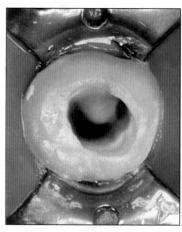

7.69 'C'-shaped canal in mandibular second molar

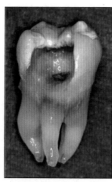

7.70 Extracted mandibular third molar

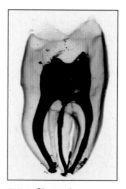

7.71 Cleared mandibular third molar

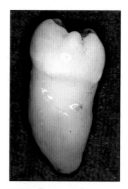

7.72 Extracted mandibular third molar

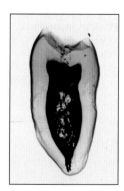

7.73 Cleared mandibular third molar

teeth the fusion of roots is common and where roots are incompletely separated interconnections are likely giving rise to the 'c'-shaped canal (**7.69**). It would seem that teeth with 'c'-shaped roots do not always have 'c'-shaped openings. Those with 'c'-shaped orifices do not always have continuous 'c'-shaped canals.

Reference

Fanibunda KB (1986) A method for measuring the volume of human dental pulp cavities. *Int Endod J* 19, 194–7.

Mandibular third molars

The roots and root canals of these teeth tend to be short and poorly developed (**7.70, 7.71**). The anatomy tends to vary and where there is root fusion the canals also fuse (**7.72, 7.73**).

Chapter 8

Root canal system preparation

K Gulabivala and C J R Stock

PRINCIPLES OF ROOT CANAL SYSTEM PREPARATION

The treatment of choice for periapical disease is elimination of microorganisms and their products from the root canal system. Microorganisms may be found in suspension in the root canal system in the apical part but they mostly colonize canal walls and dentinal tubules to a variable degree up to the apical foramina. A microbial biofilm with a variable thickness and properties coats the dentinal wall (**8.1**). Bacteria penetrating the dentinal tubules may be considered to be extensions of the main canal biofilm resulting in a three-dimensional form that may resemble a 'hairy worm'! The complex three-dimensional form of root canal systems adds to the difficulty of the task of decontaminating its surface.

It is in fact impossible to sterilize the root canal system. It is therefore fortunate that sterility is not a precondition to successful outcome of root canal treatment. Root canal treatment procedures work because the reduction in microbial content of canal systems together with that in its collective pathogenicity is sufficient to promote periradicular healing. In rare cases, the change to an altered and less pathogenic flora may account for periapical healing (**8.2, 8.3**). The precise mechanisms by which the biofilm is eliminated are not understood. It is likely that in a very crude way both the mechanical and chemical components of preparation play a role.

Root canal system preparation may therefore be thought of as:

- Mechanical intra-radicular preparation;
- Chemical intra-radicular preparation;

    1. intra-appointment (covered in this chapter)
    2. inter-appointment (covered, for convenience, in Chapter 9)

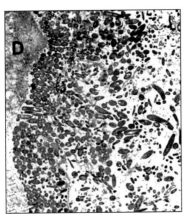

8.1 Multilayered nature of microbial colonies on root canal wall: D = dentine

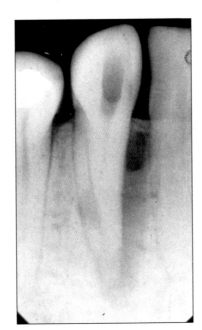

8.2

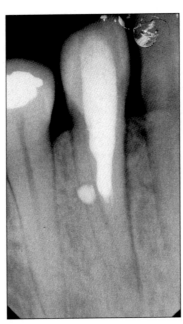

8.3

8.2–8.3 Periradicular healing despite inability to negotiate full length of canals

Mechanical intra–radicular preparation

The purpose of the *mechanical* aspect of root canal system preparation is to create an access to the root canal system. The aim of this extension of the coronal access cavity or to name it by its function, the *radicular access cavity* (conventionally known as canal preparation) is to *obtain and retain* 'patency' to the apical part of the root canal anatomy (**8.4, 8.5**). The shape of the radicular access cavity is a general tapering form that may have a circular (**8.6**) or slightly eccentric cross-sectional (**8.7**) form. The final form depends on the instruments and the manner in which they are manipulated. The mechanical preparation involves using metal instruments of graded sizes to:

- *negotiate* instruments of a sufficient size to the apical part of the root canal system without losing patency;
- *shape* the radicular access to a predefined taper and size to allow antibacterial agents and root-filling materials to be delivered to the full extent of the root canal system in a controlled way.

These goals should be achieved by *controlled* removal of intracanal dentine such that the original shape and curvature of the main root canal(s) are retained (**8.8, 8.9**). This together with a relatively conservative final preparation size helps to ensure that the root is neither weakened nor perforated. In narrow uncomplicated canal systems, the mechanical preparation may be sufficient to effect the almost complete removal of the microbial biofilm. However, this is a rare achievement even in anterior, single rooted teeth (**8.10, 8.11**). The truth is that there is always a variable proportion of non-instrumented surface in the root canal system (**8.4, 8.12**).

Chemical intraradicular preparation

It is necessary to use *chemical agents* delivered through the radicular access cavity to disrupt the microbial biofilm on the uninstrumented surface. Wider and larger radicular access cavities may allow better delivery of chemical agents to the uninstrumented surface, especially the all-important apical anatomy. However, a balance has to be struck between the desire to improve delivery of chemical agents and that to maintain the strength of the tooth (**8.13, 8.14**).

The process of bacterial biofilm disruption by antibacterial fluids and dressings is fraught with problems. The problems are two-fold:

1. To ensure that the irrigant *is* delivered to the narrow and distant apical anatomy as well as the remaining ramifications along the root canal system.
2. That, despite effective irrigant delivery, the multi-layered, three-dimensional nature of the microbial biofilm together with its polysaccharide matrix may protect the deeper layers of organisms (**8.1**).

The first problem may be overcome by enlarging and shaping the radicular access sufficiently to allow the irrigant to the apical anatomy using an appropriately sized, narrow-gauge hypodermic needle (**8.15, 8.16**) or ultrasonic agitation. The inference is that in wide, straight canals, minimal mechanical preparation should be required (**8.17**). The second problem may be overcome by using a high enough concentration or alternatively sufficient volume of irrigant to give long-lasting chemical potency. The combined action of mechanical and chemical cleaning is more efficient than either method alone, and allows a more conservative canal preparation as

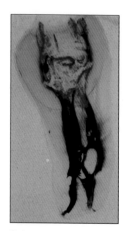

8.4

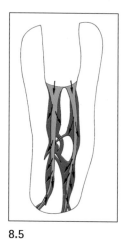

8.5

8.4–8.5 Canal preparation as a radicular access

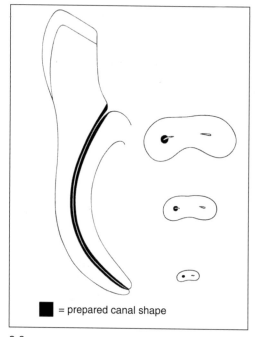

= prepared canal shape

8.6

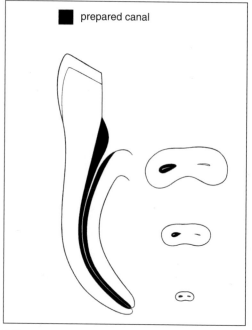

prepared canal

8.7

8.6–8.7 Longitudinal and transverse sections showing the canal before and after preparation

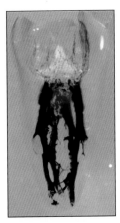

8.8 Cleared molar tooth showing complex canal system

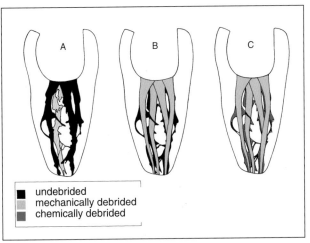

8.9 Effect of original canal anatomy and canal preparation on the final shape of the root canal system: A = before preparation; B = after mechanical preparation; C = after chemical debridement

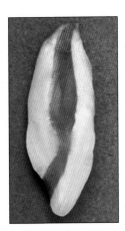

8.10 Irregular wide-root canal in maxillary canine

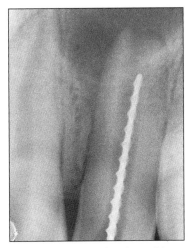

8.11 Wide, 'blunderbuss' canal in an incompletely formed root

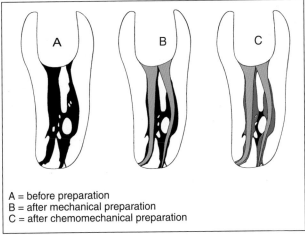

A = before preparation
B = after mechanical preparation
C = after chemomechanical preparation

8.12 These diagrams are reproduced from the cleared tooth shown in **8.4**: A = before preparation; B = after mechanical preparation; C = after chemomechanical preparation

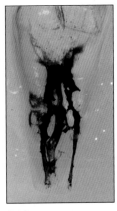

8.13

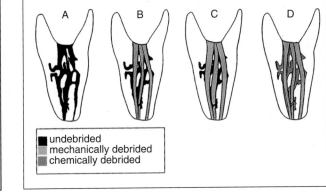

8.14

8.13–8.14 Effect of narrow and widely tapered preparations on complex canal anatomy: A = before preparation; B = after narrow-taper preparation; C = after wide-taper preparation; D = after mechanical preparation and use of irrigant with ability to dissolve debris and destroy bacteria

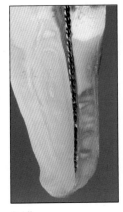

8.15

8.16

8.15–8.16 Preparation to facilitate needle placement

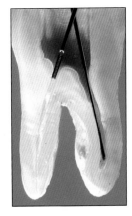

8.17 Deep penetration of irrigant needle in wide unprepared canal

reliance on dentine removal for decontamination (a forlorn hope) is reduced. This is the chemo-mechanical method of root canal system preparation.

Canal preparation in teeth requiring pulpectomy, that is vital pulp removal, has similar but not identical aims. The concern in such teeth is to remove not microorganisms but pulp tissue, which may in due course become necrotic and infected (**8.18, 8.19**). In the case shown, the uninstrumented apical portion of the distal canal has resulted in the development of periapical disease. It is therefore useful if the selected irrigant both dissolves organic tissue and destroys microorganisms.

This chapter discusses the objectives of root canal system preparation and reviews the advantages and disadvantages of the various approaches. In order to achieve satisfactory canal preparation, the entry point to the root canal system should be suitably prepared. The design of the coronal access cavity to the pulp chamber is therefore discussed first.

CORONAL ACCESS CAVITIES

Principles of cutting a coronal access cavity

These are:

1. To remove the roof of the pulp chamber so as to provide good visual and tactile access to the entrances of the main root canals (**8.20, 8.21**). It is a common fault to leave remnants of the pulp chamber roof together with some pulp remnants (**8.22–8.24**).
2. To provide straight-line access to the first curve in the root canal (**8.25**). The walls of the coronal access cavity should not deflect an instrument placed into a canal.
3. To avoid damage to the floor of the pulp chamber. This will avoid perforation of the pulp chamber floor and make it easier to locate the canal entrances (**8.26**). The natural shape of the floor tends to guide an instrument into the canal orifice.

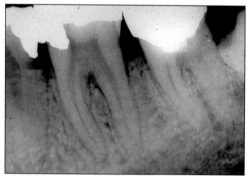

8.18

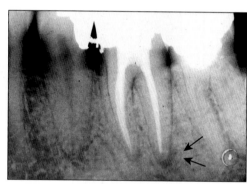

8.19

8.18–8.19 Development of periradicular area around distal root following vital extirpation

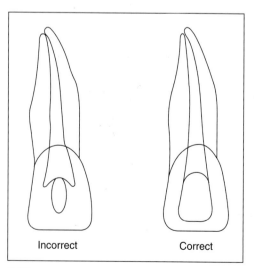

8.20

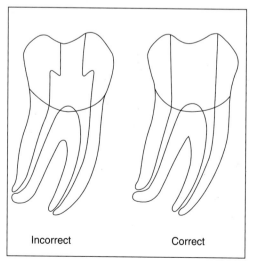

8.21

8.20–8.21 Removing the roof of the pulp chamber

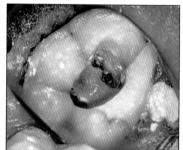

8.22 Mandibular first molar with incomplete removal of pulp chamber roof

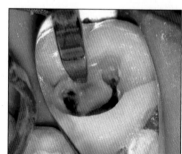

8.23 Roof of pulp chamber being removed by sickle

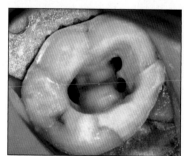

8.24 Roof of pulp chamber removed

4. To conserve as much tooth substance as possible to prevent weakening and fracture of the remaining tooth consistent with above aims (**8.27, 8.28**).
5. To provide coronal and apical resistance form so that the temporary access cavity seal remains intact until the final restoration is placed (**8.29**).

Cutting the coronal access cavity

Initial penetration is made with a tungsten-carbide, domed-fissure, crosscut bur aimed towards the largest part of the pulp chamber.

When a porcelain crown or enamel is present a round diamond bur is used followed by a tungsten-carbide bur to cut through the metal or dentine beneath (**8.30**). Once the roof of the pulp chamber has been penetrated a safe-ended, tapered, diamond bur, or similar-shaped tungsten-carbide bur, is used to reduce the risk of damaging the pulpal floor while the roof is removed. The depth of penetration is judged by holding the hand-piece containing the bur against the preoperative radiograph (**8.31**). Older teeth have smaller pulp chambers and therefore require a smaller access cavity, additionally the floor may have calcified pulp tissue attached and care must be taken to remove it (**8.32, 8.33**). Thought must be given to the type

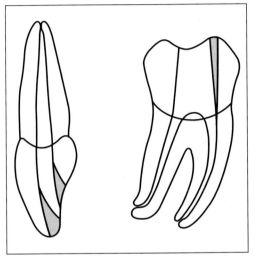
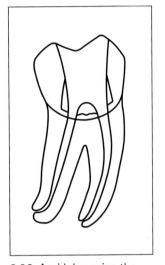
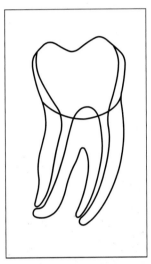

8.25 Straight line access

8.26 Avoid damaging the floor of the pulp chamber

8.27 Conserve tooth substance

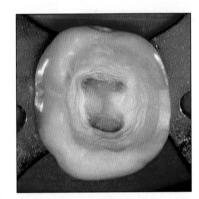

8.28 Access cavity too large

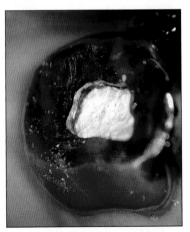

8.29 Lack of resistance form leads to intracoronal displacement of temporary filling

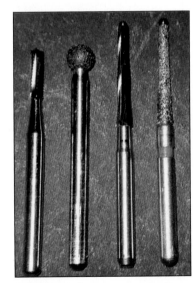

8.30 Access burs

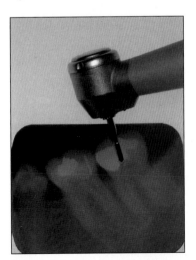

8.31 Judging access cavity depth

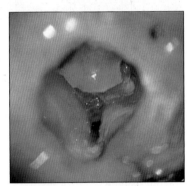

8.32 Calcified tissue and pulp remnants

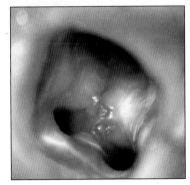

8.33 Pulp chamber thoroughly cleaned and canals prepared

of permanent restoration that will be used afterwards as this will alter the shape and approach to cutting the coronal access cavity. For example, in the case of an onlay the walls of the access may be reduced before the root treatment is carried out, or in the case of an anterior tooth which is to be crowned and is lingually inclined consider access from the buccal (**8.34, 8.35**). Radiographs (**8.36, 8.37**) show that straight-line access can be just as effective from the buccal aspect as from the lingual.

Outline shape

The outline shape of the coronal access cavities is dictated by the shape of the pulp chambers, which in turn follow that of the tooth in cross-section. The standard shapes of coronal access cavities for different tooth types are given in **Figures 8.38–8.43**. The size of the cavity is dictated by the size of the pulp chamber and will therefore tend to become smaller in older patients.

In anterior teeth straight-line access into the canals of incisors and canines means that the cavity must be cut high up on the tooth near the incisal edge. This type of access cavity will leave the cingulum intact, which provides the maximum retention for a full crown.

The shape of the pulp chamber, and therefore the coronal access cavity, of the maxillary first molar is rhomboid due to a widening

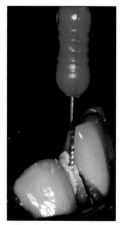
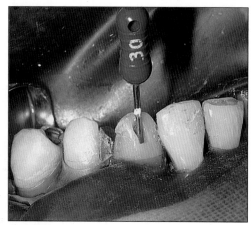

8.34   **8.35**
8.34–8.35 Buccal access in mandibular anterior tooth

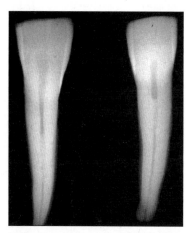

8.36 Buccal view of mandibular anterior teeth

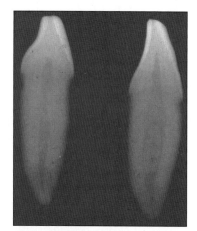

8.37 Approximal view of mandibular anterior teeth

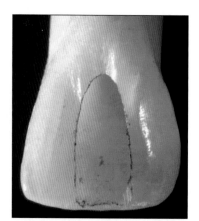

8.38 Maxillary incisor

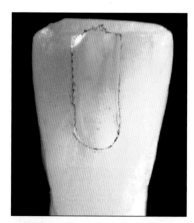

8.39 Mandibular incisor

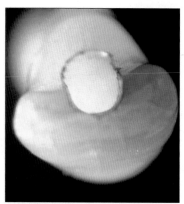
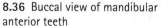

8.40 Mandibular incisor looking from incisal edge

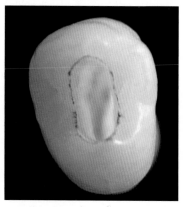

8.41 Maxillary and mandibular premolars

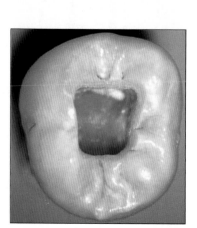

8.42 Mandibular molar

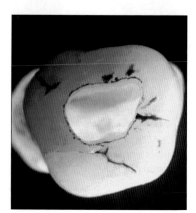

8.43 Maxillary first molar

over the palatal canal orifice. The second and third molars show a mesio-distal flattening of the pulp chamber which also lies nearer the mesial aspect of the tooth.

The access to the mandibular first molar is also rhomboid in shape because the distal canal is either broad bucco-lingually or because there are two separate canals. The second and third molar access cavity is more triangular as there is usually only one distal canal.

DETERMINATION OF CANAL AND WORKING LENGTH

Point of termination of canal preparation

It is impossible to determine the extent of contamination of a root canal clinically; it is best to assume contamination up to the apical foramina in all cases with necrotic pulps and to clean the canal to this point. It is safest to clean to the apical termination of root canals even in cases where the tooth is vital. However, it is important to ensure that instrumentation and treatment materials do not extend beyond the root canal system as this may reduce the success rate.

Clinical determination of position of root canal system terminus

The exact determination of the position of the apical termini of the root canal system is not possible. Several methods are used to estimate the termination of the root canal system, they include:

- radiographic;
- electronic apex locators;
- tactile;
- paper point.

Each of the methods is analysed independently first and then a way of combining them offered.

Radiographic method

The first problem is that the root canal system often ends in an apical delta so that there is not just one but several apical foramina. The diagnostic endodontic file usually finds only one of these (**8.44–8.46**). The second problem is that the radiographic view with a file in the canal provides a two-dimensional picture of a three-dimensional root-end in which the file may be disposed in any plane. Unless a single root canal system exit is disposed at exactly right angles to the X-ray beam and film, radiographic technique can never estimate the position of the apical foramen accurately.

The traditional protocol for canal length determination using radiographic technique alone is as follows. An estimate of the approximate length of the tooth is made from a preoperative parallel radiograph (**8.47**). A file is placed in the root canal about 1 mm short of this estimated length, ensuring that a coronal reference point is selected that is reproducible and durable. The file should be large enough to be visible on the radiograph (e.g. size 10). A parallel radiograph is then taken (**8.48**). In teeth with multiple canals, diagnostic files

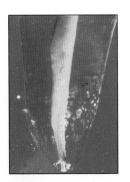
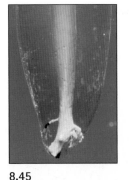
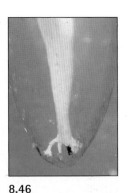

8.44   8.45   8.46

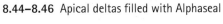

8.44–8.46 Apical deltas filled with Alphaseal

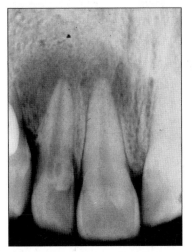
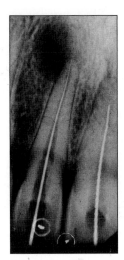

8.47 Preoperative parallel view radiograph

8.48 Periapical radiograph with diagnostic files

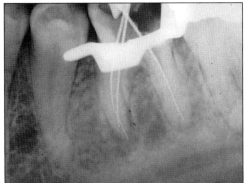

8.49 Angled periapical radiograph with diagnostic files

should be placed in all canals and a single, view taken to minimize exposure to radiation (**8.49**). Canals may exit on the root surface at a variable distance and position from the root tip and it is impossible to judge the position of apical foramina satisfactorily from radiographs (**8.50, 8.51**). This pair of photographs shows three roots, with files that appear flush with the radiographic root tip but which

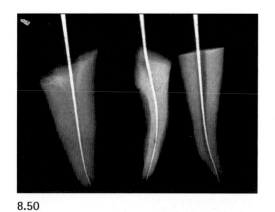

8.50

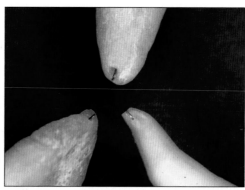

8.51

8.50–8.51 Discrepancies between radiographic images of files and reality in relation to the root apex

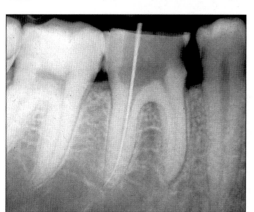

8.52

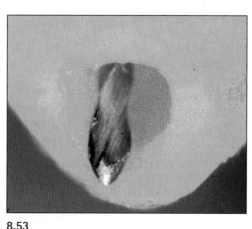

8.53

8.52–8.53 Discrepancy between radiographic images and reality (taken from a clinical study)

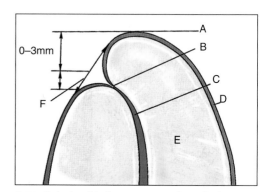

8.54 Relationship between root tip, apical foramen, and apical constriction: A = root apex; B = apical constriction; C = root canal; D = cementum; E = dentine; F = apical foramen

are actually extended past the apical foramina. **Figures 8.52 and 8.53** show a case taken from a clinical study in which a cemented file that is apparently flush with the root tip is actually extended well beyond the apical foramen. An average distance of 1 mm short of the radiographic apex is widely accepted as a reasonable estimate of the terminal position of the canal, but this may be inaccurate by up to 3.0 mm (**8.54**).

Once a parallel periapical radiograph of the tooth with diagnostic file(s) in the canal has been obtained, working length is calculated.

1. In most cases the tip of the file will be short of the radiographic apex. This is often accepted as the length of the canal if the distance is within 1 mm (as in the lateral incisor: **8.55**). If the discrepancy is greater than 1 mm, then the distance between the file tip and the radiographic apex should be measured and 1 mm subtracted from this measurement (as in the central incisor: **8.55**). This figure is added to the length of the diagnostic file to give the length of the canal (**8.56, 8.57**).

2. In some cases the file may be longer than the radiographic apex, in which case the distance between the file tip and a point 1 mm short of the radiographic apex should be measured (**8.58, 8.59**). Subtracting this figure from the length of the diagnostic file will give the length of the canal.

Electronic apex-locator method

The reliability of contemporary electronic apex locators (EALs) has increased to a point where many clinicians rely almost exclusively on them although they do not give 100% reliability.

Electronic apex locators (**8.60**) in theory enable the location of the true position of the apical terminus or foramen, utilizing the fact that root canals, in common with other tubes with one end immersed in an electrolyte solution, exhibit certain electrical characteristics that are relatively constant.

The parameter of importance is the sudden change in impedance of the root canal as the apical foramen is approached. The impedance in question is measured between a point along the length of the root canal and the oral mucosa (**8.61**). Introduction of electrolytes into the root canal causes the impedance to drop and the gradient of impedance along the canal to decrease. The impedance value at the apical foramen, that is between the periodontal ligament and the oral mucosa measured via the root canal is a relative constant. This value is used to calibrate commercial EALs, but the impedance characteristics given for the canal coronal to the apical foramen cannot be calibrated accurately. EALs should therefore always be used to achieve the 'zero' reading for greatest accuracy and not any point short of this, even if the manufacturers recommend it.

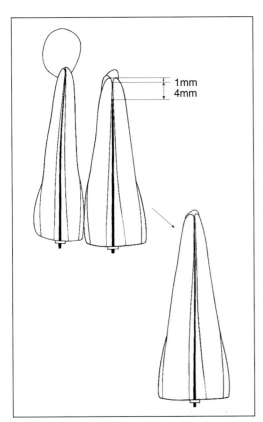

8.55 Diagram reproduced from **8.48**. Correct length in 12 accepted. Short length in 11 is corrected

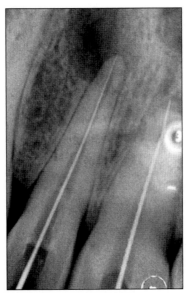

8.56

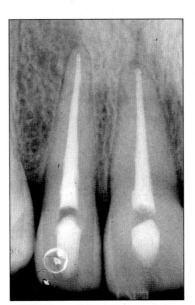

8.57

8.56–8.57 Adjusted diagnostic files and final root fillings

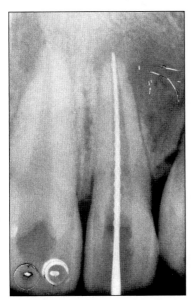

8.58 Overextended file

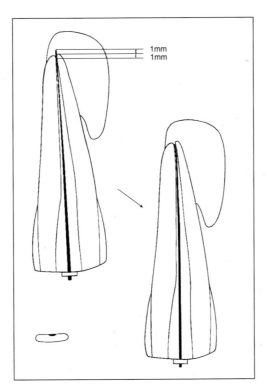

8.59 Diagram reproduced from **8.58** shows corrected length

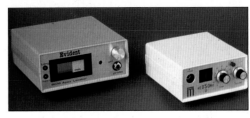

8.60 Electronic apex locators

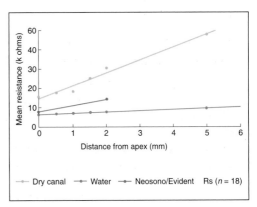

8.61 Electrical impedance of root canals at different distances from the apical foramen with water-filled and dry canals. Also shown is the average calibration of a typical apex locator.

EALs work by applying an alternating current between two electrodes, one of which is attached to the file and the other via a clip to the lip or cheek mucosa (**8.62, 8.63**). The frequency of this current, which also influences impedance, is usually fixed in a given make of instrument but differs between makes. As the file is passed down the canal the EAL measures the impedance and compares the value with its calibrated standard. A countdown scale indicates a 'zero' or 'apex' reading when the calibrated value is matched (**8.64, 8.65**). All currently available conventional EALs use this principle but display the information differently (**8.66**). The current generation of EALs have overcome the problem with electrolytes in root canals by measuring the impedance at two different current frequencies. One of these, the Apit (also known as Endex: **8.65**), uses the difference in impedance at two frequencies to calculate the position of the apical foramen. Another (the Root ZX: **8.66**) compares the ratio of impedance at two frequencies to make a similar calculation. Yet another model, the AFA (Dentsply), claims to derive the information from five different frequencies.

The accuracy of different models of EALs has been tested clinically and shows slightly variable results for the same EALs in different studies and for different EALs in the same study. These differences may be attributed to many factors, including conditions of use and calibration of the instrument. Each instrument requires practice in use to become familiar with its idiosyncrasies before it can be used with confidence. EALs are reliable but should not be relied upon in all circumstances. If there is any doubt about the reading a radiograph must be taken. Potential problems in use include short-circuiting if the file touches a metal restoration or if the canal contains excessive moisture. Clinicians are advised to use an EAL for a period of at least three months by placing a diagnostic file at the 'zero' length indicated by the EAL and taking a check radiograph (**8.67**).

Tactile method

Some clinicians claim that it is possible to gauge the apical constriction of the root canal system by tactile sense. There are several

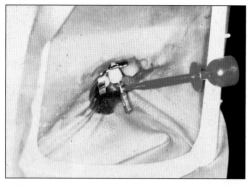

8.62

8.62–8.63 Connection of electrodes to file and cheek

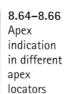

8.63

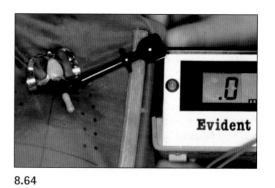

8.64

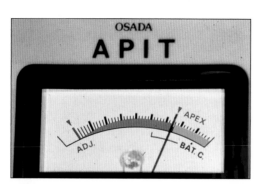

8.65

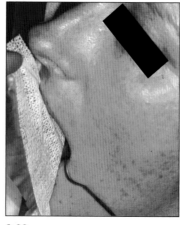

8.66

8.64–8.66 Apex indication in different apex locators

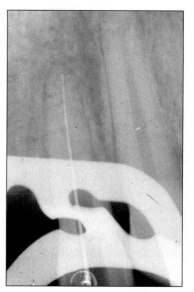

8.67 File placed to length indicated at 'zero' by apex locator

problems with this claim. First, not all teeth possess an apical constriction due to the presence of apical resorption. Second, the ability to gauge the apical constriction relies on the presence of a natural canal taper that has a minimal constriction only at the termination of the canal. Third, the tactile detection of the apical constriction relies upon the selection of a file size that will first bind only at the apical constriction. Given that the size of the apical constriction varies considerably, the method is reliant upon several preconditions as well as the fortuitous selection of the correct instrument size. Taking these factors collectively it is highly unlikely that tactile sense alone can be used to gauge the position of the apical terminus.

Paper-point method

Another recommended method is the use of a sequence of paper points that show the position of the apical foramen by the junction of blood-wetted and dry tip of the paper point. Although this can aid apical foramen location in some cases, it is unreliable by itself because of seepage of exudate or blood into the canal and by capillary action along the paper point.

Combined method for determining position of canal terminus

None of the methods described so far are infallible. The recommended approach to determination of the terminus of the root canal system is to first use an EAL to obtain the 'zero' reading. The diagnostic file should not fit too loosely in the canal otherwise a less accurate reading will be obtained. The length of the file at this reading is recorded from a stable reference point on the crown. The file(s) is replaced to the *same* length and a radiograph taken using a parallel radiograph. The file should appear to be within the confines of the root apex. If it appears to be longer, the length of the file should be rechecked. A final judgement should be made about the true position of the canal terminus by comparing the indicated lengths using tactile sense and paper points as well.

Determination of working length

The *working length* is the length to which each instrument is used in the root canal. It is not necessarily the same length as that of the canal from the reference point to the canal terminus. Some instruments may be used to the full length of the canal, while others may be used at various predetermined lengths short or long of it.

Once the length of the canal has been determined, it is necessary to decide whether the series of root canal instruments will be set to that length or short of it. Many factors dictate the length to which instruments will be used in the canal. The goal of the negotiation phase of canal preparation is to enlarge the canal to at least size 30 (ISO) *just short of the canal terminus*. That is, to preserve the original size of the apical foramen as far as possible. If the canal is to be prepared to a non-ISO taper, then it is considered that preparation to size 20 or 25 may be sufficient. If the operator is very meticulous, the length to which the canal is prepared can be controlled to 0.25 mm and the files may be set to 0.25 mm short of the canal length. If, on the other hand, the operator has poorer control it may be prudent to set the instruments up to 1 mm short of the canal length. The former is always preferable and good endodontists will strive for such accuracy. In addition, the following factors may further affect the decision to modify the length to which the canal is instrumented:

1. When apical root resorption is evident the canal terminus may be 'blunderbuss' shaped and therefore allow extrusion of endodontic materials (**8.68, 8.69**). One school of thought suggests that instrumentation should be shorter. Another suggests that the resorption is caused by microbial infection in the site and so requires vigorous apical preparation up to the full length.
2. When the root tip is very narrow there may be a risk of root perforation if the root is prepared to a significant diameter to the full length (**8.70**).

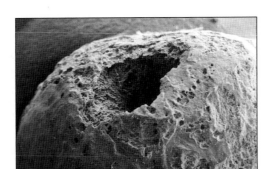

8.69 Apical root resorption: SEM view

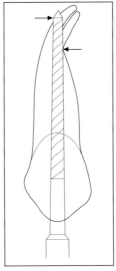

8.70 Risk of apical perforation in narrow root tips

8.68 Apical root resorption: histological view

3. When in addition to the narrow roots they also exhibit a sudden apical curve (**8.71**, **8.72**). In these cases, small flexible files may be used to the full length but larger files (above size 25) should be used to shorter lengths.

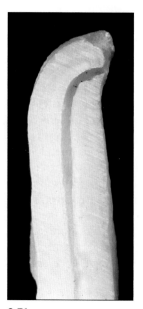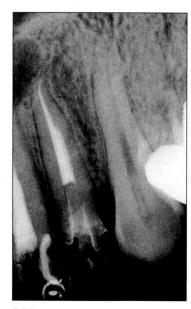

8.71   8.72

8.71–8.72 Sudden apical curve in root canal

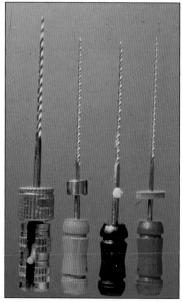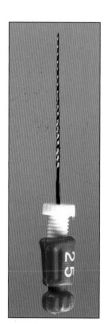

8.73   8.74

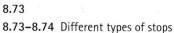
8.73–8.74 Different types of stops

Different files may therefore be used to different (working) lengths. All of this, of course, presumes that the operator has exceptionally good control of the instruments, is conscious of the attention to detail necessary in measuring the files (up to 0.25 mm) and of problems such as 'stop slippage' and parallax in judging the position of the file in relation to the coronal reference point. Lack of adherence to these basic principles is a common fault exhibited by inexperienced operators.

Displacement of the (rubber) stops on the files, which designate length, is a problem that must be prevented by selecting tightly fitting stops. Some stops are more susceptible to displacement than others (**8.73**, **8.74**). Loss of the reference point is another important cause of error. It may occur either because of lack of care in properly recording it in the record notes or because the original reference has been lost due to breakage of tooth or restoration. In either case, the length must be re-established before proceeding further.

Maintaining canal instrumentation to its terminus

In addition to operator-induced errors in maintaining canal length, operators should also be aware that the length of the curved canal will inevitably change as it is prepared. This is because as the canal is prepared, its increased width allows the rigid metal instruments to take a straighter and shorter path to the apical terminus (**8.75**). If the coronal part of the canal is prepared before the definitive measurement of the canal length, then the change in canal length during preparation is minimized. Given the ease of use of EALs, it is best to maintain constant vigilance over changes in length by frequent checking of length.

Relationship between the radicular access, its dimensions and root canal anatomy

Historically the mechanical aspect of root canal treatment has been considered the most important part of bacterial debridement. The current hypothesis may be considered to be a paradigm shift, in that the mechanical preparation is no more than an extension of the coronal access cavity into the root (radicular access cavity).

It has traditionally been held that canals should be prepared by controlled dentine removal so as to produce a regular taper with the minimum diameter at the apical constriction and the maximum diameter at the coronal end, at the same time maintaining the original shape of the canal as far as possible to preserve the strength and integrity of the root. Its original shape, therefore, also dictates the overall shape of the prepared canal.

The width or degree of taper to which the canal should be prepared has been a subject of much debate. The choice is usually based on personal preference and individual clinical experience rather than on sound scientific rationale. Widely tapered canals may allow better irrigant penetration, better debridement and probably

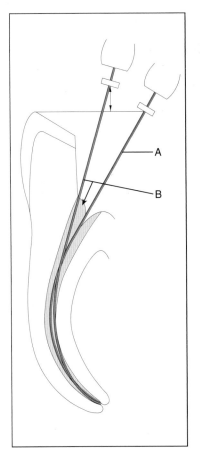

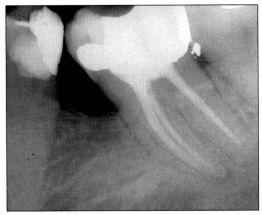

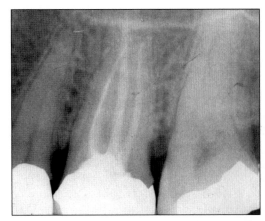

8.76 Narrowly prepared and obturated lower molar

8.77 Narrowly prepared and obturated upper molar

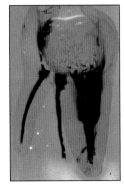

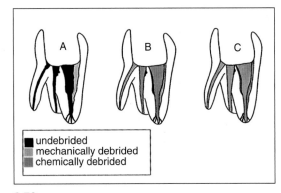

undebrided
mechanically debrided
chemically debrided

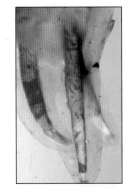

8.75 Change in length of canal as it is prepared: A = file before instrumentation; B = file after instrumentation

8.78

8.79

8.78–8.79 Simple tubular canals encompassed by tapered canal preparation: A = before preparation; B = after mechanical preparation; C = after chemical irrigation with sodium hypochlorite

8.80 Root-filled tooth with tapered canal preparations completely encompassing the root canal system

better obturation if using the cold lateral condensation technique, but these benefits are achieved at the expense of root strength and possibly long-term survival of the tooth. Advocates of narrowly prepared canals argue that a taper that allows irrigant penetration using narrow needles is sufficient for debridement and that obturation of such canals can be satisfactorily achieved with the new thermoplasticized gutta-percha techniques. Narrowly tapered preparations, if they allow adequate cleaning and obturation are more desirable as they do not compromise root strength (**8.76, 8.77**).

Simple canal systems

When the canal system is simple, consisting of *narrow main canals*, preparation to a regularly tapered radicular access cavity may entirely (or almost entirely) encompass the original canal system (**8.78, 8.79**). **Figure 8.80** shows a root-filled tooth with regularly tapered

canals completely encompassing the original canal anatomy. In such cases, cleaning may be achieved almost wholly by mechanical preparation with little reliance on the irrigant.

In contrast, where the canals are wider (such as canines and premolars, distal and palatal roots of molars), despite their simplicity, they may not allow complete debridement solely by mechanical preparation (**8.10**). The lack of direct access for instrumentation places greater reliance on the use of irrigants for cleaning. Access for irrigation is excellent in such teeth and, therefore, only minimal filing of the canal walls is necessary.

Mechanical debridement of teeth containing simple main canals with fins and ramifications extending off them would remove most microbes and organic tissue but not from the uninstrumented accessory anatomy (**8.81, 8.82**). **Figure 8.83** shows a root-filled tooth in which the main canals have been prepared to a taper and filled but the accessory anatomy remains undebrided.

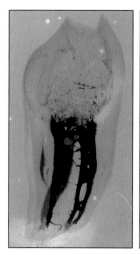

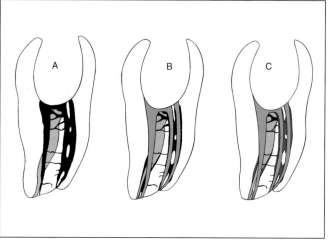

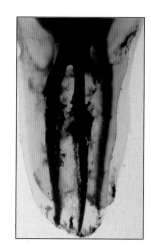

8.83 Root-filled tooth with tapered main canals but undebrided accessory anatomy

8.81   **8.82**

8.81–8.82 Simple main canals with complex intercommunications: A = before preparation; B = after mechanical preparation, C = after chemomechanical preparation

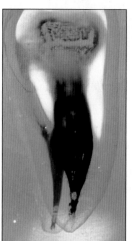

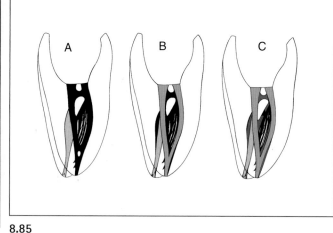

8.84–8.85 Simple main canals with complex intercommunications: A = before preparation; B = after mechanical preparation; C = after chemomechanical preparation

8.85

8.84

Complex canal systems

In teeth with more complex, irregular canal systems, the prepared radicular access cavity is encompassed by the original canal system to a greater or lesser degree and may only be partly discernible or not at all. **Figures 8.84 and 8.85** show an example where the prepared radicular access cavities would be partially discernible. **Figures 8.86 and 8.87** show an example where two of the original canals would be completely embraced by the prepared radicular access, whereas the final canal would encompass the prepared radicular access cavity. In fact this wide distal canal may require two adjacent radicular access cavities to sufficiently allow adequate irrigation. **Figures 8.88, 8.89, 8.4 and 8.12** show examples in which the original anatomy would subsume the radicular access cavity.

Examples of cleared teeth that have been root-filled show the relationship between the instrumented radicular access cavity and the uninstrumented portion of the root canal system (**8.90–8.94**). **Figures 8.95 and 8.96** show an example of a case in which the radicular access cavity is barely visible as the original canal anatomy encompasses the prepared shape.

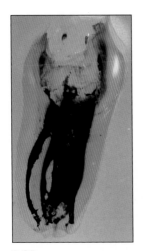

8.86

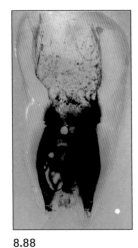

8.88

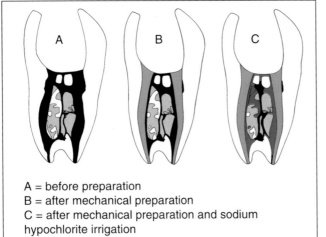

A = before preparation
B = after mechanical preparation
C = after mechanical preparation and sodium

8.87

A = before preparation
B = after mechanical preparation
C = after mechanical preparation and sodium
hypochlorite irrigation

8.89

8.86–8.89 Effect of mechanical and chemical cleaning on complex irregular canal systems:
A = before preparation;
B = after mechanical preparation;
C = after mechanical preparation and sodium hypochlorite irrigation

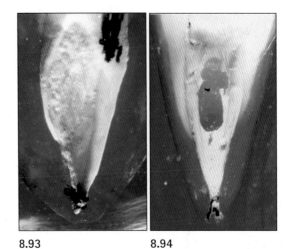

8.93   8.94

8.93–8.94 Filling of ramifications between canals with thermoplasticised gutta-percha

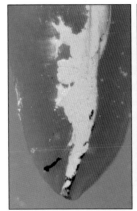
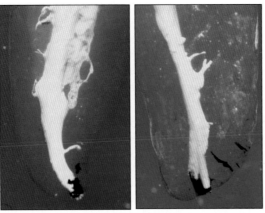

8.90   8.91   8.92

8.90–8.92 Root-filled canals showing instrumented and uninstrumented canal walls

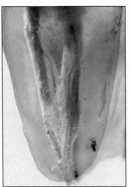
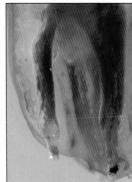

8.95   8.96

8.95–8.96 Root-filled teeth in which the tapered canal preparation is encompassed by the original canal shape

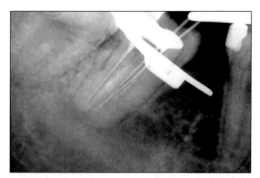

8.97 C-shaped canal in mandibular second molar with diagnostic instruments in place

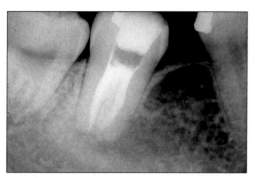

8.98 C-shaped canal obturated to reveal two overlapping tapers (Courtesy of Dr Melody Chen)

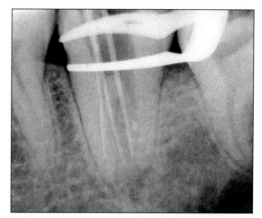

8.99 C-shaped canal in mandibular second molar with diagnostic instruments in place

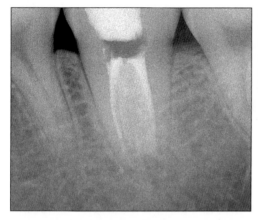

8.100 C-shaped canal obturated to reveal continuous single canal (Courtesy of Dr Melody Chen)

'C'-shaped canals would be treated as broad distal canals in lower molars that may result in two separate or overlapping tapers (**8.97**, **8.98**) prepared to allow sufficient access for irrigation. Alternatively, if filing is used then a continuous shape may be created (**8.99**, **8.100**).

Mechanical preparation of the tapered radicular access cavity

The tapered radicular access cavity may be prepared either with hand-instruments, rotary automated instruments or a combination of the two. In contemporary practice it is common to use a combined hybrid approach. It is an attractive proposition to prepare the tapered access using automated instrumentation. While root canal instrumentation has seen tremendous advances, hand-instruments have not become redundant. The advances in rotary automated instrumentation now enable much easier *shaping* of root canals although the instruments must be used with great care in fine curved canals to avoid breakage.

The skills the operator needs to develop by constant practice are:

- the ability to gauge the diameter and curvatures in the root canal system by tactile exploration to form a three-dimensional mental image of it;

- the ability to modify and refine the three-dimensional mental image using clues from radiographs and information about common anatomical traits in various tooth types;
- the tactile awareness to cut dentine either by filing (push-pull) motion or rotary (clockwise and counter-clockwise) motion in a controlled way that maintains the original canal curvatures.

Mechanical preparation of the radicular access by hand-instrumentation

Mechanical preparation of the radicular access requires the controlled removal of dentine by manipulation of root canal instruments. Acquisition of such skills requires dedicated practice under the guidance of an effective coach.

The two basic motions of the hand-instrument that remove dentine, work in essentially different ways.

Rotary motion In rotary motion the instrument cuts best when the cutting edge is oriented almost parallel to the long-axis of the instrument, such as in the reamer (**8.101**). The progressive decrease in the pitch of the flutes by making the twists in the metal shank tighter renders the cutting edges at a greater angle to the long-axis and closer to the perpendicular of the long-axis, as in a file (**8.102**). This means that the latter instrument is suitable for both rotary use as well as push-pull filing. The closer the cutting edges are to being perpendicular to the long-axis of the instrument, the better suited it is to use for filing or push-pull action (**8.103**). In addition to the orientation of the cutting flutes, the manner in which the edges engage dentine and cut it, is different in the two motions.

In rotary motion, the cutting is reliant upon engaging the dentine by apical feeding into the canal. The file engages dentine much in the same way as a screw would engage wood. The threads or cutting edges wind into the dentine. No lateral forces are involved. The operator has only to gauge the torque required to engage the dentine. The amount of dentine engaged depends on the relative mismatch in the diameter of the instrument and that of the

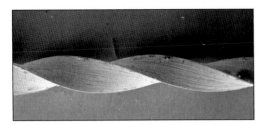

8.101 Kerr K-reamer No. 25

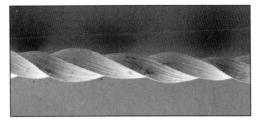

8.102 Kerr K-Flex file No. 25

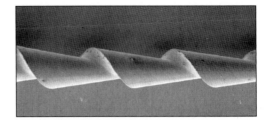

8.103 Micro Mega Hedstroem No. 25

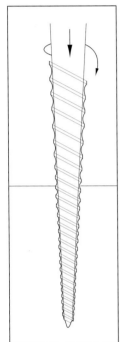

8.104 Threaded screw entering a piece of wood

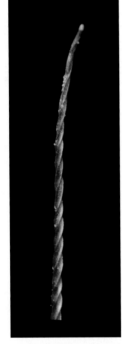

8.105 Deformed hand instrument

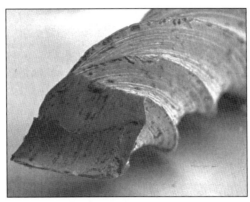

8.106 Fractured K-Flex tip

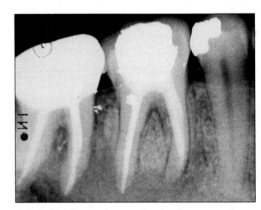

8.107 Ledging and excessive dentine removal

canal. As the instrument is tapered, a greater degree of apical feed ensures an increasing amount of mismatch at any level. Therefore the amount of dentine engaged is a function of the degree of apical feed of the instrument. Many technique manuals erroneously give instructions on the degree of clockwise or anticlockwise rotation without any mention of the degree of apical feed or torque that should be used. As a consequence, rigid pursuit of such instructions may lead to procedural errors. The operator must balance the degree of apical feed with the degree of torque required and this 'knowledge' can only be acquired by vigilant practice. To understand how the instrument cuts dentine in rotary motion, imagine a screw being rotated clockwise into a hole in a piece of wood (**8.104**). As it screws in, it engages the substrate. Rotation in the anticlockwise direction will allow it to unscrew out of the wood. If, however, apical force is applied while the screw is rotated anticlockwise, instead of removing the screw, the 'threads' in the wood are fractured. This is the principle of the *balanced force technique*. Its correct practice

requires an understanding of the torque forces that the instrument and dentine can tolerate. In unpracticed hands, there is a potential for overstressing the metal instrument with its consequent deformation (**8.105**) or fracture (**8.106**) or, alternatively, excessive dentine removal and procedural errors (**8.107**). One way of reducing the amount of force applied in torque is to limit the degree of apical feed and, therefore, the amount of dentine engaged. The file is only fed in until some slight resistance is met, then the file is turned anticlockwise with or without apical force. Rapid cycling clockwise and anticlockwise without heavy torque in a stem-winding or watch-winding motion enables the gentle negotiation of the canal without risk of procedural errors. As in all rotary techniques, the flutes of the instruments should always be cleaned frequently.

Push-pull filing   In contrast, in push-pull filing the entire circumference of the instrument can rarely be engaged for more than one stroke. In this method of cutting, the sharp edges are ideally oriented perpendicular to the direction of file movement. Other than in the situation where the file is *rotated* into engaging the dentine and then pulled (also a valid approach to cutting), push-pull filing requires the application of a lateral or interfacial force to enable the file to engage dentine. This is akin to using a wood-file on a piece of wood. A wood-file held lightly against the wood will remove few wood shavings. Pressing on the wood-file harder will allow it to engage the wood surface more effectively and remove more wood shavings. In the same way an endodontic file is more effective when it is rigid enough to engage dentine when interfacial force is applied. A flexible file will tend to bend away from the dentine surface on application of an interfacial force.

This produces contradictory requirements of a file when a curved canal has to be instrumented because only flexible instruments will negotiate the canal without producing procedural errors. The apical portion of the file, therefore, cannot be controlled effectively without pre-shaping the coronal part of the canal and learning the tactile sensation of what it feels like to engage the tip of the file. In order to control dentine removal along the entire length of the instrument, the interfacial force must be controlled over its entire length. Other strategies to overcome this problem are discussed below.

Design of hand instruments A skilled operator must understand and know the tools(s) he/she uses. The manner of manipulation has to be based on the cutting properties of the instrument. The mode of manufacture, orientation and sharpness of the cutting edges, as well as the response to use and sterilization on the cutting properties, should be aspects the operator should be familiar with.

The root canal instruments available may be manufactured from metal wires of different alloys (stainless steel, carbon steel, titanium, nickel-titanium), cross-sectional shapes and diameters. These alloys have different physical and chemical properties: carbon steel is the most brittle, rigid and susceptible to corrosion; stainless steel is more resilient; titanium is more flexible; and nickel–titanium is the most flexible. The cross-sectional shapes may be square (K-file – **8.108**), triangular (K-reamer – **8.109**), rhomboid (K-Flex-file – **8.110**), circular (Hedstrom file – **8.111**) or S-shaped (Unifile).

These shapes have a bearing on the physical properties of the instruments. The cutting edges may be generated by twisting the metal shaft along its long axis or by machining it. When twisted, the square blank produces the most rigid instrument; the triangular shape is more flexible and the rhomboid more flexible still. When machined, the depth of cut used to produce the flutes dictates the flexibility and strength of the instrument. The rake angle thus produced, influences the optimal mode of use (rotational or push-pull). Machined instruments generally tend to be more susceptible to fracture.

Twisted instruments These instruments are designed to meet the requirements of the American National Standards Institute (ANSI) for endodontic K-type files and reamers, which lay down the dimensional formulae for size, taper, length of cutting blade and tip angle (**8.112**). A number of companies manufacture instruments to these specifications and include the K-file (Kerr), K-reamer (Kerr), K-Flex file (Kerr), Flexofile (Maillefer) and Zipperer Flexicut (Anteos).

Machined instruments A number of conventional and new generations of instruments are machined. Only the H-type instrument is governed by the ANSI specification (No. 58) (**8.113**). Several companies manufacture H-files all of which have different designs and properties despite the specification. The H-file is manufactured from a blank of circular cross-section. The flutes are produced by machining a single helix into the metal stock, producing a series of intersecting cones which increase in size from tip to handle (**8.114**).

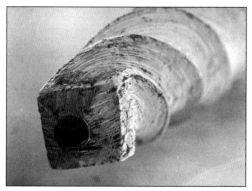

8.108 Kerr K-file No. 25

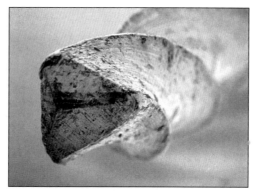

8.109 Kerr K-reamer No. 25

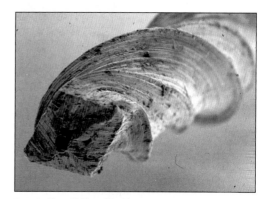

8.110 Kerr K-Flex file No. 25

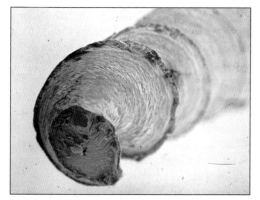

8.111 Kerr Hedstroem No. 25

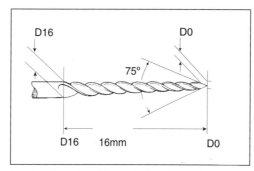

8.112 Dimensional formula for files and reamers: D = diameter

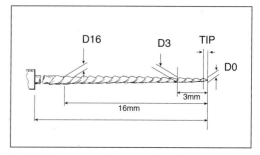

8.113 Dimensional formula of an H-type instrument (ANSI specification No. 58: D = diameter)

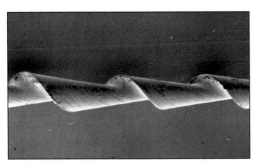

8.114 Bayer Hedstrom No. 25

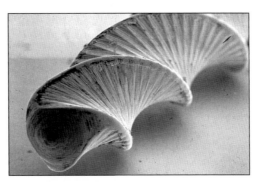

8.115 Flex R-file No. 25

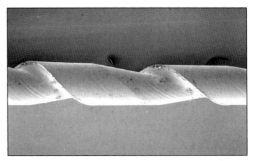

8.116 McSpadden engine-driven nickel–titanium file No. 25

The depth of flute or the residual bulk of metal in the central portion of the file determines the strength and flexibility of the instrument. The blades thus formed are virtually at right angles to the dentine surface and so the most efficient cutting motion is a pulling stroke; no dentine will be removed by the push stroke. Rotating the instrument with the tip of the instrument engaged in dentine is a common cause of its fracture.

Other examples of machined instruments include the Flex-R file (8.115). Although machined, it resembles a conventional K-type file. The Heliapical, Canal Master, Light Speed and Sonic shaper instruments are other examples of machined instruments. Nickel–titanium instruments are also all machined. This is because they cannot be twisted, given their structural memory (8.116).

Mechanical preparation of the radicular access by automated devices

Most operators are attracted by the idea of using an automated instrument that will make root canal preparation easier and quicker. Many automated devices have been introduced onto the market through the years and we have seen reciprocal, vertical, and random movement and both sonic and ultrasonic oscillation. Nickel–titanium rotaries (non ISO taper) since their introduction in 1995 have taken an increasing share of the market. There are many advantages to these instruments but many improvements are still necessary before they will have universal acceptance. The reason why nickel–titanium has been chosen is that it is five-times more flexible and more resistant to fracture when compared to stainless steel.

In the final radiograph of a root filling, where the preparation has been carried out with nickel–titanium rotaries, the walls of the root canals look smooth and show a gradual even taper but this may be, in part, due to the action of a rotating file packing debris into the crevices. The importance of removing microorganisms and debris is paramount, so a system that uses both a reciprocating and oscillating movement may be more appropriate (Endo-Eze manufactured by Ultradent). Such a movement may be able to clean the asymmetric shapes found in root canals more effectively.

Table 8.1 shows the advantages and disadvantages of rotaries over hand instrumentation.

Table 8.1 Nickel-titanium rotary instruments

Advantages	Disadvantages
• A gradual evenly tapered radicular access is produced in the root canal system that facilitates its obturation • Fewer instruments are required to achieve the desired shape • It takes less time to shape the radicular access into the root canal system • Using the instruments in a hand-piece allows better vision particularly with the small headed hand-pieces now available	• Attempting to negotiate narrow curved (especially double curved) canals, without preparing a pilot channel with hand instruments will cause instrument fracture • Fracture may occur unexpectedly without any sign of permanent deformation • More expensive than stainless steel • Become dull quicker than stainless steel • Shape memory makes it more difficult to access root canals in posterior teeth and to negotiate acute curves and double curves

Nickel–titanium rotary instruments

There are many different nickel–titanium rotary instruments available on the market. The first generation had many design faults, but better designs are gradually appearing. All of these instruments are prone to fracture and most are technique sensitive. Nickel–titanium rotaries require a light touch, with a slow in and out movement within the canal and must be run at the recommended speed.

All the nickel–titanium rotaries are machined by computer-controlled grinders from a round blank, which allows complicated designs to be manufactured. The original concept was to produce a screw type design similar to a wood screw but with radial lands (8.117).

Radial lands In the first generation of instruments the radial lands were spaced equally apart so that when the instrument rotated it tended to be pulled into the root canal. The result was that the apical portion of the instrument bound in the root canal and increased the chance of fracture. Breaking up the screw design by

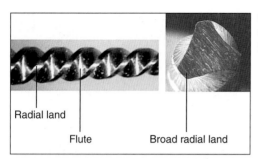

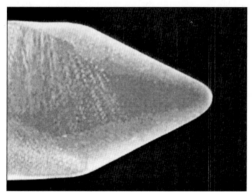

8.117 Early design for nickel–titanium rotaries

Radial land

Flute   Broad radial land

8.118 Non-end-cutting or safety tip

Flutes   The flute is the cut-away portion of the shank in between the radial lands. Debris removed from the canal or cut from the wall lies within the flutes. If the flutes become tightly packed with debris while the instrument is rotating there is an increased chance of fracture. The design of the shape of the flute is important. A gradual increase in the depth of the flutes from the tip of the instrument up the shank means that when the instrument is rotating the debris will be forced into the larger flute spaces. Debris is, therefore, removed from the root canal.

Safety tip   The majority of nickel–titanium instruments have been designed so that they do not cut at the tip (**8.118**). It is obvious that if the tip had an aggressive cutting action the instrument would tend to cut into the wall of the root canal when a curve was reached.

Figures **8.119–8.130** show both side views and cross-sections of Profile, Quantec, K3, Hero, Pro Taper, and RaCe nickel-titanium rotary instruments.

Initially, the disadvantage of automated instruments is the loss of tactile sense but with time and practice this can be acquired. It has been demonstrated that experience results in fewer instrument fractures and better-shaped canals. The tactile skills required are different from those required for hand instruments. Which automated device is 'best' is a matter of personal preference.

Preparation of the radicular access in curved canals

The controlled, regularly tapered, radicular access preparation in curved canals is the ultimate challenge in endodontics. Many ingenious strategies have been devised to enable the achievement of this goal using rigid metal instruments.

The majority were devised to overcome the problem of uneven preferential contact during push-pull filing. The advent of the rotational mode of instrument manipulation and the flexibility of non-ISO-taper nickel–titanium instruments have revolutionized the approach to *negotiation* and *shaping* of curved canals, respectively. Hand-instrumentation skills are still a requisite feature of root canal treatment because of the need to negotiate and prepare acutely and

varying the distances between the radial lands reduced the screw-in effect and helped to prevent breakage. The wide radial land, although providing more metal and therefore strength behind the cutting edge, also increased the area of metal in contact with the wall of the canal. To reduce friction against the wall the radial land may be relieved (see **8.121**). A more recent approach has been to reduce the width of the radial land to just a cutting edge, which further reduces the frictional resistance against the wall of the canal. Several manufacturers have produced a triangular cross-section; one of them adding an alternating cutting edge (see RaCe **8.124**). A coke bottle effect has also been devised where the diameter of the instrument varies in a waveform up the shank to reduce resistance with the wall.

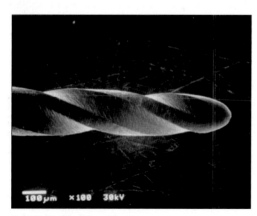

8.119 Profile GT – side view

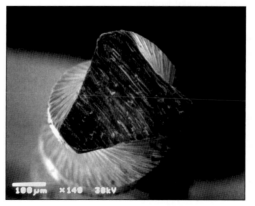

8.120 This instrument has been based on the original ProFile so it shows wide radial lands

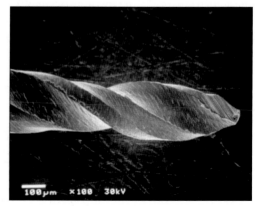

8.121 The Quantec – side view

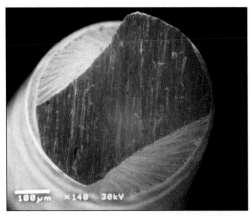

8.122 The Quantec has two radial lands which are relieved to reduce friction against the root canal wall

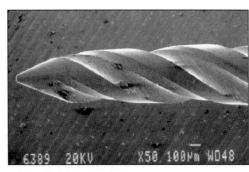

8.123 The K3 – side view

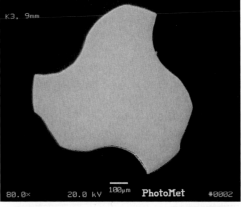

8.124 The K3 shows three radial lands in cross-section, two of which are relieved. The flutes increase in depth towards the top of the shank, the shallower flutes near the tip impart additional strength to the instrument. The radial lands are spaced at varying distances apart reducing the pull-in effect.

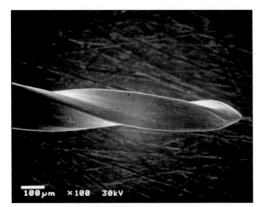

8.125 The Hero – side view

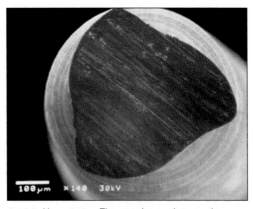

8.126 Hero 642 – The numbers relate to the tapers. The coronal and middle portion of the canal is prepared to 06 and 04 taper respectively and the apical portion to 02. Note narrow radial lands

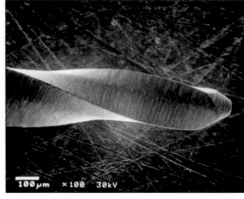

8.127 Pro Taper – side view

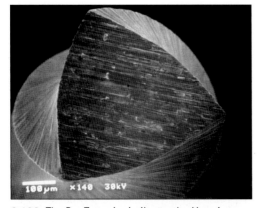

8.128 The Pro Taper is similar to the Hero in cross-section. It has a variable taper along the shank. The cutting action is fairly aggressive

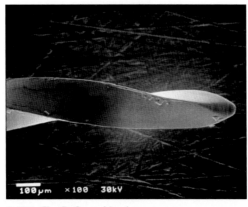

8.129 The RaCe – side view

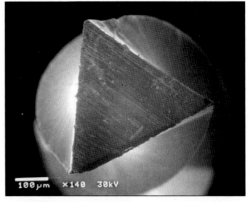

8.130 RaCe stands for reamer with alternating cutting edge. The alternating cutting edge reduces the tendency for the instrument to be pulled into the canal. The instrument cuts aggressively and may make a clicking sound when being used

double-curved canals. Automated instrumentation may facilitate easier shaping of canals. It is therefore necessary to be aware of how to maintain canal curvatures using both modes of instrument manipulation. Although in theory rotational manipulation of instruments should enable more effective maintenance of canal curvatures, the authors have witnessed that those with established *filing* habits may find it difficult to adapt to rotary skills. Clearly a different set of tactile skills is required.

Maintaining curvature with a push-pull filing mode of instrument manipulation

As already described, the only situation in which *even* dentine removal can be guaranteed during filling is when the file engages tightly around its entire circumference (**8.131**). However, immediately after the first stroke and thereafter with each subsequent stroke, the file becomes loose and a lateral force has to be applied to the file in numerous different directions (traversing 360°) as the file is moved circumferentially around the canal (**8.132**). Once the file is loose in a curved canal, however, its natural tendency to straighten up will only allow preferential contact at certain points along its

length (**8.133**). These points are predictably at the outer aspect of the major curve apical to the curve, on the inner aspect of the curve at the height of the curve and either at the inner curve or outer curve coronal to the curve depending upon the direction in which the lateral force is applied. The contacts result in procedural errors such as ledging (**8.134**), zipping (**8.135**), transportation of apical foramen (**8.136, 8.137**), and perforation (**8.138, 8.139**). Strategies to avoid such uneven preferential contacts involve ways of reducing them. There are two elements to such uncontrolled dentine removal:

- the file contacts areas apical to the curve with sufficient interfacial force to cut dentine purely as a result of its tendency to straighten to its normal shape;
- it is difficult to control dentine removal along the entire length of the file during push-pull filing.

These problems may be overcome by:

- reducing the restoring force with which straight files tend to lean against the curved dentine surface;
- reducing the length of the file that is actively cutting at any given time.

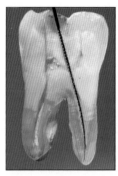

8.131 File fitting tightly in the canal

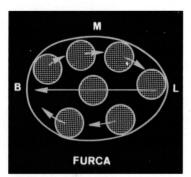

8.132 Circumferential filing: anticurvature filing: 3 × on B, M, L; 1 × furca

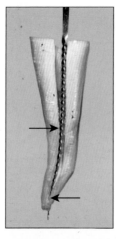

8.133 File fitting loosely in the canal

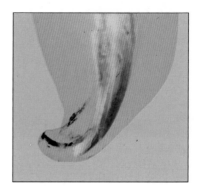

8.134 Ledging

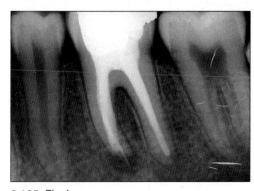

8.135 Zipping

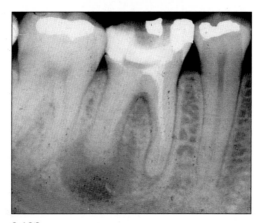

8.136

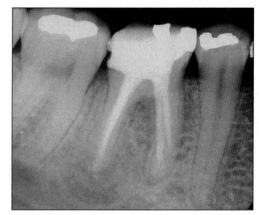

8.137

8.136–8.137 Transportation of the apical foramen

Reducing the restoring force This can be achieved in a number of ways:

1. *Pre-curving the file* – the restoring force may be reduced by achieving a closer match in the curvature of the instrument with that of the canal. Assuming that an accurate match is obtained, this match is true only in one position (**8.140**). The greater the amplitude of the filing stroke the greater the mismatch at the extremes of the filing stroke. The amplitude, therefore, must

also be reduced. Files may be precurved by using a cotton wool roll or using commercial devices (**8.141, 8.142**). The curve perpendicular to the X-ray beam is estimated from the radiograph and any curve in the planes parallel to the X-ray beam must be estimated by tactile sense and the curvature on initial explorer files (**8.143–8.145**). Files that are to be used at different lengths in the canal relative to the curvature should be appropriately precurved (**8.146**).

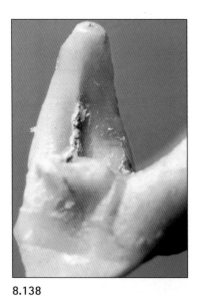

8.138

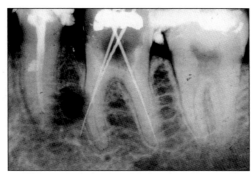

8.139

8.138–8.139 Perforation

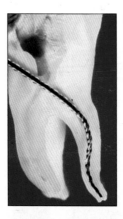

8.140
Precurved file matches canal curvature in only one position

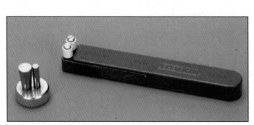

8.141

8.141–8.142 Commercially available devices for precurving files

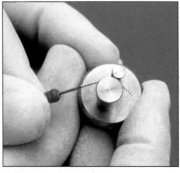

8.142

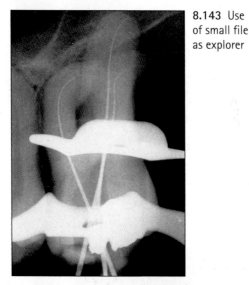

8.143 Use of small file as explorer

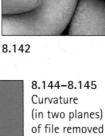

8.144

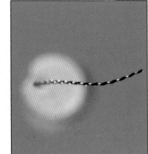

8.145

8.144–8.145 Curvature (in two planes) of file removed from the mesiobuccal canal in 8.143

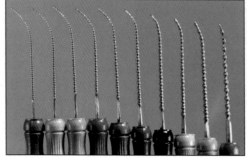

8.146 Files are precurved at different levels depending on the depth of insertion into the canal

2. *Use of flexible files* – the restoring force in more flexible files is naturally lower. Some makes of instruments are more flexible by virtue of their cross-section shape (**8.147, 8.148**) or material of construction such as nickel–titanium.

3. *Greater use of smaller files* – smaller instruments (size 20 and below) are more flexible and so their use until larger instruments are able to negotiate without force may reduce adverse dentine removal (**8.149, 8.150**).

4. *Use of intermediate sized files* – The transition from one file to the next can also be made easier by the use of half sizes,

e.g. sizes 12, 17, 22, 27 and 32 (**8.151**). This reduces the force required to negotiate the files apically and also the probability of procedural errors.

Reducing the length or area of file actively engaged in cutting
This can be achieved in a number of ways:

1. *Modified canal preparation techniques* – preparing the coronal part of the canal first in a corono-apical or crown-down approach removes coronal binding and allows more controlled preparation of the apical part of the canal with the apical part of the file (**8.152, 8.153**).

2. *Modified manipulation of instruments* – the manner in which the instruments are manipulated can allow a restricted part of the canal or instrument to be engaged, increasing the control over dentine removal.
   - *Anticurvature filing* – denotes filing preferentially away from the inner curve or furcal aspect of the root canal, the site of potential perforation (**8.154–8.156**). This method, which

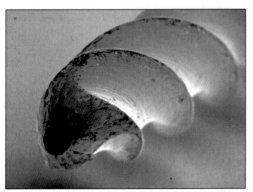

8.147 Maillefer 'Golden Medium' No. 27

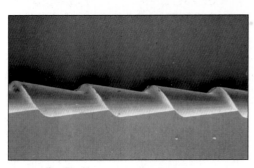

8.148 Girofile No. 25

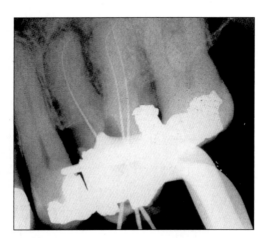

8.149

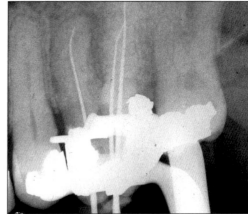

8.150

8.149–8.150 Loss of length caused by forcing large instruments into canals too early

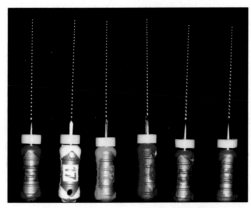

8.151 'Golden medium' intermediate files (12, 17, 22, 27, 32, 37)

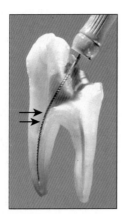

8.152

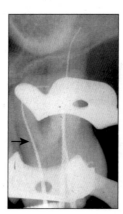

8.153

8.152–8.153 Preflaring allows more direct apical access

involves filing the buccal, mesial and lingual walls of the root canal with more strokes than the furcal wall by a ratio of 3 : 1, is effective (**8.132**). However, simply following the prescription without regard for tactile feedback, flexibility of the file and controlled manipulation of the file will render it ineffective. The technique does not work with files that are too flexible and a degree of straightening may be inevitable (**8.157**).

● *Modified use of files* – files may be used in such a way that their area of contact is reduced. For example, in the crown-down-pressure-less technique, only the tips of the instruments are used for cutting. The file is placed in the canal until it binds (**8.158**) and is then rotated twice without apical pressure to remove dentine at this point.

3. *Modified instruments* – the idea of only using the apical part of instruments has been extended by the development of instruments that have cutting edges only in their apical part, such as Light Speed (**8.159**). These instruments are particularly useful for gauging the apical size of the canal.

Maintaining curvature with a rotational mode of hand instrument manipulation

The mechanics of rotational action of hand instruments were described before. The approach is inherently conducive to maintenance of canal curvatures. However, this cannot be taken for granted. It is possible for some operators to lose control and straighten curved canals even with this technique (**8.160**). Furthermore, operators

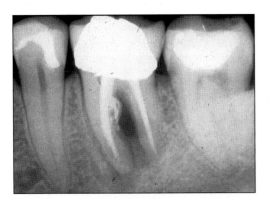

8.154 Severe strip perforation

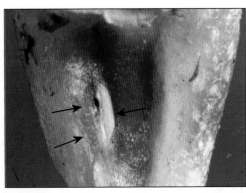

8.155 Furcal view of mesial root of extracted tooth

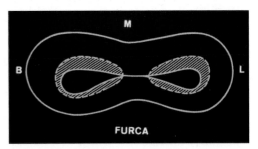

8.156 Cross-section of a mesial root. Ideal removal of dentine during preparation (shaded area): B = buccal; M = mesial; L = lingual

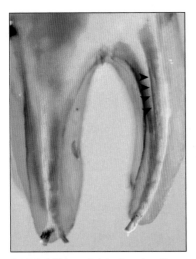

8.157 Mild straightening despite anticurvature filing

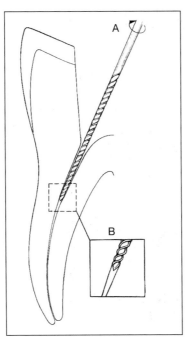

8.158 Modified use of files: A = circular movement of file; B = only the tip of the instrument engages and cuts dentine

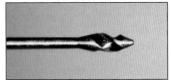

8.159 Light Speed instrument tip

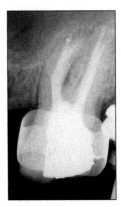

8.160 Loss of canal curvature in mesiobuccal root of maxillary molar using a rotational technique

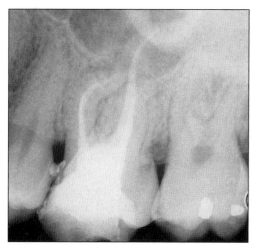

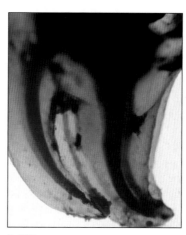

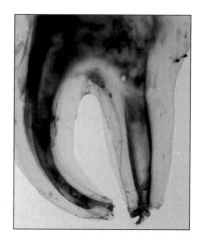

8.161 Mesiobuccal canal with narrowly tapered radicular access

8.163   **8.164**

8.163–8.164 Prepared and filled root canals with curvature maintained

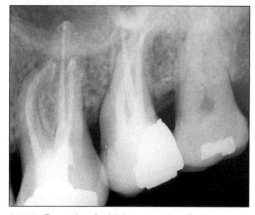

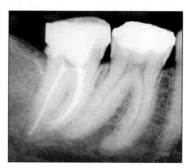

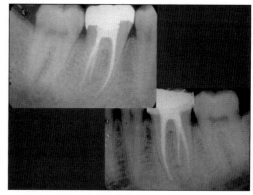

8.162 Example of widely tapered radicular access

8.165   **8.166**

8.165–8.166 Radiographs of treated case where the natural canal contour has been maintained

often have to practice the method to achieve satisfactory canal widening. When minimal instrumentation is performed, the tendency is to produce narrowly tapered radicular access cavities (**8.161**). However, some operators are able to produce widely tapered radicular access cavities using supposedly identical protocols (**8.162**). The difference lies in the degree of instrument manipulation and the amount of apical feed and force used. Unlike the filing technique, the numbers of variables that require control are limited. They are:

- degree of apical feed of the instrument (synonymous with degree of rotation when visualized as feeding a screw into a hole);
- frequency of clockwise and anticlockwise rotation (without or with apical pressure on anticlockwise rotation – file may rotate out, stay at the same level or be pushed further apically);
- the degree of apical pressure accompanying the anticlockwise torque affects the degree of dentine cutting;
- the degree of rotational torque (in both clockwise and anticlockwise rotation) affects the depth of dentine cut.

These are all inter-related quantities. A combination of aggressive apical feed and rotational torque, especially with larger rigid instruments can lead to loss of curvature in the radicular access.

The degree of widening is controlled by the size of the instrument used, as well as the degree of manipulation (rotational cycling).

A combination of any of the above strategies may be used to prepare radicular access cavities that maintain the original curvature of the root canals (**8.163–8.166**).

Maintenance of double curves

Root canal systems often contain main canals that exhibit two or more curvatures. Most of the time the second curves are not visible because they occur within the plane of the X-ray beam. The operator tends to act on the curve visible from the radiograph but will ignore the other plane. Therefore when the filing technique is used that curve may be straightened and if the root dentine is thin it may

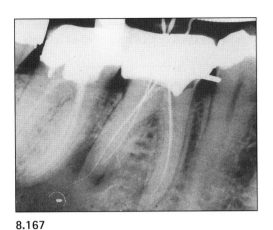

8.167

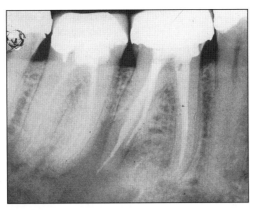

8.168

8.167–8.168 Straightening coronal curve in the distal root

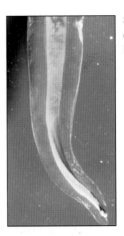

8.171 Curvature in opposite directions in the same plane

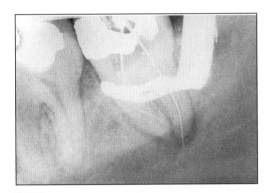

8.169

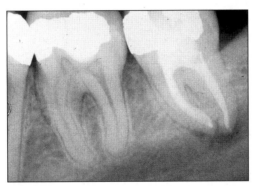

8.170

8.169–8.170 Straightening apical curve on the mesial root

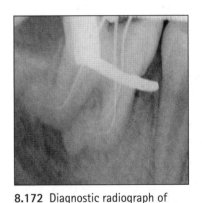

8.172 Diagnostic radiograph of severe curves in two planes

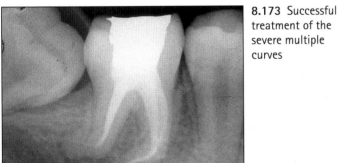

8.173 Successful treatment of the severe multiple curves

result in a strip perforation in the furcation. The use of a rotational technique is more likely to retain the curve.

Sometimes the double canal curvatures will be evident in the same radiographic plane. These are difficult to maintain using a filing technique. Either the coronal (**8.167, 8.168**) or apical curve (**8.169, 8.170**) may be straightened. The preparation of such curves with automated nickel–titanium rotary instruments is only possible if the curves are gentle (**8.171**). When more severe curves in two planes are present, only hand instrumentation with a rotational technique will achieve the desired result (**8.172, 8.173**). The size of the taper will have to be limited but greater reliance should be placed on the chemical preparation.

Gauging the taper of the radicular access

The ability to prepare a well and regularly tapered radicular access is based on two factors:

- knowing when to stop using a given instrument. Under-use of an instrument may leave the taper too narrow and over-use, too wide;
- knowing how to gauge the canal taper.

Gauging the canal taper is the most under-rated aspect of learning to prepare canal systems to a consistent and predictable shape. Unlike the taper of a crown preparation, that of the canal cannot be seen. It can only be *felt* using a series of instruments. Gauging a radicular access cavity, therefore, means placing accurately measured instruments into the radicular access and *feeling* the tightness or looseness at its appropriate length. In order to prepare a regular taper, it is essential that each instrument at its respective length (whether 1 mm or 0.5 mm step-back) *feels* loose or tight by exactly the same amount.

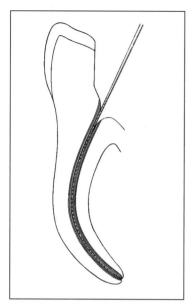

8.174 Apical-coronal preparation techniques

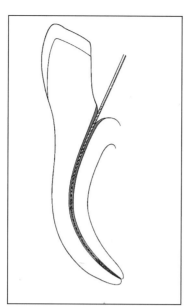

8.175 Coronal-apical preparation techniques

Colour code for file sizes:
Purple = 10, White = 15, Yellow = 20, Red = 25, Blue = 30, Green = 35, Black = 40, White = 45, Yellow = 50, Red = 55.

The design of the Light Speed instrument lends itself very well to canal gauging.

The advent of non-ISO taper nickel–titanium instruments with a predetermined taper has meant that a single instrument, that is, the one used to finish the entire radicular preparation can be used to gauge the canal taper. However, if the same instrument is over-used, the same problem of loss of taper control may arise even with these instruments.

Recommended approach to preparing the radicular access

There are an almost infinite number of techniques to prepare the radicular access cavity. Various strategies have been invented to help dentists to learn how they reach the end-point of preparation. The techniques have been divided into two groups:

- apico-coronal techniques (e.g. standardized, step-back techniques) (**8.174**);
- corono-apical techniques (e.g. step-down, double flared, crown-down-pressureless techniques) (**8.175**).

These simply describe the order in which instruments are used to prepare either the coronal part of the canal first or the apical part first (though together with the coronal part).

The preparation of the radicular access is divided into three phases:

1. *Preparation of coronal flare* to the beginning of the canal curve or to two-thirds the estimated length of the canal.

8.176–8.180 Coronal preflaring – progressive enlargement at same length using a push-pull filing motion and refined by planing motion of rotating Gates Gidden drills

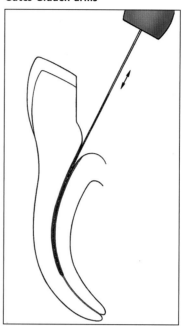

8.176 File with size 10 to 16–18 mm or beginning of the curve

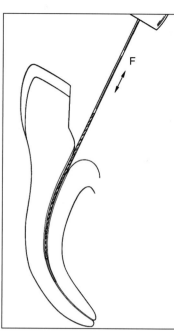

8.177 File using Hedstrom size 15 to same length: F = filing

2. *Negotiation* of hand instruments to the full canal length after accurate confirmation of the length, using a rotational mode of manipulation. Preferably a gentle stem-winding technique.
3. *Final shaping* to achieve a regular taper.

Coronal preflaring

The benefits of coronal preflaring are usually quoted as follows:

- it allows early debridement of the coronal part of the canal that contains the bulk of organic and microbial debris, reducing the risk of carrying this material to the apical end and its extrusion through the apical foramen;
- early coronal widening enables better and deeper penetration of irrigant early in the preparation, which reduces the risk of apical blockage with dentine mud and pulp tissue;
- preparation of the coronal portion of the canal tends to shorten the effective canal length and determining the working length after such enlargement will reduce the problem of its alteration during preparation;
- it allows better control over apical instrumentation.

The preflaring can be achieved in any one of a number of ways according to personal preference. One approach is by filing the coronal part of the canal using either Hedstrom or K-type files and then refining with Gates Glidden drills as in the step-down technique (**8.176–8.180**). It is important to maintain patency beyond the point of instrumentation.

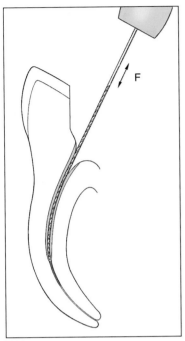

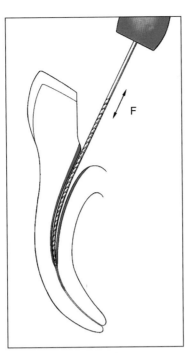

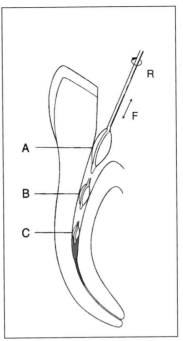

8.178 Hedstrom file size 20 to 16–18 mm: F = filing motion

8.179 Hedstrom file size 25 to 16–18 mm: F = filing motion

8.180 Refine coronal flare with Gates Glidden drill sizes 1–3 used in a planing motion: A = Gates Glidden 3; B = Gates Glidden 2; C = Gates Glidden 1: R = rotational motion

8.181–8.184 Coronal preflaring – using rotational instrument manipulation in a progressive step down approach

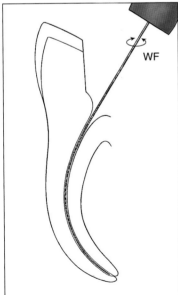

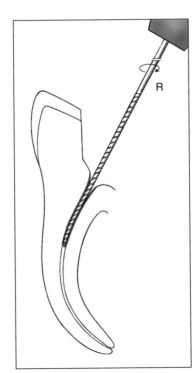

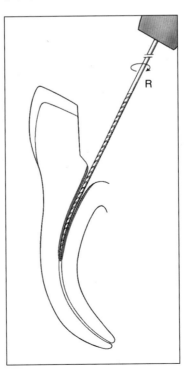

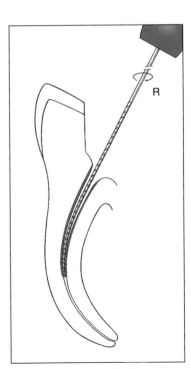

8.181 Introduce small file (No. 10) to full WL to establish patency: WF = without filing

8.182 Instrument to size 35 at about 14 mm: R = rotational motion

8.183 Instrument with file 30 to 1 mm deeper than size 35

8.184 Instrument with size 25 to 1 mm deeper than size 30

The instrumentation may also be performed in a step-down approach using rotational manipulation to achieve a similar result, as in the double-flare technique (**8.181–8.184**).

Alternatively, the coronal part of the canal may be opened and flared with nickel–titanium orifice openers or rotary instruments (**8.185, 8.186**). This is an efficient and effective means of achieving this goal.

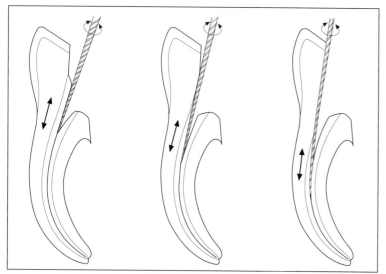

8.185 Coronal flaring achieved using nickel–titanium orifice shapers using a pecking motion; each narrower instrument advancing further than the last

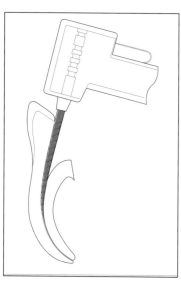

8.186 Coronal flaring achieved using increased taper nickel–titanium rotary instrument; note the desired straightening of the outer curve

Negotiation to the full length of canal

Having preflared the canal, its full length is determined as previously described. The apical part of the canal should now be negotiated with a series of hand instruments of increasing size up to 20, to the full length without deviating from the canal curvature. Again a number of approaches are available but the safest way is to use a gentle stem-winding technique that does not remove excessive amounts of dentine. The instruments may be used in a step-down (**8.188–8.192**) or stepback (**8.193–8.196**) sequence according to preference. Alternatively, nickel–titanium rotary instruments may be used for negotiation of full length of canals (**8.187**). However caution should be exercised if canals are narrow or severely curved.

Where the canal system is relatively wide at the outset and does not require negotiation as such, the apical part of the canal should be gauged to determine its size after length determination. The process of shaping may then be commenced directly, bypassing the negotiation step.

Final shaping of the radicular access

This may be achieved by using hand instruments to gauge the canal taper in a stepback filing approach (**8.197–8.202**) or a stepback rotational motion approach (**8.203–8.208**). Alternatively, the instruments may be used in step-down fashion.

Another option is to use nickel–titanium rotary instruments for final shaping of the radicular access (**8.209**).

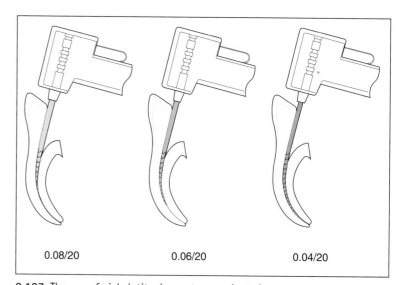

0.08/20   0.06/20   0.04/20

8.187 The use of nickel–titanium rotary graduated tapers

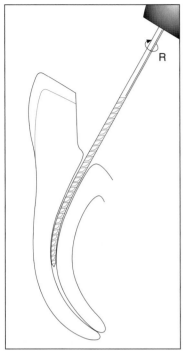

8.188 Size 40

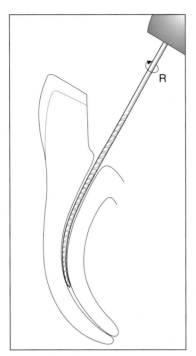

8.189 Size 35

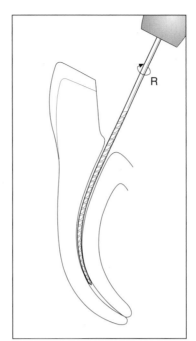

8.190 Size 30

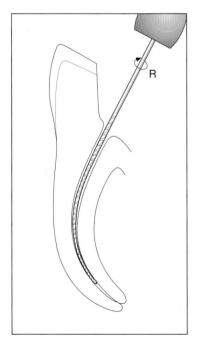

8.191 Size 25

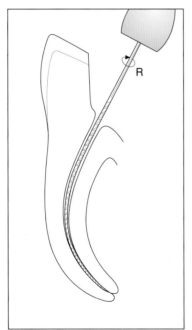

8.192 Size 20 at full WL. Apical enlargement may be continued to desired size by adopting another 'wave' of instrumentation starting with a larger sized instrument

8.188–8.192 Negotiation of full length of canal: using step-down rotational instrumentation

8.193–8.196 Negotiation of full length of canal: using the 'stepback' or apico-coronal rotational approach

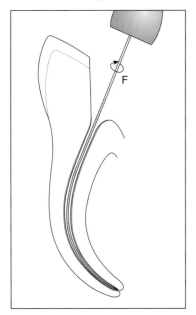

8.193 File with size 10 to WL

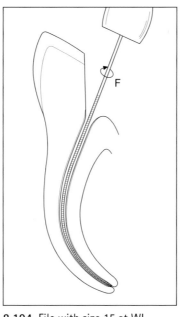

8.194 File with size 15 at WL

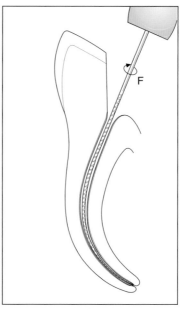

8.195 File with size 20 at WL

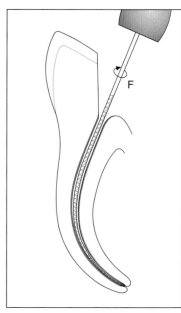

8.196 File with size 25 at WL

8.197–8.202 Final shaping of canal: stepback filing approach

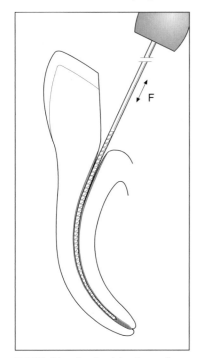

8.197 Stepping back by 1 mm from WL at size 30

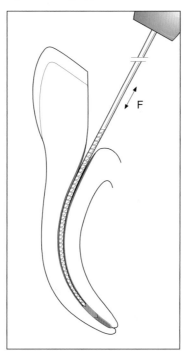

8.198 Stepping back by 2 mm from WL at size 35

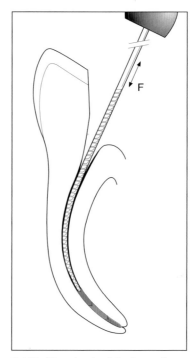

8.199 Stepping back by 3 mm from WL at size 40

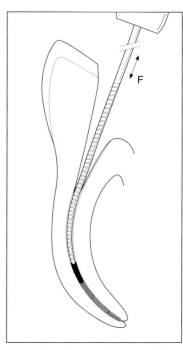

8.200 Stepping back by 4 mm from WL at size 45

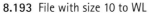

8.203–8.208 Final shaping of canal: using the stepback rotational approach

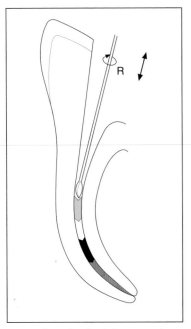

8.201 Stepping back by 5 mm from WL at size 50

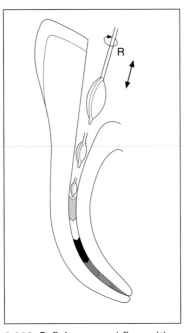

8.202 Refining coronal flare with Gates Glidden if necessary

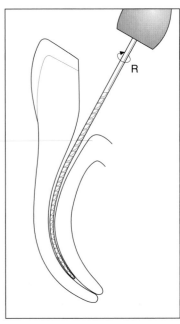

8.203 Size 25 at full WL

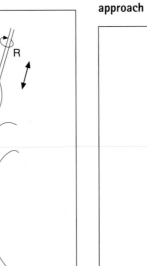

8.204 Size 30

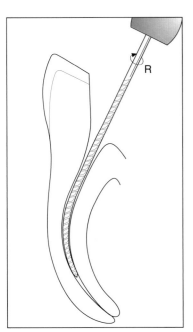

8.205 Size 35

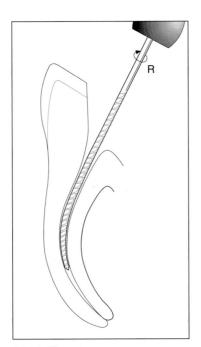

8.206 Size 40

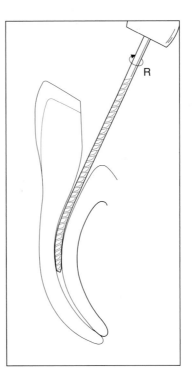

8.207 Size 45

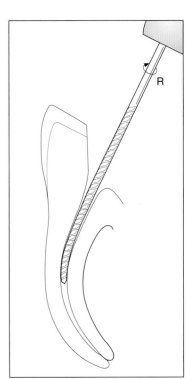

8.208 Size 50

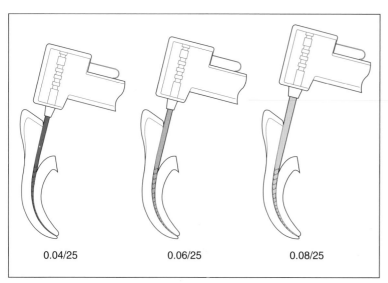

0.04/25   0.06/25   0.08/25

8.209 The use of rotary nickel–titanium instruments to achieve final shaping

Chemical preparation of root canal systems

This phase of root canal system preparation, of course, does not begin as a separate step to that of the mechanical phase. Both commence at the same time but are described separately purely for the convenience of describing them. The purpose of the radicular access cavity is to facilitate delivery of the antibacterial irrigants that will help to debride the uninstrumented surfaces free of the microbial biofilm. In order that access to the entire root canal system is maintained during the radicular access preparation, the dentine filings, chips and pulp debris generated must be flushed out of the system. The debris generated during instrumentation may be pushed into the accessory anatomy, through the apical foramen or, preferably, flushed out of the coronal access. Preflaring enables easier delivery of the irrigant but the selection of a good delivery system and good wetting characteristics of the irrigant are also important. The solution should be delivered using a hypodermic needle and syringe (**8.210**). In most canals, preparation is required to achieve placement of the needle tip near the apical part of the canal (**8.15, 8.16**). However, in some canals, apical delivery may be limited by various factors even after preparation, for example in severely curved canals or the example in **Figures 8.211 and 8.212**. A narrow-gauge needle (27) is recommended for deeper irrigant placement (**8.213**). Use of a smaller needle may slow injection and make control difficult because of the force required to extrude it. Some space is required adjacent to the needle to prevent extrusion through the apical foramen (**8.214**). Several needle designs are available to resolve the problem; most include a perforation in the side of the needle shank (**8.215**). Despite these aids, replacing irrigant in the apical portion of the canal system may be difficult, yet it is *most important*. A strategy for ensuring that irrigant replacement takes place apically is called '*recapitulation*.' This is illustrated in **Figures 8.216–8.219**. *This is about the single most important aspect of canal preparation.*

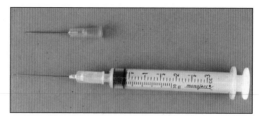

8.210 Hypodermic needle and syringe

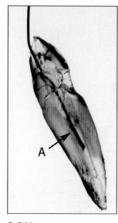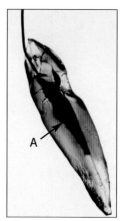

8.211   8.212

8.211–8.212 Hypodermic needle in cleared canine tooth: A = irrigant

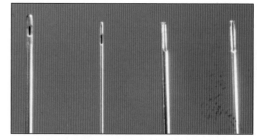

8.213 Different gauges of needle are available in all types

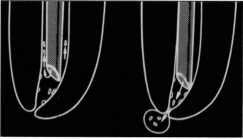

8.214 Needle binding encourages extrusion of irrigant

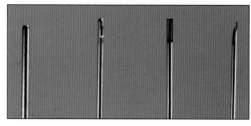

8.215 Needle designs

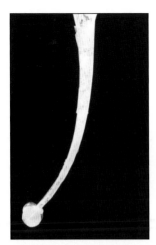

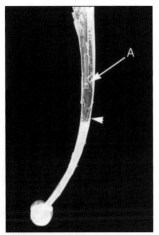

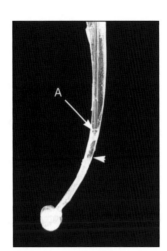

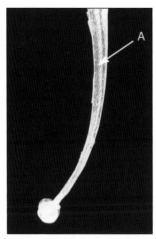

8.216 Canal containing dentine-saturated irrigant

8.217 Fresh irrigant replaces coronal saturated irrigant (arrowed): A = needle tip

8.218 Deeper needle placement allows deeper replacement of irrigant (arrowed): A = needle tip

8.219 Recapitulation to mix apical dentine-saturated irrigant with coronal fresh irrigant: A = small file

As the canal is instrumented, more and more dentine debris is generated which will be loosely suspended in the irrigant fluid in the canal system (**8.216**). As it becomes saturated, the dentine may start to form a 'dentine mud' that has the potential to block the canal apically and the exits to accessory anatomy. The irrigant fluid must, therefore, be replaced frequently. As preparation of the apical portion of the canal nears completion it is necessary to mix the fresh coronal solution with the saturated apical solution in order to dilute it (**8.219**). This process of dilution is called recapitulation and simply involves placing a small file (size 8 or 10) in the canal to its full length and agitating it.

Given that the apical anatomy may contain several apical exits in a delta, it is important that the entrance to it is not blocked. It is therefore considered prudent to pass a small file (size 8) just beyond the apical foramen to ensure its patency. This is called *patency filing*. It also allows the periapical status of infection and inflammation to be gauged by virtue of the presence of pus or exudate. Blocked apical foramina at the first appointment is the same as single visit obturation even though the root filling may not have been placed. Both recapitulation and patency filing should be performed frequently.

Functions of the irrigant

These may be considered to be as follows:

- lubrication of the instruments;
- flushing out of root canal debris;
- chemical degradation of residual pulp tissue;
- chemical degradation of the smear layer on the instrumented surface;
- chemical degradation of the microbial biofilm both on the instrumented and, more importantly, on the uninstrumented surface;
- antibacterial action against the root canal microbial flora.

The first two points have already been discussed and rely on the irrigant having low surface tension so that it wets the instruments, canal surface and debris adequately to allow lubrication and flushing. Specific agents to lubricate instruments and canal walls include EDTA pastes such as RCPrep and File-eze. Other agents, such as Glyoxide or Glyde contain carbamide peroxide (an oxidizing agent).

Degradation of pulp tissue The best solution for degrading pulp tissue is sodium hypochlorite (**8.220–8.223**). These figures show degradation of an extirpated pulp over 10 minutes when the tissue is fully exposed in a large volume container. The access to unreacted sodium hypochlorite is unimpeded. In the root canal system, the access is far more restricted. It is therefore necessary to ensure that unreacted solution reaches the tissue in all parts of the root canal system. This is done through the radicular access, during and after its preparation. Diffusion of unreacted molecules, however, demands very frequent replenishment of the solution in the radicular access. Higher concentration solutions (5%) will enable better diffusion along a gradient but its use must be balanced against the problem of over-weakening the tooth. Concentrations up to 3% are sufficient for antibacterial effect and tissue-degradation effect in most cases. Higher concentrations may be used intermittently in the case of non-responding infections or where canal patency is difficult because of compacted apical debris. Sodium hypochlorite is a caustic solution and has the potential to corrode equipment (**8.224**), bleach clothes and cause a severe reaction if extruded through the apical foramen. A good rubber dam seal must be ensured (**8.225**). It is also prudent to check prior to treatment whether the patient is allergic to household bleach.

Degradation of the smear layer Some operators consider this to be a very important aspect of root canal treatment because the smear layer is thought to harbour bacteria and prevent sufficient adaptation of the root-filling material. There is, however, no definite proof for

8.220–8.223 Dissolution of pulp tissue in sodium hypochlorite immediately after extirpation

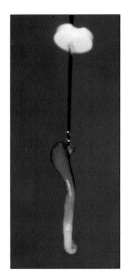

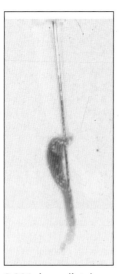

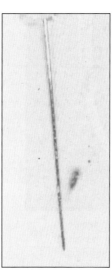

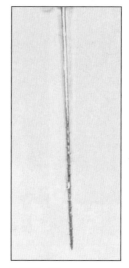

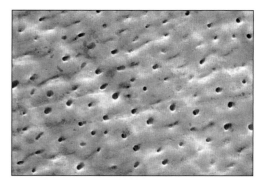

8.220 Extirpated pulp

8.221 Immediately after placement in sodium hypochlorite

8.222 After 5 minutes

8.223 After 10 minutes

8.224 Corrosion of Endosonic handpiece with sodium hypochlorite

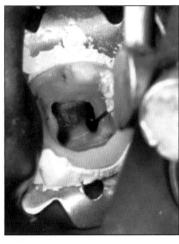

8.225 Well-sealed rubber dam

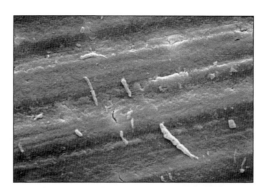

8.226 Smear layer formed by instrumentation

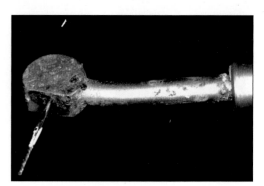

8.227 Smear layer removed

this. Weak organic acids may remove the smear layer. The one recommended is ethylenediamine-tetra-acetic acid (EDTA) 17%. Irrigation with this will help to remove the smear layer if it reaches and reacts with the layer in all parts of the canal (**8.226, 8.227**).

Degradation of the microbial biofilm The microbial biofilm contains an aggregate of microbes and extra-cellular polysaccharide matrix. The two are highly adherent to the canal wall. Given their multiple cellular thickness, biofilm removal is not an easy task. It is certainly facilitated by organic tissue solvents such as sodium hypochlorite and also EDTA. The EDTA helps by chelating and sequestering heavy metal ions which normally act as bridges to bond bacteria together. EDTA is routinely used in microbiology laboratories to wash bacterial cells free of the extracellular polysaccharide and

to separate them. EDTA probably plays an important role in degrading the biofilm on the uninstrumented walls of the root canal system.

Another agent that has recently been considered for its potential to break down bacterial biofilms is electrochemically activated water (ECA). That is, saline water that has been electrolysed under specific conditions to create various hypochlorous ions. A recent study showed ECA to be bactericidal with the ability to remove biofilm. It was not, however, as effective as sodium hypochlorite.

Antibacterial action against the root canal flora Perhaps the most significant action of the irrigant must be its ability to kill all elements of the root canal microbial flora. A number of different antibacterial agents have been used and exhibit a different range of actions against the different bacteria. The agents include:

- sodium hypochlorite – most effective;
- iodine in various solvents, e.g. alcohol or povidone-iodine;
- chlorhexidine – smaller range of action but longer-lasting effect.

Other agents suggested include ozone in gaseous or soluble form and ECA. However, neither of these has shown any comparability with sodium hypochlorite.

As stressed earlier, the agents will reach the radicular access in sufficient concentration but their penetration to the accessory and peripheral anatomy will be restricted by diffusion along a concentration gradient or else bulk flow delivery by agitation with a file or one that is sonically or ultrasonically activated. Once again, constant replenishment by fresh agents is essential as some of the molecules will have reacted and become spent by the time they reach their peripheral site. Replenishment with fresh agents takes time and therefore adequate time should be allowed for the irrigants to act, even if the radicular access preparation has been completed quickly.

If the antibacterial agents reach the bacteria in subinhibitory doses, there is a high chance of inducing resistance to them. This has been demonstrated not only for antibiotics but also for the antiseptic agents mentioned above.

It is clear that although sodium hypochlorite is able to perform most of the tasks and is clearly the favoured irrigant, it may be supplemented by all or some of the other agents according to the individual need of the case. Chemical preparation of the root canal system then begins with the use of a series of chemical agents before, during and after the radicular access preparation. In infected cases, unfortunately, this may not be adequate and the process must continue during the interappointment phase. This aspect of the chemical preparation is described in Chapter 9.

Chapter 9

Intracanal medication and temporary seal

K Gulabivala

INTRACANAL MEDICATION

Since the beginning of the practice of root canal treatment, a variety of chemically active materials have been placed into the root canal space either temporarily (antiseptics and antibiotics) or permanently (formaldehyde-containing materials) for various reasons. Many of these practices were not based on proper rationale. In modern endodontics, the placement of specific chemicals during the inter-appointment period between visits of a multivisit procedure forms part of the chemical preparation of the root canal system prior to placement of a permanent seal by obturation.

Rationale for intracanal medication

The main rationale for using such medication is to help fulfil part of the aim of root canal system preparation, that is to help degrade residual microbial biofilm and organic tissue and to kill remaining bacteria. The medicament should, therefore, also prevent bacterial recolonization of the root canal system, from either those bacteria left behind after preparation or new invaders through lateral communications or the coronal access. In addition it would be useful if the medicament possessed a range of other properties that would suppress pain and facilitate apical healing. A root canal medicament should therefore ideally:

1. Be able to kill all root canal bacteria.
2. Have long-lasting antibacterial effect.
3. Not be inactivated by the presence of organic material.
4. Be able to help degrade residual organic tissue.
5. Be able to help degrade residual microbial biofilm.
6. Not be irritating to periapical tissues or have systemic toxicity.
7. Be able to induce regeneration of periapical tissues.
8. Not affect the physical properties of the temporary access cavity restoration.
9. Not be able to diffuse through the temporary seal.
10. Be easily placed and removed.
11. Be radiopaque.
12. Have anodyne properties.
13. Not stain the tooth.

No single root canal medicament has proved capable of meeting all of these requirements and it is therefore not surprising that a vast range of different materials have been tried. Many agents have been tried empirically or in laboratory tests only. There is little clinical research on the efficacy of most of these, and use of particular materials tends to be propagated on the basis of personal preference. The vast array of materials may be divided for analysis into groups of like chemical structures and mode of function.

PHENOL-BASED AGENTS

These, which were once the most commonly used agents, include phenol, parachlorophenol, camphorated parachlorophenol, camphorated monoparachlorophenol, metacresyl acetate, cresol, creosote, eugenol and thymol. Gradually over the years more dilute solutions have been adopted but the antibacterial efficacy was based only on laboratory tests that did not involve biofilm phenotypes. The laboratory tests generally involved intimate contact between the agent and the planktonic phenotype of the bacteria, thereby allowing effective killing. It is, however, difficult to achieve such intimate contact in the root-canal environment where the bacteria may also be embedded in a biofilm matrix. A pledget of cotton wool soaked in the solution and placed in the pulp chamber is not sufficient. The characteristic strong-smelling vapours are not concentrated enough to kill bacteria. The solutions are only likely to kill bacteria when used in sufficient volume and concentration; by flooding the canals. Furthermore, their antibacterial effect is not long lasting. These solutions are also able to diffuse through the temporary filling material and cause a bad taste in the mouth while some even soften the filling material.

Phenol and camphorated monochlorophenol (CMCP)

Pure phenol was not used much because of its toxicity but its chemical modification monochlorophenol was adopted because of its lower toxicity and improved bactericidal effect. A solution of CMCP may be made by dissolving monochlorophenol crystals in camphor.

Metacresyl acetate or cresatin

This has been favoured by some clinicians because it was thought to have low irritation potential and anodyne action but the latter is unproven. These materials are now largely out of favour because of their limited antibacterial effect (in both range and duration), toxicity and absence of other positive features. However, they continue to be used in by some operators.

ALDEHYDES

These materials (formaldehyde-containing preparations, formocresol, gluteraldehyde) have mainly been used in paedodontics, and their efficacy in this aspect is covered in Chapter 17. They have no role in the treatment of permanent teeth. Formaldehyde-containing materials have been used for their antimicrobial and fixative properties but they are very toxic to the periradicular tissues and, furthermore, fixed tissue is potentially antigenic.

Gluteraldehyde also has the potential to cause hypersensitivity.

HALIDES

These include sodium hypochlorite, iodine-potasium-iodide, and a combination of iodine and calcium hydroxide preparation (Vitapex®).

Sodium hypochlorite fulfils the most important criteria of antibacterial effect and tissue dissolution, but its efficacy as a medicament is limited because chemical reaction depletes its effect rapidly. In addition, since the canal would need to be flooded there may be an interaction with the temporary filling material.

Iodine-potassium iodide has low toxicity and good antibacterial effect *in vitro*. It is easily made by mixing 4 g of potassium iodide with 2 g of iodine and 94 mL of water. The canal needs to be flooded but its long-term effectiveness is not known. It has probably not gained favour because of its potential for allergic responses and tooth staining.

Vitapex® is a recently introduced medicament with little information from controlled clinical studies. It appears to combine the best effects of iodoform and calcium hydroxide. Its support is currently mainly anecdotal.

ANTIBIOTICS

Because of a few uniquely favourable properties, topical application of antibiotics (such as bacitracin, neomycin, polymixin, chloramphenicol, tyrothricin and nystatin) in the root canal has been popular with some clinicians. The substances are not toxic to the periapical tissues, do not stain teeth and are active in the presence of organic material. Since no single antibiotic is active against all the bacteria found in the root canal, a combination of antibiotics with different ranges of activity is used, usually in the form of a paste. The most commonly used antibiotics include neomycin, bacitracin, polymixin, nystatin and tyrothricin.

Objections raised to the use of antibiotic pastes include the possibility of developing resistant strains, possible sensitization of the patient and development of an allergic response. Although all of these are possibilities, and a few cases of allergic response have been recorded, there is no overwhelming evidence against their use. However, their efficacy has not been thoroughly tested in properly controlled clinical studies. Where they have been tested (clindamycin and penicillin) the results have been reasonably favourable but not comparable to calcium hydroxide.

There has been a renewed interest in the use of topical antibiotics in the root canal system, following the recent interest in their topical use in localized periodontal pockets. A number of commonly used systemic antibiotics have been tried in combination including metronidazole, ciprofloxacin and minocycline. No definitive evidence of its efficacy is available.

STEROIDS

Steroids (prednisolone, triamcinalone, hydrocortisone) have been used in root canals mainly for pain relief and there is limited clinical evidence of their anodyne action. These materials have no other beneficial quality and, therefore, they may be mixed with other antibacterial agents such as calcium hydroxide. The commercially available paste popularly used in this manner is Ledermix, which also contains the antibiotic tetracycline. However, mixing these materials may reduce the effect of individual components rather than provide synergism. The disadvantage of the use of these substances is the depressive effect they have on the defence mechanisms including inflammation. Their use may also bring the risk of a bacteraemia, a particular hazard in patients susceptible to infection of damaged tissue or prosthetic replacements, e.g. those with infective endocarditis and prosthetic heart valves.

CALCIUM HYDROXIDE

This material has now gained wide popularity and acceptance as an intracanal medicament as it is effective against most root-canal bacteria and additionally has the ability to degrade residual organic tissue, making it more susceptible to dissolution by sodium hypochlorite at a subsequent appointment. The duration of the antibacterial effect is dependent upon the concentration and volume of the material but it has lasting effect because of its low solubility. A saturated solution effectively provides a store of unreacted ions ready to go into solution as the dissolved ions are removed. The material is quite irritating if extruded and can cause localized necrosis that is self-limiting. Extrusion may be accompanied by severe pain lasting 12–24 hours. It is for this reason that some clinicians prefer to mix it with a steroid paste. This ability to cause localized necrosis may help to form a hard calcific barrier at the junction with the periapical tissues. It is, therefore, a useful intracanal medicament for closure of immature apices (**9.1, 9.2**), intracanal perforation repairs (**9.3–9.5**) and horizontal root fractures (**9.6–9.8**) before obturation.

Calcium hydroxide is also readily available, inexpensive, simple to place and simple to remove from the root canal system. It does not stain the tooth or affect the temporary restoration. Another benefit attributed to calcium hydroxide is its ability to dry weeping canals. The reason for this is unclear but it is probably related to the antibacterial effect of the material and possibly the inactivation of toxins. Calcium hydroxide has been recommended for treatment of external inflammatory and internal resorption. Its action is probably related to its antibacterial properties. **Figures 9.9 and 9.10** show both external inflammatory resorption (right lateral incisor) and external replacement resorption (left central incisor); the latter does not respond to calcium hydroxide treatment as demonstrated by the case shown (**9.11–9.13**). One recently raised concern is that, in common with sodium hypochlorite, it may affect the physical properties of dentine adversely, particularly when used long term. According to some early studies, it does appear to make teeth more susceptible to fracture.

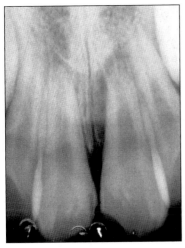
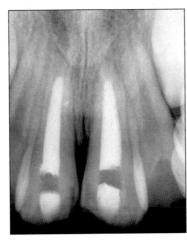

9.1

9.2

9.1–9.2 Closure of wide apices

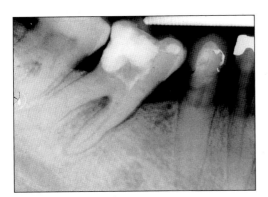
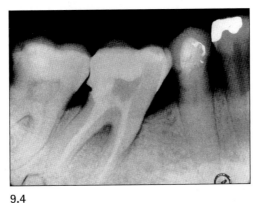
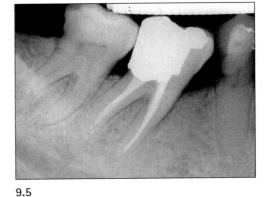

9.3

9.4

9.5

9.3–9.5 Intracanal repair of perforation in the furcal aspect of the mesial root of lower molar

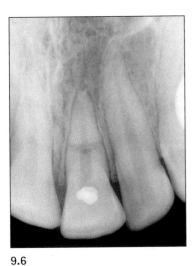
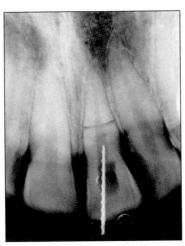
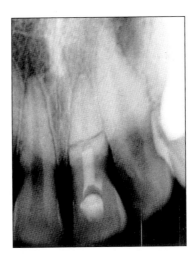

9.6

9.7

9.8

9.6–9.8 Treatment of horizontal fractures where apical fragment has vital pulp tissue

Calcium hydroxide preparations

Many commercially available products (e.g. Multical, Pulpdent, Hypocal, Rootcal, Reogan) contain calcium hydroxide together with other ingredients. The constituents of these commercial products vary widely: the calcium hydroxide content is about 34–50%; barium sulphate 5–15%. The remainder is water and methyl or hydroxyl-methyl cellulose. Other antiseptic materials such as chlorothymonol may be added.

The disadvantages of commercially available materials are that the most important ingredient (calcium hydroxide) is diluted and the pastes may be difficult to place with any degree of control. Many clinicians prefer to use the pure-grade calcium hydroxide powder, which can be mixed in a ratio of 7:1 with barium sulphate powder for radiopacity. The resultant mixture should be stored in an air-tight bottle. It may be mixed with water, saline or local anaesthetic (without vasoconstrictor) to a paste of the required consistency (**9.14**). The consistency of the paste can be changed on demand even within the canal by simply absorbing water with a paper point or adding more. It is, therefore, very versatile in placement. The powder may also be added as a thickener to commercial products but this may adversely affect its rheological properties.

Placement of calcium hydroxide

The method of placement of calcium hydroxide is usually a matter of personal preference. A range of manual and automated techniques may be used depending upon the consistency of the preparation. The more fluid, commercially available, pastes may be applied with files or paper points but the material is unlikely to reach all aspects of the root canal system. Some recommend the use of spiral fillers or an ultrasonically activated file as the most effective means of placement.

The stiffer pastes mixed to requirement may be loaded using amalgam carriers such as the Messing Gun (**9.15**). The paste can be packed down to the position required using pluggers or files (**9.16–9.19**). As above, the consistency is very easily modified as per the requirement of the case. Packing large pellets of hard mix may

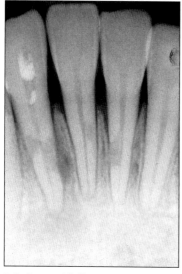

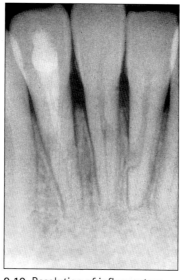

9.9 External inflammatory resorption in mandibular right lateral incisor and replacement resorption in left central incisor

9.10 Resolution of inflammatory resorption following canal debridement and calcium hydroxide dressing in right lateral incisor

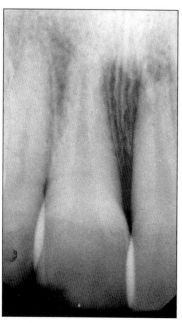

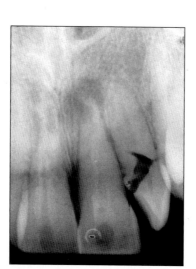

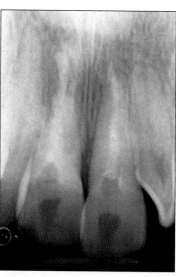

9.11–9.13 Non-resolution of replacement resorption, despite root canal treatment

9.11

9.12

9.13

cause periapical discomfort if air is trapped apical to the calcium hydroxide. It is better to break up the dressing into smaller portions within the canal before packing these apically.

Removal and replacement of calcium hydroxide

Calcium hydroxide is relatively easily removed by washing and irrigating with water or sodium hypochlorite. The latter is preferable because it will allow further dissolution of residual organic debris. Sometimes, the calcium hydroxide may become very well compacted in a narrow canal giving the impression of a blockage. It is important then to use sufficient water and a small file to negotiate past it. An ultrasonically activated file is very effective at removing calcium hydroxide dressings.

The duration of dressing with calcium hydroxide is dependent upon the objective of dressing. If used as a routine antibacterial dressing, then a week is sufficient. If the objective is to arrest a weeping canal, then it may be necessary to dress with a stiff paste for a period of 2 weeks. If it is found that a substantial amount of the paste has been resorbed (**9.20, 9.21**) more frequent dressings with stiffer pastes may be required. Dressing and irrigation are continued until weeping is stemmed.

The use of calcium hydroxide to induce calcific repair at the periapex requires longer periods of dressing. In the first instance the dressing is changed at 2 weeks to evaluate the degree of loss or contamination of the calcium hydroxide. It also allows a further opportunity to irrigate the canal with sodium hypochlorite and reduce the bacterial and organic contamination. The dressing may then be left in place and healing reassessed at three to four monthly intervals.

Criteria for assessment of healing include absence of intracanal bleeding or exudates, absence of symptoms, tactile evidence of a barrier and radiographic evidence of bone resolution adjacent to the site of calcific repair (**9.22, 9.23**). Incompletely formed apices can take up to 24 months before a complete barrier forms, but most are complete by 9 months.

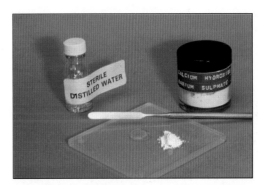

9.14 Preparation of calcium hydroxide paste with powder and water

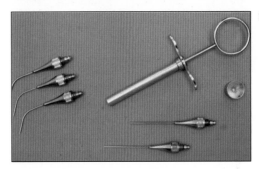

9.15 Messing gun

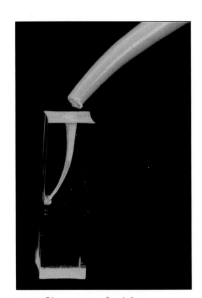

9.16 Placement of calcium hydroxide with amalgam carrier

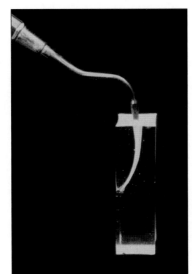

9.17 Placement of calcium hydroxide. Coronal compaction into the canal with a narrow amalgam plugger

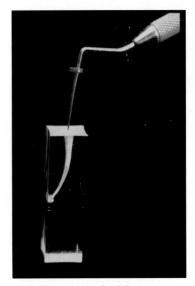

9.18 Placement of calcium hydroxide. Breakage of calcium hydroxide mass in canal into small pellets with a plugger

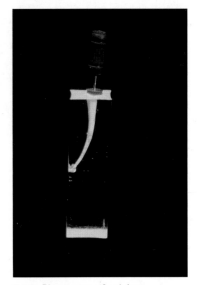

9.19 Placement of calcium hydroxide. Small pellets from **9.18** carried apically with a file or plugger

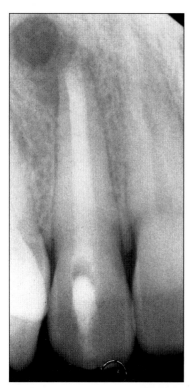

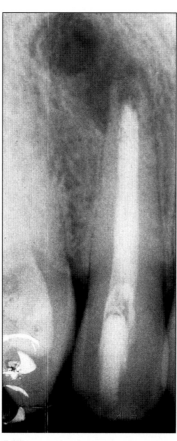

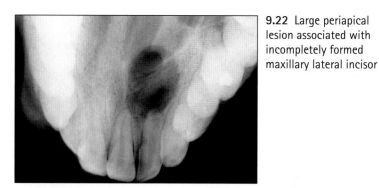

9.22 Large periapical lesion associated with incompletely formed maxillary lateral incisor

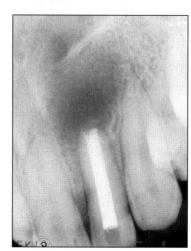

9.23 Periapical resolution following canal debridement and calcium hydroxide dressing

9.20
9.20–9.21 Resorption of calcium hydroxide paste with time

9.21

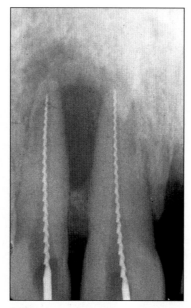

9.24
9.24–9.25 Canal debridement and dressing with calcium hydroxide may aid diagnosis of a perio-endo lesion

9.25

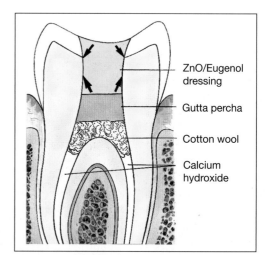

ZnO/Eugenol dressing

Gutta percha

Cotton wool

Calcium hydroxide

9.26 Retention and resistance form of an access cavity

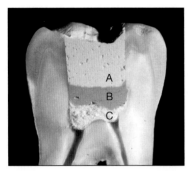

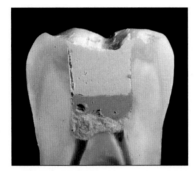

9.27 Double-layered dressing of access cavity: A = zinc oxide/eugenol dressing; B = gutta-percha: C = cotton wool

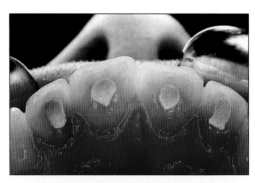

9.29 IRM dressing with a high powder: liquid ratio after two years

9.28 The IRM dressing tends to pull away from the cavity wall opposite to that being adapted unless adapted with apical pressure

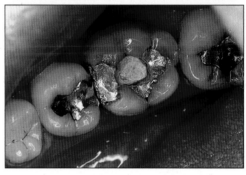

9.30 IRM dressing with a low powder: liquid ratio after three months

There is no definitive guidance on the duration of dressing in case of dental trauma and root resorption. These should be gauged on the basis of the requirement of the case. For further guidance see Andreasen & Andreasen (1994).

Calcium hydroxide may also be used as a long-term dressing or as a short-term root filling if treatment cannot be completed for logistical reasons or if the tooth needs to be left on review to assess the possible outcome of treatment, e.g. perio-endo cases (**9.24, 9.25**) or orthodontic cases under treatment.

It may be concluded that there are positive advantages to the routine dressing of root canals with calcium hydroxide.

TEMPORARY CORONAL ACCESS CAVITY SEAL

Following the completion of radicular access and the chemical dressing of the root canal system, it is essential to ensure that the coronal access cavity is sealed to exclude bacterial microleakage and saliva which may inactivate the medicament and allow regrowth of bacteria. Lack of an adequate temporary access cavity seal has been implicated as one of the sources of infection by *E. faecalis* that makes infection of the root canal system difficult to eradicate.

The integrity of the seal depends on the strength and durability of the temporary restorative material and the marginal seal. Access cavities should be designed to provide retention in both the apical as well as coronal directions. It is customary for the access cavity to be sealed in a double layer by applying a layer of gutta-percha over some cotton wool, prior to applying the definitive sealing material (**9.26, 9.27**). This enables the seal to be condensed against a relatively firm material that is easily removed.

The materials available for temporary seal include, zinc oxide/eugenol (preferably reinforced), Cavit, glass ionomer cements, polycarboxylate cements, composite resins and zinc phosphate cement.

Zinc oxide/eugenol cement

The material of choice is zinc oxide/eugenol because it has proven ability to seal against microorganisms. It is not very strong or

durable and, therefore, reinforced cements (such as IRM or Kalzinol) should be used. These materials are best used to restore a conventional access cavity rather than a larger defect.

To effect a good seal, proper manipulation of this sticky material is essential. It should be adapted with apical pressure from the centre of the cavity outwards or it may pull away from the margin (**9.28**). When mixed to a high powder/liquid ratio the material is very durable (**9.29**). In the case shown, the patient did not attend for two years after placement but the IRM dressings were still intact. In the second case (**9.30**), a low powder/liquid ratio resulted in surface loss of material over a period of three months.

The only disadvantage of using zinc oxide/eugenol is its incompatibility with composite resins. If this is likely to be a problem, a non-eugenol dressing may be used.

Glass ionomer cements

Glass ionomer cements have been recommended because of their adhesive properties. However, the need to use the material in bulk means that the setting contraction may be significant and can cause the integrity of at least part of its margin to be compromised.

Resin reinforced glass ionomer appears to have good antibacterial properties.

Other materials

Other cements, such as *zinc phosphate* and *zinc polycarboxylate*, provide durable restorations and reasonable marginal integrity at high powder/liquid ratios but do not possess the same antimicrobial activity as zinc oxide/eugenol.

Cavit is popular because it is available in a ready-to-use form. It is essentially 'plaster', and can give a reasonable seal over periods of about a week, but is not very durable. It does possess some antimicrobial effect but is not as strong as zinc oxide/eugenol. Its so-called 'self-repair' capacity is related to its ability to absorb moisture and expand. Because of its lack of physical strength it needs to be used in adequate depth, considered to be about 3–4 mm. Restoration of large cavities with Cavit results in cracks within it accompanied by leakage.

The most recent generation of access restorative materials consist of resins. One example is *Term*, which is also a hygroscopic material, and which may be useful for larger cavities.

References

Andreason JO, Andreason FM (1994) *Text book and colour atlas of traumatic injuries to the teeth*, 3rd edn. Mosby, Copenhagen, Denmark.

Bender IB, Seltzer S (1952) Combination of antibiotics and fungicides used in treatment of the infected pulpless tooth. *J Amer Dent Assoc* **45**, 293–300.

Bystrom A, Claesson R, Sundqvist G (1985) The antibacterial effect of camphorated paramonochlorophenol, camphorated phenol and calcium hydroxide in the treatment of infected root canals. *Endod Dent Traumatol* **1**, 170–5.

Gilbert P, Allison DG (1999) Biofilms and their resistance towards antimicrobial agents. In Newman HN, Wilson M (eds) *Dental Plaque Revisited – oral biofilms in health and disease*. Bioline.

Goldman M, Pearson AH (1969) Post-debridement bacterial flora and antibiotic sensitivity. *Oral Surg, Oral Med, Oral Pathol* **28**, 897–905.

Hoshino E, Ando-Kurihara N, Sato I, Vematsu H, Sto M, Kota K, lwaku M (1996) *In vitro* antibacterial susceptibility of bacteria taken from infected root dentine to a mixture of ciprofloxacin, metronidazole and minocycline. *Int Endod J* **29**, 125–30.

House of Lords Science and Technology Committee (1998). *Resistance to antibiotics and other antimicrobial agents*, seventh report from the Science and Technology Committee: session 1997–98 (HL81; Vol. 1). London: Stationery Office.

Le Goff A, Bunetel L, Mouton C, Bonnaure-Mallet M (1997) Evaluation of root canal bacteria and their antimicrobial susceptibility in teeth with necrotic pulp. *Oral Microbiol Immunol* **12**, 318–22.

Longman LP, Preston Al, Martin MV, Wilson NHF (2000) Endodontics in the adult patient: the role of antibiotics. *J Dent* **28**, 539–48.

McDonnell G, Russell D (1999) Antiseptics and disinfectants: activity, action and resistance. *Clin Microbiol Rev* **12**, 147–79.

Molander A, Reit C, Dahlen G (1990) Microbiological evaluation of clindamycin as a root canal dressing in teeth with apical periodontitis. *Int Endod J* **23**, 113–18.

Ørstavik D, Kerekes K, Molven O (1991) Effects of extensive apical reaming and calcium hydroxide dressing on bacterial infection during treatment of apical periodontitis: a pilot study. *Int Endod J* **24**, 1–7.

Reit C, Molander A, Dahlen G (1999) The diagnostic accuracy of microbiologic root canal sampling and the influence of antimicrobial dressings. *Endod Dent Traumatol* **15**, 278–83.

Sato I, Ando-Kurihara N, Kota K, lwaku M, Hoshino E (1996) Sterilization of infected root-canal dentine by topical application of a mixture of ciprofloxacin, metronidazole and minocycline *in situ*. *Int Endod J* **29**, 118–24.

Sjogren U, Figdor D, Spangberg L, Sundqvist G (1991) The antimicrobial effect of calcium hydroxide as a short-term intracanal dressing. *Int Endod J* **24**, 119–25.

Chapter 10

Root canal system obturation

J D Regan

INTRODUCTION

To obturate is to occlude or fill a cavity. Historically, obturation of the root canal system has been viewed as the most critical part of the whole treatment. As a result, extensive efforts have been devoted to the development of the ideal root canal filling techniques and filling material. However, it must be stated that the success of the non-surgical root canal treatment is more dependent on the debridement of the root canal system.

RATIONALE FOR OBTURATION

Bacteria are undoubtedly the main aetiological factors in the development and progression of pulpal and periradicular disease. Following debridement of the root canal system it would appear logical to attempt to prevent movement of microorganisms into the periradicular tissues. Obturation of the root canal system along with an adequate coronal restoration aim to prevent this recontamination by establishing a barrier to the passage of microorganisms and their products.

In the past, the main emphasis was placed on establishing an apical 'seal'. However, in recent years the importance of the coronal seal has been appreciated more fully and it is now believed that the coronal seal is as important, if not more important, than the apical seal. Cases have been reported which demonstrate that it is possible to achieve resolution of periradicular lesions following root canal preparation and coronal seal alone or even spontaneous resolution of a lesion following caries removal and placement of a coronal restoration! Therefore, obturation of the root canal system should begin with the root canal filling and finish with an integrated, well designed and executed coronal restoration (**10.1**).

AIMS AND OBJECTIVES OF OBTURATION

The aims and objectives of the obturation are:

- to establish a barrier to the passage of microorganisms from the oral cavity to the periradicular tissues;
- to 'entomb' and isolate any microorganisms that may survive the cleaning and shaping process;

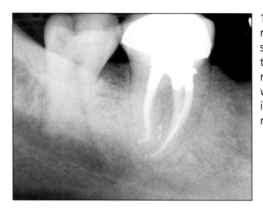

10.1 Postoperative radiograph of non-surgical root canal treatment on lower molar tooth with well-designed and integrated coronal restoration

- to prevent leakage into the canal system of potential nutrients that would support microbial growth;
- to reduce the risk of bacterial movement or fluid percolation into the canal system space from the gingival sulcus or periodontal pockets.

The concept of an 'hermetic' or 'airtight' seal in endodontics is erroneous as it is now understood that all restorative materials leak to some extent. It suffices to say that all efforts should be made to hinder the invasion of microorganisms.

WHEN SHOULD THE ROOT CANAL SYSTEM BE OBTURATED?

It appears that non-surgical endodontic treatment performed in multiple visits may be associated with a greater chance of failure than those completed in a single or two visits (Siren et al., 1997, Cheung & Chan, 2003). This may be due to contamination of the canal system with microorganisms between visits. However, an on-going debate, fuelled by the occasional research publication, concerns endodontists at present. The issue to be resolved is whether root canal treatments should be completed in a single visit or not. There are numerous advantages to completing treatments in a single visit and it is generally accepted that certain cases, such as vital cases, are best treated in a single-visit therapy. Many endodontists believe that, given adequate time, most cases can be completed in a single visit.

However, many are of the opinion that non-vital cases should never be treated in a single visit. This may be due to the belief that there is likely to be more postoperative pain and further complications and that the success rates associated with single-visit cases are lower than with multiple-visit therapy. To date, these beliefs have not been substantiated by research, and clinicians throughout the world are successfully performing single-visit therapies.

There are, however, a number of conditions that should exist before a root filling is placed. These include:

- absence of pain and swelling;
- absence of persistent exudate in the canal;
- thoroughly debrided root canal system;
- adequate time to complete the procedure.

Completion of the treatment in a single visit has a number of advantages for both the patient and the clinician. These include the following:

- the root canal system will never be 'cleaner' than immediately after shaping and debridement;

- there is potential for recontamination between visits;
- single visit therapy provides no opportunity for temporary restorations to leak;
- there is less opportunity for teeth to fracture as definitive restorations can be placed earlier;
- the clinician is most familiar with the root-canal morphology at the completion of the preparation;
- there are both financial and temporal savings;
- single-visit treatments are particularly beneficial for medically compromised patients whose conditions necessitate antibiotic premedication.

WHERE SHOULD THE ROOT FILLING END?

A second controversial issue is the question as to where to end the root filling. Prognostic studies published in the last fifty years all agree that overfilling the canal will result in a reduced success rate. According to these studies, the optimal result is to end the root filling one to two millimetres short of the radiographic apex at a point corresponding to the apical constriction or the point at which the

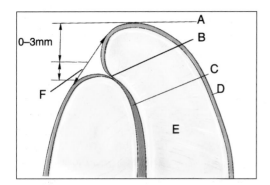

10.2 Relationship between root tip, apical foramen and apical constriction: A = root apex; B = apical constriction; C = root canal; D = cementum; E = dentine; F = apical foramen

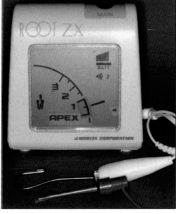

10.3 Contemporary impedance-type apex locator Root ZX

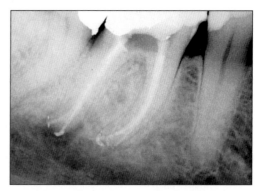

10.4 Overfilling of the root canal system

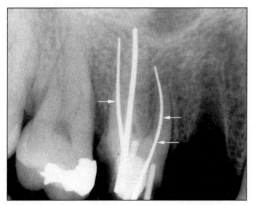

10.5 Overextension of the root canal system – note the voids alongside the silver cones (arrows)

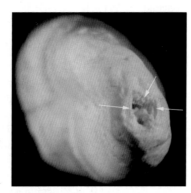

10.6 External apical root resorption: resorbed root surface arrowed

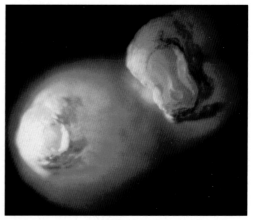

10.7 Arrested root formation resulting in an open apex

canal dimensions are at their smallest (**10.2**). However, it is important to remember that many factors other than the obturating material influenced these results.

Ideally, all root-filling material should remain within the confines of the root canal system. The apical extent of the root canal system is designated by the dentine–cemental junction. Beyond this point the root canal system ends and the periodontal structures begin. The dentine–cemental junction is approximately 0.5–0.7 mm from the external aspect of the apical foramen but it is sometimes very difficult to determine the position of the dentine–cemental junction. "*It is sometimes very difficult to know where the root canal ends and the rest of the body begins*" (Hasselgren, 1994). Radiographic interpretation of this point is unpredictable and fraught with difficulties. However, the use of apex locators (**10.3**), or, possibly more correctly, 'apical foramen locators', has greatly facilitated the location of the end point for instrumentation and obturation.

In practice, the extrusion of small amounts of sealer beyond the confines of the root canal system can affect the success but not adversely: it is actually viewed by some endodontists as a desirable indication of the adequacy of obturation of the complete canal system. It is important to appreciate the difference between overfilling (**10.4**) and overextension (**10.5**) of an obturation. An overextended obturation is one that has been extruded beyond the confines of the canal system but does not completely fill the canal system while an overfilled canal is completely obturated and has, in addition, been extended beyond the confines of the root canal system.

Difficulties frequently arise in canal systems with incomplete apices or in cases where resorption (**10.6**), incomplete apical development (**10.7**) or iatrogenic causes have destroyed the normal apical anatomy. In these cases modifications may have to be made during both the preparation and obturation of the canal system.

THE IDEAL ROOT-FILLING MATERIAL

Unfortunately the ideal root-filling material does not exist. The required properties of an ideal material include the following. It would:

- induce or at least support regeneration of damaged tissues;
- be antimicrobial;
- not irritate periradicular tissues;
- be toxic neither locally nor systemically;
- be adhesive and be easily adapted to the canal walls;
- have good flow characteristics;
- not stain dentine;
- have good handling characteristics;
- be radiopaque;
- be impermeable to tissue fluids;
- be dimensionally stable;
- be cheap and have a long shelf-life;
- reinforce and strengthen the root structure.

Historically, a plethora of materials have been used to obturate the root canal system. Effective use requires an understanding of the properties of the material and an appreciation of the anatomy and morphology of the root canal system. Many obturating techniques and materials were designed and used based on misunderstandings of this morphology.

Solid obturators such as silver or acrylic cones were designed to fit snugly into a canal 'machined' to an equivalent dimension. However, the irregular nature of the root canal system was not fully appreciated and these solid cores fitted only where they actually touched the canal walls (**10.8**). The remaining spaces were filled with cement or sealer. Over time tissue fluids percolated into the canal system as the sealer was gradually washed out. In cases obturated with silver cones this frequently resulted in formation of corrosion products such as silver sulphites and silver chlorides (**10.9–10.11**). These corrosion products leaked into the periradicular tissues thereby provoking an inflammatory response ultimately resulting in failure of the case.

Many 'paste' materials have been formulated in order to simplify obturation and have been recommended for use alone or in combination with a master obturation cone. As it is not possible to compact a paste it is virtually impossible to ensure complete obturation of the root canal system with paste materials unless they expand on setting (**10.12**). On the other hand, if expansion on setting is a property of the material, then the main difficulty encountered will be confinement of the material to the root canal system. Extrusion of obturation materials beyond the confines of the root canal system is undesirable and, in the case of some paste materials, can result in permanent damage to adjacent structures such as neural tissue.

The most commonly used obturating material is 'gutta-percha' (trans-polyisoprene) (**10.13**). It has been used in endodontics as the core filling material for well over 100 years. The 'gutta-percha' used in dentistry is composed of approximately 19–22% of the actual trans-polyisoprene gutta-percha molecule and 59–75% zinc oxide filler with other additives (**Table 10.1**). These additives include waxes or resins, which enhance the plasticity of the material and metal salts, which are used to increase the radiodensity of the material. The exact composition of the commercially available product varies from manufacturer to manufacturer.

Table 10.1 Percentage composition of conventional gutta-percha points

Gutta-percha	20
Zinc oxide	60–75
Metal sulphates	1.5–17
Waxes/resins	1–4

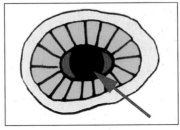

10.8 Cross-sectional diagram of silver cone obturation showing poor adaptation of cone to irregular canal outline: silver cone arrowed

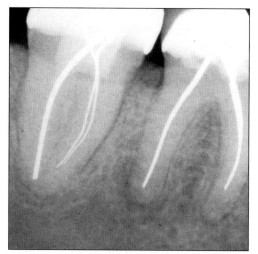

10.9 Preoperative radiograph of symptomatic lower molar tooth with prior silver cone obturation

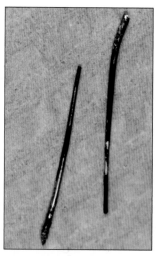

10.10 Corroded silver cones removed during the retreatment – note the black corrosion products formed on the cones

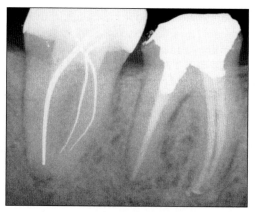

10.11 Case immediately after retreatment with gutta-percha

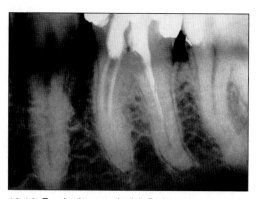

10.12 Tooth obturated with Endomethasone paste

10.13 Structural formulae for isoprene, rubber, gutta-percha (α and β phases)

Stereochemistry of polyisoprene

Isoprene monomer

cis-polyisoprene = natural rubber

trans-polyisoprene = Alpha gutta-percha

trans-polyisoprene = Beta gutta-percha

The gutta-percha molecule is the mirror image of the natural rubber molecule (a trans-isomer of rubber) and it exists in three different forms; two crystalline forms (α and β) and an amorphous form. All three forms play a part in root canal obturation. Gutta-percha harvested from the *Palaquium gutta* tree is mainly the α-phase while that in gutta-percha cones available commercially exists mainly as the β-phase. The β-phase is converted to the α-phase by heating to 42–49°C. Further heating to between 53 and 59°C results in loss of the crystalline form and formation of an amorphous melt (**10.14**). The relevance of these structural changes is the fact that they are associated with volumetric changes that in turn has an influence on the clinical procedures during obturation. Manufacturers of some thermoplasticized obturating systems such as Thermafil® stress the importance of maintaining vertical compaction pressures on the molten gutta-percha in the coronal portion of the canal system while the material cools and undergoes contraction and shrinkage. This vertical pressure is necessary to compensate for the volumetric contraction associated with cooling of the gutta-percha in the root canal system.

Commercially available dental gutta-percha demonstrates several of the properties of the ideal root-filling material but does not fulfil all of the properties by any means. It is not toxic and is cheap. It is possible to encourage flow by thermoplasticizing it and it adapts fairly well to the canal wall, but does not bond to dentine. It does not stain dentine; it is radiopaque (due to added radiopaque agents) and has good handling characteristics and has a relatively long shelf-life.

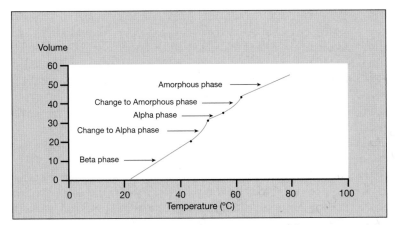

10.14 Volumetric and phase changes associated with heating gutta-percha

Clinically, it is not very irritating to periradicular tissues but histologically provokes a chronic inflammatory response. In addition, it neither induces nor supports regeneration of damaged tissues. Despite its many drawbacks it remains the material of choice at the beginning of the new millennium. The following discussion on obturation techniques relates to the use of gutta-percha as the obturation material.

OBTURATION TECHNIQUES

Gutta-percha has been presented to the profession in many forms for use in combination with a variety of obturating techniques. These include:

- lateral compaction;
- warm vertical compaction;
- thermocompaction and hybrid technique;
- thermoplasticized gutta-percha supported on a solid core;
- injectable thermoplasticized gutta-percha.

Comparisons have been made between the different gutta-percha obturating techniques but, despite a large body of research papers, there is no definite evidence to support one technique in favour of another. Historically, lateral compaction has been used as a 'gold-standard' comparison in order to evaluate new obturating techniques and lateral compaction remains the most widely taught and practised technique worldwide. The term 'compaction' is used throughout this chapter and is considered more accurate than 'condensation' as examination of the physical properties of gutta-percha demonstrates that the material cannot be condensed.

LATERAL COMPACTION

The lateral compaction technique involves placing tapered gutta-percha cones in the canal and compacting them under pressure against the walls of the canal with a metal spreader (**10.15**). The first gutta-percha cone called the 'master cone' is an ISO standardized cone and should be chosen to match the size of the master apical file

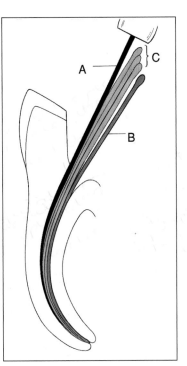

10.15 The taper of the canal should be matched with spreader and accessory points: A = spreader; B = master point; C = accessory points

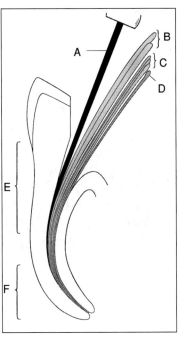

10.16 The taper of the canal should be matched with spreader and accessory points: A = spreader; B = wide accessory points; C = narrow accessory points; D = master point; E = wide taper; F = narrow taper

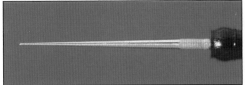

10.17 Magnified image of hand spreader (Miller Inc, York, PA, USA)

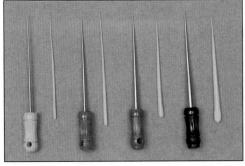

10.18 Non-standardized gutta-percha points should be used with matching spreaders

(**10.16–10.21**). Ideally, the master cone should fit accurately in the apical few millimetres at the predetermined length. Unfortunately, a mismatch frequently exists between the sizes of the master apical file and the corresponding gutta-percha cone and this may prevent accurate adaptation of the master gutta-percha cone. It should not be easily forced beyond the final preparation point and may demonstrate a slight resistance to removal called 'tug-back'. The concept of 'tug-back' has been widely cited as a requirement for a well-fitting master cone. However, this feeling of 'tug-back' is often due to the binding of the gutta-percha cone to the walls of the preparation at any point along its length. The master cone may be customized by dipping the apical 1 mm in chloroform for one second and placing it into the wet canal (**10.22**, **10.23**). An impression of the apical preparation is made on the softened gutta-percha. The canal is then dried. Following application of sealer the waster cone is reinstated. Subsequent cones are called 'accessory cones' and are usually non-standardized cones demonstrating a range of tapers. The metal spreaders are made in a variety of sizes corresponding to the accessory cones and can be either finger or hand spreaders. The spreader is placed in the canal and the master cone is compacted (**10.24**, **10.25**). The spreader should be left in place for a few seconds to allow the gutta-percha time to deform and flow under pressure. Following removal of the spreader, the first accessory cone is placed and compacted into place. This process is repeated until the canal is filled (**10.26–10.29**).

It is important that the spreader reaches at least to within 1 mm of the working length in order to ensure adequate compaction of the gutta-percha against the canal walls. In addition, a regularly tapered canal is essential to ensure adequate obturation. It is recommended that finger spreaders be used as hand spreaders very easily generate forces that may fracture roots.

In order to enhance the adaptation and compaction of the gutta-percha to the walls of the root canal system heat is frequently applied. This can be done in a number of ways. Originally, instruments were heated in an open flame and then rapidly applied to the gutta-percha mass. More sophisticated heat-delivery systems have now been developed which allow heat to be safely and easily applied to the mass of gutta-percha within a few millimetres of the working length. Endotec or Touch n' Heat can be used (**10.30–10.33**). The use of heat improves the homogeneity of the final obturation in comparison to cold lateral compaction where the cones essentially retain their integrity. In addition, heating the gutta-percha reduces the compaction pressures necessary to ensure adaptation thereby reducing the risk of root fracture.

WARM VERTICAL COMPACTION

No compaction technique is exclusively lateral or vertical in nature. All techniques will have both vertical and lateral components. Vertical compaction was first described many years ago but was made popular in 1967 by Schilder. The technique described involves placement of a fitted non-standardized master cone in the canal with a minimal amount of sealer. The master cone tip is adjusted to ensure a close fit apically either by cutting off the tip or by using

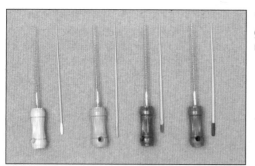

10.19 Stanardized gutta-percha points match files

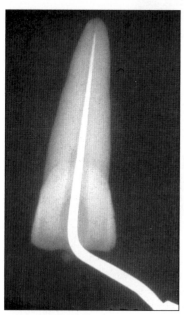

10.20 Radiograph showing prefitting of spreader

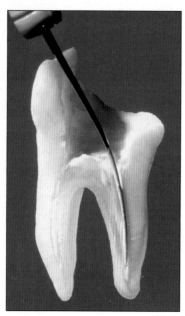

10.21 Application of sealer to canal wall

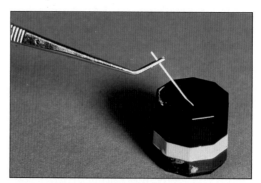

10.22 Chloroform dip technique

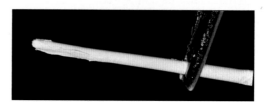

10.23 Impression of apical foramen

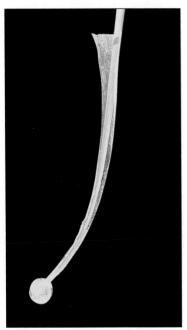

10.24 Selection of master gutta-percha point (A) to occlude apical foramen

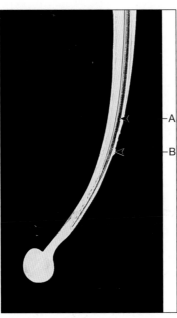

10.25 Compaction of gutta-percha point with spreader: A = spreader; B = gutta-percha

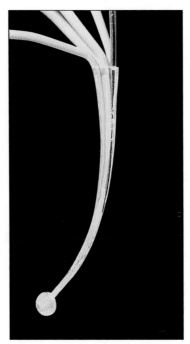

10.26 Longitudinal view – three accessory points compounded into place apically

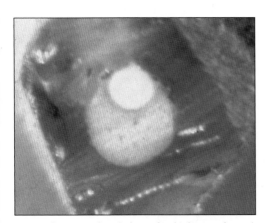

10.27 Cross-sectional view of apical part of canal showing master point and one accessory point

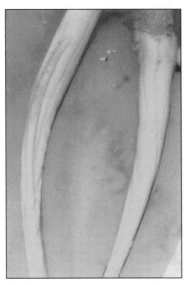

10.28

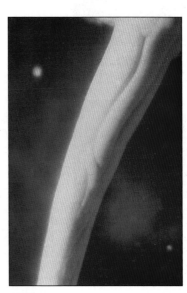

10.29

10.28–10.29 Cleared extracted tooth showing morphology of a lateral compaction obturation

solvent to soften the tip, which can then be more easily adapted to the apical portion of the canal. The gutta-percha is warmed with heat carriers and a series of flat-ended pluggers are used to compact the gutta-percha starting initially in the apical portion. It is important that the pluggers are prefitted at 5 mm intervals (**10.34–10.36**) so that at each level of the canal the appropriate plugger captures the maximum cross-sectional area of softened gutta-percha (**10.37,** **10.38**) without binding on the canal walls. Binding of the pluggers on the canal walls (**10.39**) could cause facture of the root. Too small a plugger (**10.40**) would simply plunge through the gutta-percha. The smallest plugger should fit to within 5 mm of the working length to achieve good apical compaction without extrusion. The width and rigidity of the pluggers necessitate a more widely tapered canal preparation than for lateral compaction.

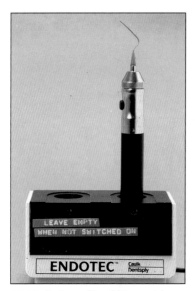

10.30 Endotec (Caulk/Dentsply)

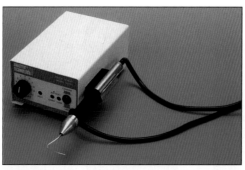

10.31 Touch 'n Heat (Analytic Technology)

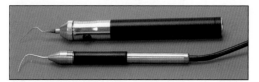

10.32 Comparison of Endotec and Touch 'n Heat spreaders

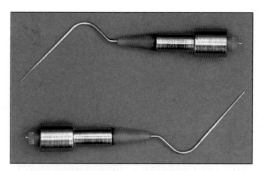

10.33 Spreader tips (small, large) for Endotec

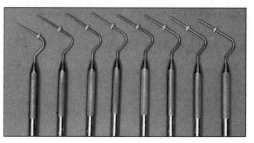

10.34 Premeasured pluggers

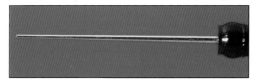

10.35 Magnified image of finger plugger (Miller Inc, York, PA, USA)

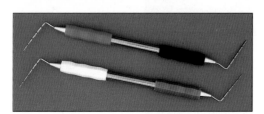

10.36 Double ended Dovgan Pluggers (Miltex Inc, York, PA, USA)

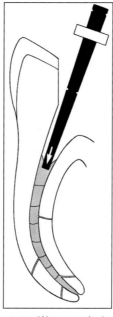

10.37 Warm vertical compaction

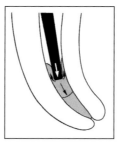

10.38 Plugger should capture maximum cross-sectional area of gutta-percha without apical binding

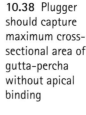

10.39 Plugger binding apically may split root

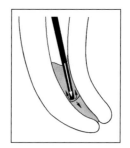

10.40 Small plugger is ineffective

The prefitted master cone is placed to the designated length in the canal, the walls of which have been coated lightly with sealer (**10.41–10.52**). The cone is seared off at the canal-orifice level with a hot instrument. A cold plugger dipped in sealer powder or wiped with alcohol is used to begin the compaction process. The coronal-most few millimetres of warmed gutta-percha are moved laterally and apically. The heat carrier is now plunged 3–4 mm into the gutta-percha and quickly removed. Some gutta-percha is removed with the heated instrument and immediately the remaining gutta-percha is compacted with the next prefit plugger. The body of the gutta-percha is warmed 4–5 mm ahead of the heated instrument and the compacting action of the cold plugger moves the gutta-percha

10.41–10.52 Procedure for warm vertical compaction

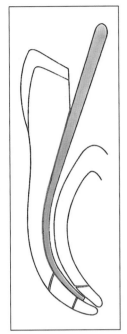

10.41 Fitting master point

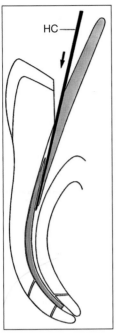

10.42 Application of heat carrier (HC)

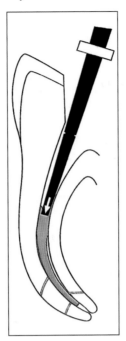

10.43 Plugging heated gutta-percha

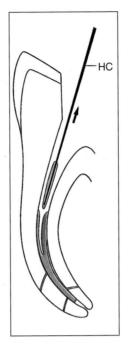

10.44 Reapplication of heat carrier (HC)

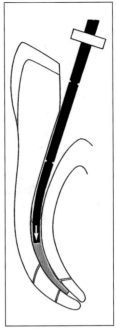

10.45 Reapplication of plugger

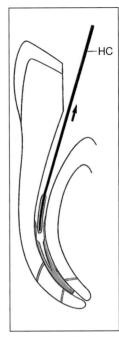

10.46 Reapplication of heat carrier (HC)

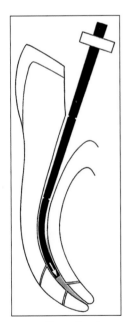

10.47 Reapplication of plugger

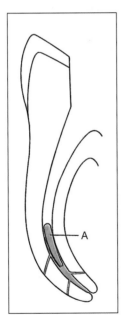

10.48 Addition of new section of gutta-percha (3–4 mm)

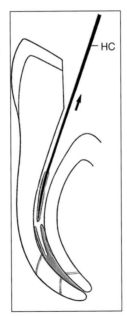

10.49 Application of heat carrier (HC)

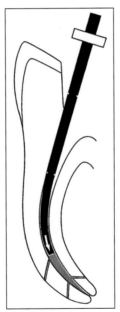

10.50 Reapplication of plugger

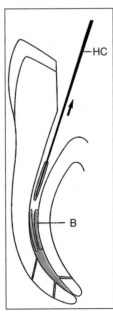

10.51 Reapplication of heat carrier (HC)

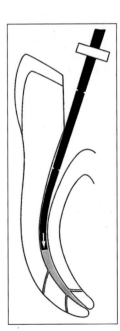

10.52 Reapplication of plugger

apically and laterally. This procedure is repeated until about 5 mm of well-compacted gutta-percha remains in the apical portion of the canal. The coronal portion is then back-filled by introducing 3–4 mm segments of gutta-percha, which are then heated and compacted in sequence.

The compaction of the heated gutta-percha encourages flow of the obturating material in canal irregularities and accessory anatomical features. Careful adherence to the step-by-step approach usually results in a dense homogenous fill (**10.53–10.55**).

Variations on the warm vertical obturation procedure have been introduced to improve and simplify the procedure. These include the use of electrically operated heat carriers such as the Touch n' Heat unit or the more sophisticated System-B unit (**10.56–10.58**). Both of these units allow for instant delivery of heat to the gutta-percha mass that can then be compacted. The System-B heating element is contained within specifically designed pluggers the tips of which are 0.55 mm in diameter. The heat carriers or 'Buchanan pluggers' have shapes that closely approximate the shapes of tapered root canal preparations. These pluggers come in four sizes or shapes; fine, fine-medium, medium, and medium-large which resemble the taper of non-standard master cones. In addition, these dead-soft stainless steel heat pluggers are quite flexible, allowing for deeper compaction especially in narrow, curved canals. An example of a technique recommended by the manufacturer for use with the System-B is illustrated in **Box 10.1**.

The System-B 'Continuous Wave' obturation technique is based on the Schilder warm vertical compaction procedure. Before the master cone is positioned, one of the four System-B pluggers is chosen. The plugger (ML, M, FM or F) is fitted to within 5–7 mm of the working length and a position on the plugger noted. The heat source is set to 200°C. The canal orifice is coated with a small amount of sealer and the cone is placed to length. The tip of the plugger is placed into the canal orifice and activated. It is driven through the gutta-percha to the predetermined length. The heat is removed, the tip cools rapidly and the plugger's position is maintained for 5–10 seconds until the apical gutta-percha has set. This apical pressure compensates for volumetric changes as the gutta-percha changes

from the amorphous melt form back to the crystalline α-form. The tip is reactivated for 1 second in order to release the plugger and to remove excess gutta-percha. At this stage the apical portion has been obturated and the remainder of the canal can be back-filled or post-space can be formed.

The 'back-fill' can be completed as described by Schilder or injectable thermoplasticized gutta-percha can be used. A number of injectable gutta-percha systems are available including the Obtura

---

Box 10.1 Recommended technique for System-B compaction

1. Fit a non-standardized (fine, fine-medium, medium, or medium-large) gutta-percha cone into a tapered root canal preparation. You can also use greater taper gutta-percha points 0.04, 0.06, 0.08, 0.10, and 0.12.
2. Choose a Buchanan plugger that matches the taper of the gutta-percha point and place a rubber stop onto the plugger 5 mm short of the working length: Fine plugger = 0.04 + 0.06 taper; Fine-medium plugger = 0.06 + 0.08 taper; Medium plugger = 0.08 + 0.10 taper; Medium-large plugger = 0.10 + 0.12 taper.
3. Prefit the Buchanan plugger to its binding point in the canal (usually 5–7 mm short of length). Adjust the stop and remove the plugger.
4. Dry the canal and cement the cone.
5. Turn the System-B unit to 'Use' position. Then, holding the button on momentarily, drive the preheated plugger smoothly through the gutta percha until it stops. Repeat this procedure until the plugger is within 0.5–1 mm of the binding point.
6. Maintain apical pressure without heat for a 10 second 'sustained push' to take up any shrinkage that might occur upon cooling.
7. Still maintaining apical pressure, push the button again for 1.5 seconds. Withdraw the plugger after cooling for 1 second. Because the Buchanan pluggers heat from their tips back, the heat burst in this portion of the procedure causes rapid severance of the instrument and the coronal surplus of gutta-percha from the already condensed and set apical mass.
8. The canal is now ready for the Obtura Backfill.

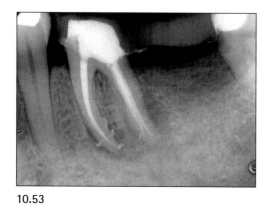

10.53

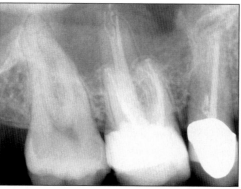

10.54

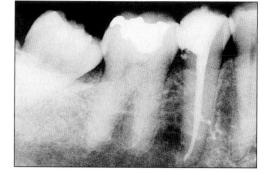

10.55

10.53–10.55 Radiograph of case obturated with the warm vertical compaction technique

('high-heat') (**10.59–10.61**) and the Ultrafil ('low-heat') (**10.62**) systems. Injectable gutta-percha allows for rapid back-filling of the canal with material that demonstrates excellent flow properties.

The Obtura® system consists of a control unit and a pistol-grip syringe designed to accept gutta-percha pellets formulated for use with the system. The gutta-percha is heated in the barrel of the syringe to 160–200°C. The molten gutta-percha is extruded through silver needles that are supplied in 20, 23 and 25 gauge sizes (**10.61**). As the gutta-percha leaves the tip of the needle, its temperature drops to between 62 and 65°C. The heating barrel reaches full operating temperature in less than two minutes thereby eliminating the need to preheat the gutta-percha.

The 'low-heat' Ultrafil system heats cannules (**10.63**) containing gutta-percha to 70°C in a heating unit. The gutta-percha is supplied in three different formulations; regular set; endoset; and firm set. The cannules must be placed in the heater at least 15 minutes before use and must be discarded after 4 hours' heating. The trigger is squeezed gently and released and the gutta-percha is allowed to flow out at its own rate (**10.64**). It is important to avoid excessive pressure in order to prevent extrusion of the material from other channels (**10.65, 10.66**).

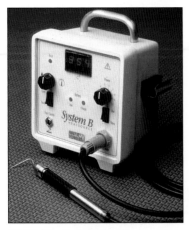

10.56 The System B unit (Sybron Endo, CA, USA)

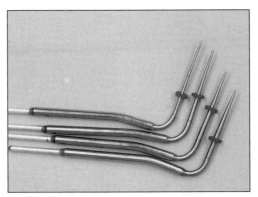

10.57 Obturator tips for the System B. Fine, Fine-Medium, Medium and Medium-Large pluggers, all with a size 55 tip

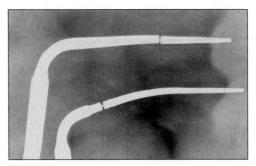

10.58 Radiograph of broken System-B tips demonstrating the heating coil in the centre

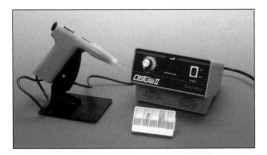

10.59 Obtura system (Texceed Corporation)

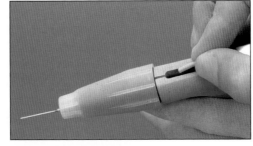

10.60 Loading Obtura gun with gutta-percha

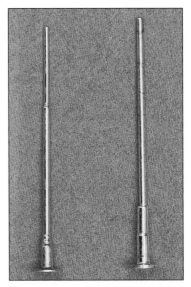

10.61 Disposable silver needles for Obtura

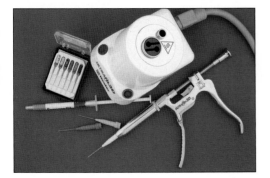

10.62 Ultrafil system (Hygenic Corp, NJ, USA)

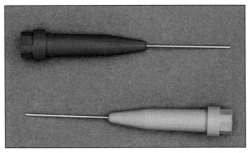

10.63 Prefilled gutta-percha cannules for Ultrafil

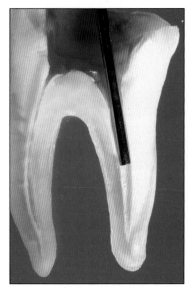

10.64 A wide canal is necessary for adequate needle placement

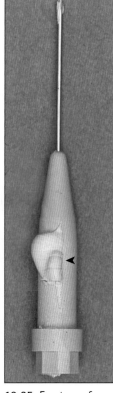

10.65 Fracture of cannule due to haste or inadequate heating

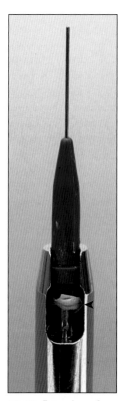

10.66 Extrusion of gutta-percha through the back of cannule

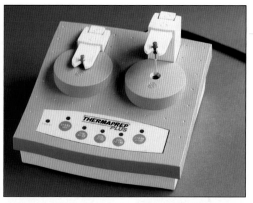

10.67 The Thermafil System (Tulsa Dentsply)

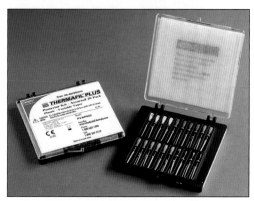

10.68 Thermafil obturators (Tulsa Dentsply)

THERMOPLASTICIZED GUTTA-PERCHA CARRIERS

In 1978 Johnson described a technique for delivery of gutta-percha to a root canal system by coating an endodontic file with thermo-plasticized α-phase gutta-percha. This concept is widely marketed as the Thermafil system (**10.67**). The original, commercially available metal carrier has now been replaced with a radiopaque plastic carrier and is available in a series of sizes from #20 to #140 (**10.68, 10.69**). Blank plastic carriers called verifiers (**10.70**) are used to gauge the appropriate size for a canal. If the selected carrier is too small the carrier may be extruded (**10.71**) and if it is too large the root canal filling may be short. The carriers must be heated in a special oven at 115°C according to the manufacturer's instructions. Maximum and minimum times should be observed in order to ensure adequate heating. However, if left in the oven longer than the designated time the obturators must be discarded. A very small amount of slow-setting sealer is applied to the walls and the heated carriers are then placed rapidly to full length in the canal. The length can be deter-mined in advance using the rubber stoppers on the carriers. In teeth with multiple canals, excess gutta-percha from the first carrier can be prevented from blocking the orifices to the other canals by placing a temporary obstruction such as damp cotton pellet or paper points into these orifices.

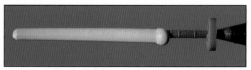

10.69 A size 40 Thermafil obturator

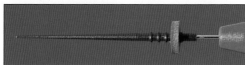

10.70 Blank plastic carriers are used to verify selection of size

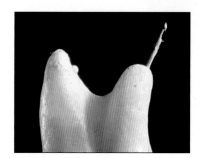

10.71 If carrier is too small it may be extruded

As with other thermoplasticized techniques it is important to compensate for the volumetric shrinkage that occurs when the gutta-percha cools by maintaining apical pressure on the cooling material. This is done by compacting the gutta-percha around the central carrier in an apical direction as it cools.

Thermoplasticized gutta-percha has been shown to obturate the canal system effectively and to flow very well into accessory anatomical spaces (**10.72–10.75**). The apical seal provided by these techniques has also proven to be as effective as any other obturation technique. However, apical control of the flow of the thermoplasticized material is difficult and constitutes a potential disadvantage of these techniques. In addition, a section of the core carrier obturators such as Thermafil or Softcore (Soft-Core, Denmark) need to be removed if the tooth has been treatment planned for a post-retained restoration. Burs specifically designed to aid removal of the plastic core have been designed by the manufacturer of the Thermafil system and are called 'Prepiburs' (**10.76–10.78**). A core carrier system called 'SimpliFil' has been designed to overcome the problem of

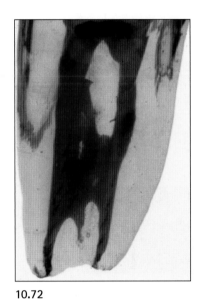

10.72

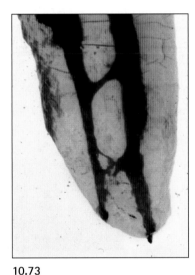

10.73

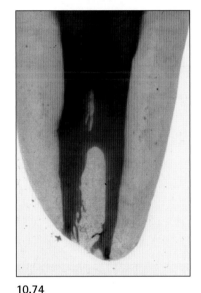

10.74

10.72–10.74 Roots rendered transparent by clearing show good filling of accessory anatomy using Thermafil obturators

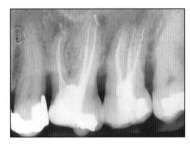

10.75 Molars filled with Thermafil obturators

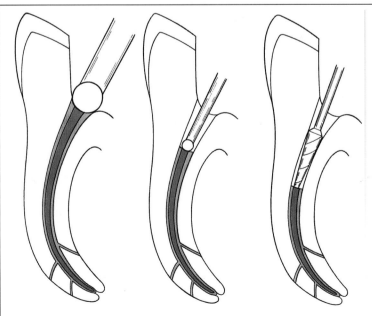

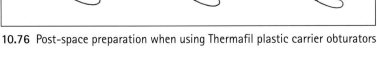

10.76 Post-space preparation when using Thermafil plastic carrier obturators

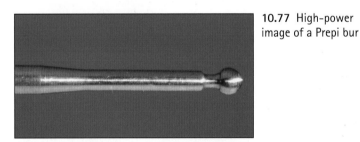

10.77 High-power image of a Prepi bur

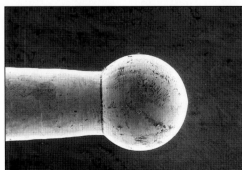

10.78 Scanning electron microscope image of Prepi bur

providing post space following obturation (**10.79–10.81**). In this technique 5 mm plugs of gutta-percha are carried to the apical portion of the preparation and sealed in place with an endodontic sealer (AH Plus Epoxy Resin is recommended by the manufacturer). The carrier can then be removed leaving the apical 5 mm of gutta-percha behind. The plugs are supplied in ISO sizes 35–90.

THERMOMECHANICAL COMPACTION TECHNIQUE

Thermomechanical compaction describes the plasticity generated within gutta-percha by heat developed by mechanical activity. A well-adapted master cone is placed in the canal with a suitable sealer. A mechanically activated rotating compactor similar to a reverse Hedstroem file (thermocompactor) (**10.82, 10.83**) is introduced into the canal, which will then heat up the gutta-percha and thermoplasticize it (**10.84, 10.85**). Accessory points may be added prior to commencing compaction if necessary. Thermocompactors available include Maillefer Gutta-condenser, McSpadden nickel–titanium thermocompactor, Zipperer thermocompactor and Quickfill

compactor. Disadvantages of the thermocompaction technique include apical extrusion of obturation material, as is common with all thermoplasticized techniques, gouging of the wall by the compactor, excessive heating of the supporting tissues surrounding the root and fracture of the instrument.

INJECTION OF THERMOPLASTICIZED GUTTA-PERCHA

This technique involves injecting molten gutta-percha into the root canal system. Theoretically simple, this technique demands considerable care and is associated with the disadvantages of any thermoplasticized material. Even though it has been recommended for obturation of the complete root canal system, it is probably prudent to use the injectable heated gutta-percha as a back-filling material or in cases where apical occlusion is assured. As with all gutta-percha obturations, a sealer must be used. Commonly used systems include the Obtura system, the Ultrafil system and a recently-introduced Inject-R Fill from Endo Solutions, York, PA, USA.

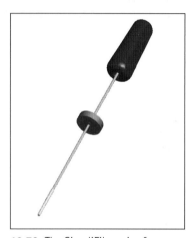

10.79 The SimpliFil carrier from Lightspeed Endodontics, TX, USA

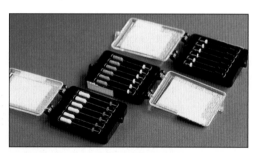

10.80 SimpliFil obturators (Lightspeed Endodontics, TX, USA)

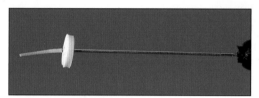

10.81 A SimpliFil obturator

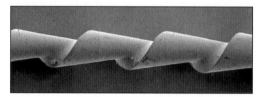

10.82 Maillefer gutta-condensor (SEM view)

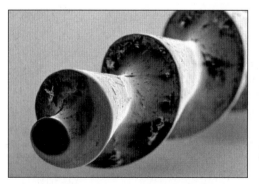

10.83 Maillefer gutta-condensor (SEM view)

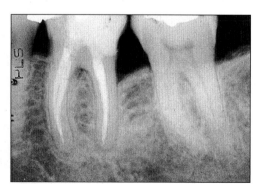

10.84

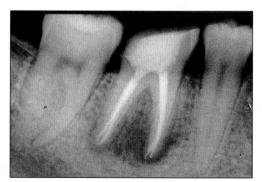

10.85

10.84–10.85 Thermomechanical compaction obturation (courtesy Dr J Woodson)

SEALERS

A root-canal sealer is radiopaque dental cement used, usually in combination with a solid or semi-solid core material, to fill voids and to seal root canals during obturation. All obturation techniques require the use of a sealer to fill minor discrepancies and voids in the obturation and to improve the seal between the core material and the walls of the canal. Sealers also act as a lubricant during gutta-percha placement of the master cone and any accessory cones. Sealers also reduce leakage.

Sealers (**10.86, 10.87**) can be divided into a number of main groups based on their constituents:

- zinc-oxide/eugenol materials (Roths, Pulp canal sealer, Wachs, Tubliseal, Procosol);
- calcium hydroxide-based materials (Sealapex, Apexit);
- combination zinc oxide/calcium hydroxide material (CRCS);
- glass ionomer (Ketac-Endo);
- resins (AH-26, AH-26 plus, Thermafil, Diaket);
- silicones (Lee Endo-Fill).

As with obturating materials the ideal sealer should be biocompatible, adhere to canal walls, be radiopaque, impermeable to tissue fluids, dimensionally stable, antiseptic, not discolour the tooth, and be easily manipulated.

SMEAR LAYER

The smear layer is a surface layer of debris formed on dentine during instrumentation (**10.88**). It is composed of organic and inorganic components and forms both a superficial, loosely adherent, layer and a deeper, tightly adherent, layer. There is some debate as to whether the smear layer should be removed or not. On the one hand, removal will eliminate the bacteria contained within the smear layer and will expose the dentinal tubules allowing close adaptation of the obturating material. Sealer and gutta-percha have been shown to flow into the tubules and bonding agents can form tags in the dentine. On the other hand, opening the tubules may provide a passage for microorganisms into the body of the dentine wall (**10.89**).

As mentioned earlier, apical resorption or iatrogenic alterations to the apical anatomy present a challenge to the clinician during all stages of treatment including obturation. Overcoming these problems frequently demands the institution of creative approaches. This may involve creation of an apical matrix or barrier in order to prevent extrusion of the obturating material. The matrix may be calcium hydroxide, ProRoot MTA (mineral trioxide aggregate) (**10.90**) or collagen (**10.91**), which can be placed to the established working length. The obturating material can then be packed against this matrix.

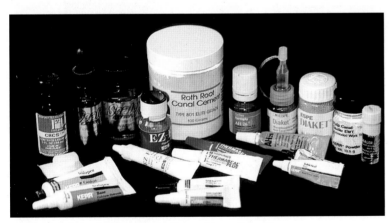

10.86 A variety of sealers currently used in endodontics

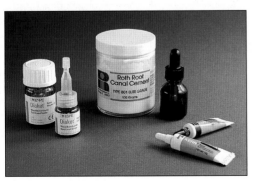

10.87 Endodontic sealers – Diaket; a resin-based sealer; Roths; a zinc oxide/eugenol-based sealer; and Sealapex; a calcium hydroxide-based sealer

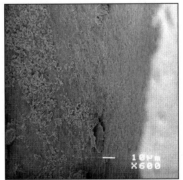

10.88 SEM of smear layer formed during instrumentation of a canal (× 600)

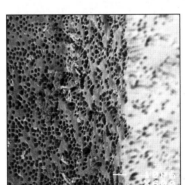

10.89 SEM of canal wall following irrigation with 5.25% sodium hypochlorite and 17% ethylenediamine-tetra-acetic acid showing exposure of the dentinal tubules (× 600)

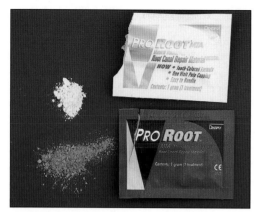

10.90 Mineral trioxide aggregate (MTA)

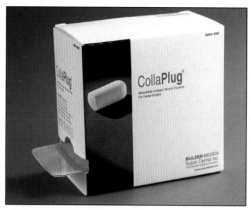

10.91 Collagen material such as CollaPlug can be used to form an apical matrix.

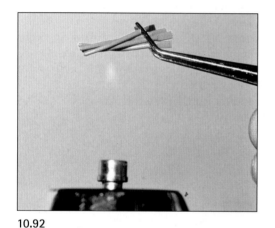

10.92

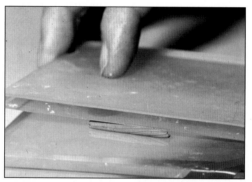

10.93

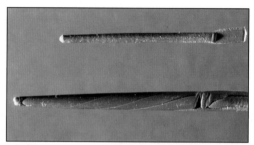

10.94

10.92–10.94 Customizing master point

Alternatively, gutta-percha cones can be custom moulded (**10.92–10.94**) to fit the apical anatomy. Large canals can also be obturated with customized gutta-percha cones.

CORONAL SEAL

Post preparation/restorative considerations

It is absolutely essential that an adequate coronal restoration be placed following obturation of the root canal system (**10.1**). It has been shown that the coronal restoration is as important, if not more important, than the root canal obturation. Placement of a permanent core restoration at this time would appear to be a sensible approach to the overall management of the case. Following obturation of the root canal system the tooth will never be 'cleaner' as it has been soaking in sodium hypochlorite throughout the preparation stage and the rubber dam remains in place. In addition, placing the core at this appointment negates the need to place a temporary restoration and reduces the number of dental appointments for the patient.

If a post space is required, the space created may be filled with a calcium hydroxide paste between visits in an attempt to reduce the chance of bacterial recontamination.

References

Cheung GS, Chan TK (2003) Long-term survival of primary root canal treatment carried out in a dental teaching hospital. *Int Endod J* **36**, 117–28.

Hasselgren G (1994) Where shall the root filling end? *New York State Dental J* **60**, 34–5.

Johnson WB (1978) A new gutta-percha technique. *J Endod* **4**, 184–7.

Siren EK, Haapasalo MP, Ranta K, Salami P, Kerosuo EN (1997) Microbiological findings and clinical treatment procedures in endodontic cases selected for microbiological investigation. *Int Endod J* **36**, 117–28.

Chapter 11

The endo–perio interface

K Gulabivala and U R Darbar

COMPARISON OF THE PRESENTATION OF APICAL AND MARGINAL PERIODONTITIS

It is a curious fact that both pulpal and periodontal diseases have their terminal effects in the periodontal tissues (cementum, periodontal ligament, alveolar bone). The difference is that the initial manifestation in periapical disease is at the apex of the root and in periodontal disease at the cervical (marginal) aspect of the tooth (**11.1**). In both cases, the periodontal tissues become chronically inflamed as a result of the establishment of an anaerobically dominated microbial flora in or on the adjacent root surface.

Marginal inflammation of the gingival tissues is preceded by the accumulation of plaque on the tooth surface, which may progress to periodontitis if the host susceptibility is compromised or altered as a result of modifying (risk) factors. The initial defence is mediated via the gingival sulcus at the level of the marginal attachment of the gingival tissues. In contrast, apical periodontitis is preceded by persistent pulp inflammation that is triggered by bacterial colonization of dentine. The initial defence is mediated at the level of the odontoblastic layer (see Chapter 1).

In periodontal disease, supragingival plaque sets the stage for subgingival microbial colonization of the root surface. This progresses apically with migration of the junctional epithelium and loss of the connective tissue attachment and ultimately bone (**11.2–11.5**). The pattern of attachment and bone loss can be site specific, varying around the circumference of the same tooth, and/or tooth specific varying around isolated sites on different teeth in the same mouth. The pattern of attachment loss may be relatively constant around all teeth in the mouth resulting in marginal bone loss such that the alveolar crest lies more than 2 mm below the cemento–enamel junction but parallel to the occlusal plane. This is commonly termed

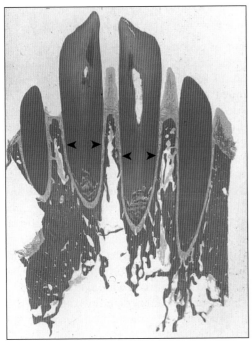

11.1 Periodontal ligament supporting teeth in alveolar bone (arrowed)

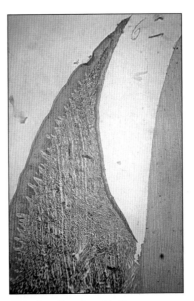

11.2 Junctional epithelium

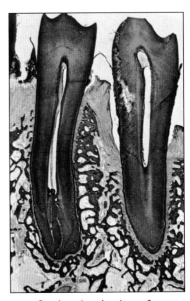

11.3 Section showing loss of marginal attachment and periodontal destruction

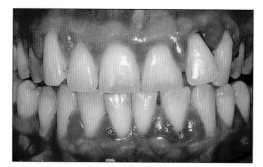

11.4 Early periodontal destruction

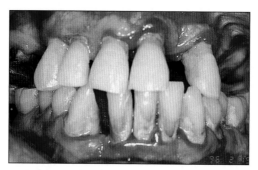

11.5 Advanced periodontal destruction

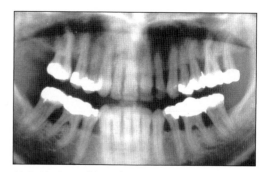

11.6 Horizontal bone loss

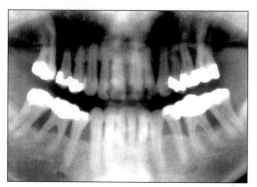

11.7 Horizontal bone loss – 4 years later

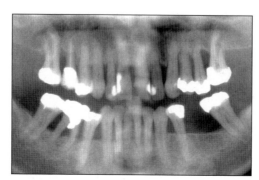

11.8 Horizontal bone loss – 12 years later

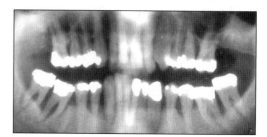

11.9 Vertical bone loss

horizontal bone loss (**11.6–11.8**). In other cases, the attachment loss may be irregular and localized to specific teeth with angular bone defects (also called vertical defects), in which the pattern of bone destruction progresses vertically along the root creating an oblique orientation of the alveolar crest with the tooth, the crest and root comprising opposite sides of the defect (**11.9**). This type of attachment loss may be associated with:

● anatomical defects on the root;
● nature of specific pathogenic flora on the root;
● necrotic (or at least partly necrotic) and infected pulp;
● defect in the host defence mechanism in the periodontium.

Such localized attachment loss may eventually encroach (**11.10**) and envelop the apex of the tooth root (**11.11, 11.12**) resulting in secondary involvement of the pulp, although this process may take years.

The extent and severity of the disease is measured by characterizing the attachment loss by periodontal probing and radiographic assessment of the pattern of bone loss.

In periapical disease, pulp infection usually begins in the crown of the tooth and progresses apically. If the pulp tissue in a lateral canal becomes necrotic and infected, a lateral periradicular radiolucency (usually enclosed by intact marginal bone) will arise, representing a localized site of inflammation (**11.13, 11.14**). As the infection in the pulp progresses further apically, the pulp tissue in the apical part of the root succumbs and further lateral and apical foramina may

become associated with adjacent bone loss (**11.15, 11.16**). The size and distribution of apical periodontitis (and thus apical radiolucency) is dictated by:

● the distribution of the lateral and apical foramina;
● the nature of the infecting microbial flora;
● the nature of the apical host defences.

The presence and extent of periapical disease is measured radiographically and also requires standardized radiography. The lesions of chronic apical periodontitis seldom result in retrograde marginal periodontitis with attachment loss. However, when this occurs, the probing depth and bone defect is usually deep and localized. Long-standing, untreated, marginal loss of attachment caused by root-canal infection may secondarily become established as a true marginal periodontitis requiring endodontic and periodontal treatment. Such lesions caused by root-canal infection may progressively widen with time and characterization of such loss of attachment requires *continuous probing* around the tooth (**11.17–11.19**), which gives a profile of both the width and the depth of the defect. Following treatment of the root canal infection, the chances of resolution of this type of localized marginal loss of attachment are high, because the infection is 'closed', that is, it is 'contained' within the tooth. In contrast, marginal loss of attachment due to periodontitis is seldom recovered due to 'the open' nature of the lesion, the immediate proximity of the infection to the marginal tissues and the role of host susceptibility and modifying factors in the initial progression of the lesion.

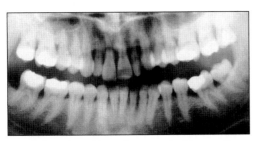

11.10 Periodontal bone loss encroaching on the apices of teeth

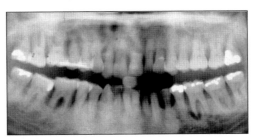

11.11 Periodontal bone loss involving the mesial root of 36

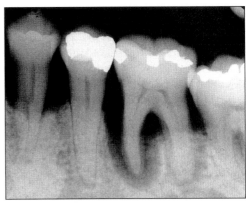

11.12 Periapical radiograph of the same as in **11.11**

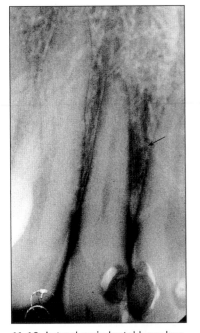

11.13 Lateral periodontal bone loss of pulpal origin (arrowed)

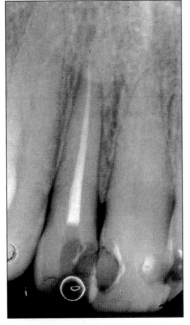

11.14 Resolution following root canal treatment

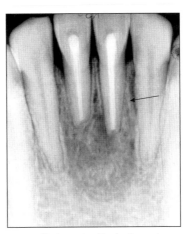

11.15 Early periradicular bone loss in 32 (arrowed)

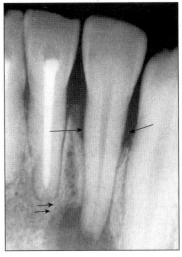

11.16 Further apical and marginal bone loss over a ten-year period in the tooth shown in **11.15**

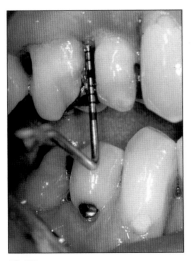

11.17

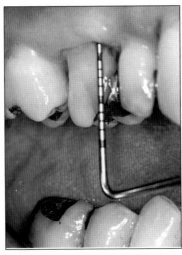

11.18

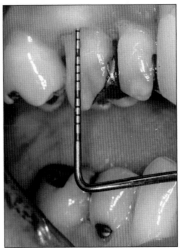

11.19

11.17–11.19 Continuous periodontal probing around maxillary molar showing sudden changes in probing depths

PATHWAYS OF COMMUNICATION BETWEEN PULP AND PERIODONTIUM

The pulp and periodontal tissues may communicate via anatomical features such as lateral or accessory canals, apical foramina, exposed dentinal tubules and developmental and cementum defects or by iatrogenic defects such as perforations or root fractures. The extent of the communication is determined by virtue of the morphology and dimension of the channel.

Lateral and accessory canals

Lateral canals are considered to be rare in the coronal third of the root and arise with a frequency of ~10% in the middle third (**11.20**) and ~25–35% in the apical third (**11.21, 11.22**) of the root. The mean prevalence of lateral canals, derived from a number of studies as shown in **Table 11.1**, is ~45%.

The prevalence of accessory canals in the furcation varies between 30 and 60%. The wide range reflects the outcome of methods used to detect them, since not all openings pass through as continuous channels.

Table 11.1 Prevalence of lateral canals

Studies	Year	No. of teeth	% with lateral canals
Rubach & Mitchell	1965	74	45
Lowman *et al.*	1973	46	59
Vertucci & Williams	1974	100	46
Kirkham	1975	100	23
Vertucci & Gegauff	1979	400	49
Total & Mean		720	44.4

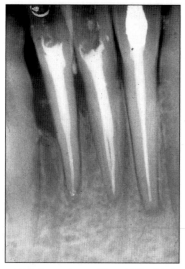

11.20 Lateral canal in middle third of mandibular incisor

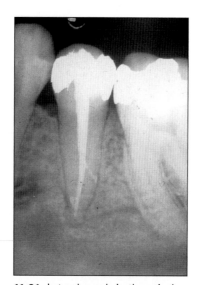

11.21 Lateral canals in the apical third of a mandibular premolar

Dentinal tubules

Provide long and extremely narrow channels of communication (see Chapter 1) but are perfectly capable of conveying bacteria and their products as well as molecular mediators of inflammation (**11.23**). Fortunately they do not communicate with the periodontium under normal circumstances. See Cementum defects below.

Development defects

Various defects such as invaginations of the coronal or radicular tissues may occur during the development of teeth. In the majority of cases, the invaginations do not allow communication between the tissues but occasionally developmental grooves, e.g. palato-gingival grooves may be deep enough to communicate with the pulp (**11.24–11.27**).

Cementum defects

In 10% of teeth (see Chapter 1), the cementum does not abut or overlap the enamel, leaving dentinal tubules open at the cervical margin of teeth. Equally such defects may sometimes arise on the root surface naturally or as a result of resorption caused by trauma or inflammation.

Iatrogenic perforations and root fracture

Iatrogenic perforations may occur in lateral walls of the roots or through the pulpal floor in a multirooted tooth as a result of root canal treatment (furcal strip perforation, apical transportation, lateral

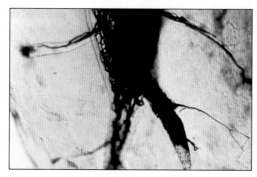

11.22 Histological demonstration of apical lateral canals

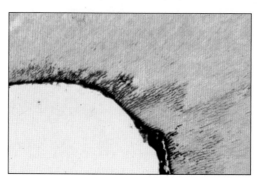

11.23 Microorganisms within dentinal tubules of infected tooth

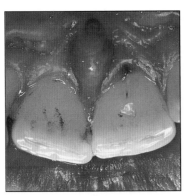

11.24 Palato-gingival groove in maxillary central incisor

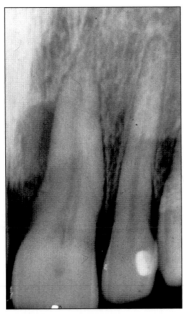

11.25 Radiograph of the tooth showing bone loss

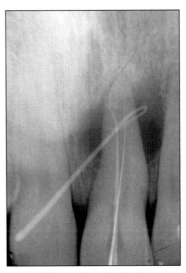

11.26 Diagnostic endodontic instruments and gutta-percha in place

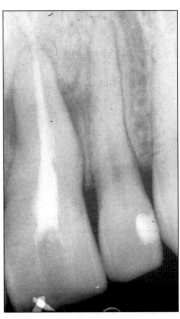

11.27 Radiograph demonstrating some infilling of bony defect

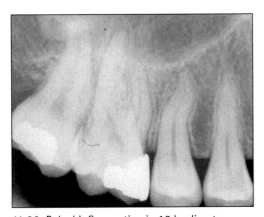

11.28 Pulpal inflammation in 16 leading to thickening of the periodontal ligament space on the palatal root

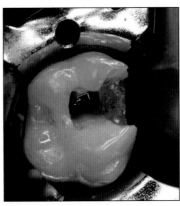

11.29 Pulpal inflammation evident on opening the pulp chamber

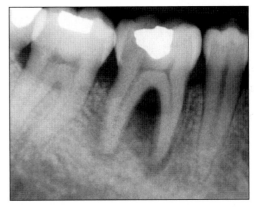

11.30 Furcal and apical bone loss in a mandibular molar

perforation) or restorative procedures (post or pin perforations). In addition, root fractures, both vertical and horizontal, create an artificial communication between the root and pulp space, the periodontal ligament, and may be associated with healthy or root-treated teeth.

EFFECT OF PULP DISEASE AND ITS TREATMENT ON THE PERIODONTIUM

Periodontal inflammation and bone loss

It is known that pulp inflammation can be transmitted through lateral communications to the periodontium, both in the furcation and apically. It is possible for the inflammation to be severe enough to manifest in submarginal bone loss, especially in younger patients (**11.28, 11.29**). Root-canal infection in addition to apical periodontitis can have a number of other effects on the periodontium. It may contribute to horizontal marginal bone loss (**11.20**) and also vertical intrabony defects (**11.16**). There is also a higher likelihood of furcation involvement in multirooted teeth with root-canal infection (**11.30**).

Periodontal wound healing

Teeth with pulps necrotized by acute trauma may have compromised periodontal healing with marginal epithelial down-growth on their roots. Periodontal wound healing after surgery may also be

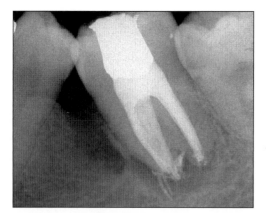

11.31 Extrusion of root-filling material in mandibular molar

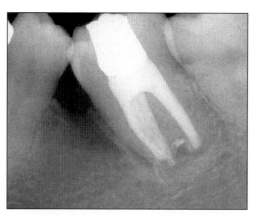

11.32 Delayed apical healing associated with the extrusion

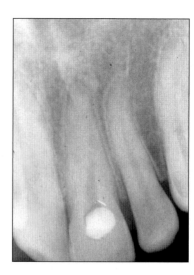

11.33 Perforation in central incisor

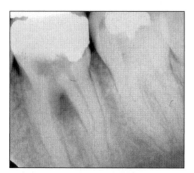

11.34 Perforation in the floor of the pulp chamber of a mandibular molar

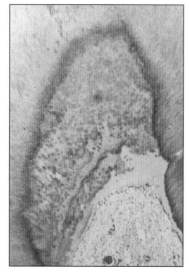

11.35 Reparative dentine defending the pulp space

compromised if root-canal infection is present. Periodontal healing after periapical surgery is often associated with postsurgical attachment loss or recession. Many factors influence this, including gingival tissue thickness, alveolar bone level, surgical trauma to the flap and effectiveness of flap repositioning. In addition, it is also known that such mean attachment loss after periapical surgery is greater when there is absence of periapical healing indicating the persistence of root-canal infection.

There is a trend among some periodontists to request root canal treatment on teeth with 'doubtful' pulp status when regenerative surgery is planned in the site. The rationale is to eliminate possible sources of infection to maximize the potential for successful outcome. This desire to eliminate root-canal infection must be tempered by the knowledge that extrusion of root canal treatment materials may have an equally negative impact on periapical healing (**11.31, 11.32**) and therefore the prognosis of subsequent periodontal surgery.

Effect of iatrogenic problems

Iatrogenic perforations create additional, and usually larger, channels of communication between the pulp space and periodontium. If previously infected these may cause insurmountable inflammation that may be treated only by root resection or tooth extraction. The larger the communication the more difficult the management (**11.33, 11.34**).

EFFECT OF PERIODONTAL DISEASE AND ITS TREATMENT ON THE PULP

Effect of periodontal disease on the pulp

Infection of the periodontium and the root surface appears to have only a limited effect on the pulp. This is probably because the pulp response tends to close off channels of communication by the laying down of secondary dentine and sclerosis of dentinal tubules (**11.35**). There may be a greater prevalence of dystrophic pulp calcification and canal narrowing in periodontally involved teeth, which can lead to technical problems during root canal treatment. Occasionally the bacterial stimulus from exposed lateral canals may be sufficient to cause localized pulp necrosis and infection, adding to the periodontal problem. The pulp may eventually succumb either because the periodontal disease reaches the root apex or the infection in the pulp spreads (**11.36, 11.37**). In either case, the long-term prognosis of the tooth is likely to be poor at this point and it should be extracted or, if a single root of a multi-rooted tooth is involved, root resection may be considered.

Effect of periodontal treatment on the pulp

Periodontal treatment consists of debridement (scaling and root planing) which may sometimes result in removal of excessive amounts

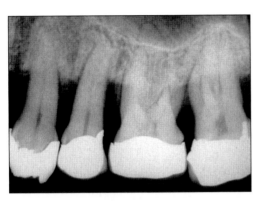

11.36 Pulpal and periodontal involvement of maxillary premolar

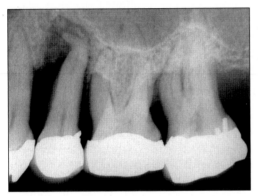

11.37 Progression of the two separate processes gives a combined lesion

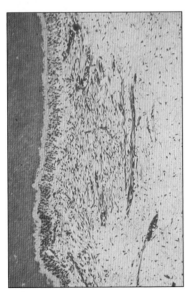

11.38 Pulp inflammation adjacent to open dentinal tubules

DEFINITION AND CLASSIFICATION OF PERIO–ENDO LESIONS

Both apical and marginal periodontitis manifest in their common borderland, the periodontal tissues. In the vast majority of patients, these two disease processes, which require entirely different treatment regimens, are easily differentiated. In a small proportion of cases, each disease process has the potential to mimic the other and in some, the two disease processes may be coexistent. If the disease in one tissue is either left untreated or is inadequately treated, it may progress to involve the secondary tissues.

Definition of perio–endo lesions

The small group of unique clinical cases mentioned above have been loosely termed 'perio–endo' lesions but precise definitions are elusive. Definition may be attempted as follows:

- an isolated, usually narrow, deep probing depth of pulpal or periodontal origin;
- lesion with submarginal or intrabony periradicular bone loss of pulpal and/or periodontal origin that communicates with the oral cavity via a probing defect;
- a *localized* periodontal probing depth of pulpal or periodontal origin.

These definitions do not allude to the apical or marginal origin of the lesions, as by their nature the origin is unknown at the time of presentation. The key aspect of the definitions is that they represent a potentially broad range of clinical presentations.

Classification

Several classifications have been proposed but none of them especially contributes to diagnosis or treatment. They do, however, serve to delineate the categories possible to encounter in practice. A simple classification is adopted here:

1. Primary endodontic lesion (with potential for true secondary periodontal involvement).
2. Primary periodontal lesion (with potential for true secondary pulpal involvement).
3. True combined lesion of dual origin.

DIAGNOSIS OF PERIO–ENDO LESIONS

Isolated 'perio–endo' lesions in patients without generalized periodontal disease are easily categorized as such, despite their variable presentation. The precise presentation features depend on the aetiology and its duration of existence. Localized, marked areas of attachment loss (often categorized as perio–endo lesions) also arise in patients with generalized periodontal disease but the number of sites involved and their presentation are more variable and complex.

Regardless of their location and number, 'perio–endo' lesions continue to challenge clinicians in arriving at a definitive diagnosis of origin. The principle reason for this is the difficulty in ascertaining

of cementum and exposure of the dentinal tubules. Microbial colonization of these exposed tubules can lead to pulp inflammation (**11.38**) that will usually resolve if the pulp is not already compromised by restorative procedures. If it is, then the microbial insult may be sufficient to tip the balance thus causing pulp necrosis and infection. Exposure of dentinal tubules inevitably leads to dentine sensitivity and with plaque accumulation may lead to hypersensitivity.

the pulp status, as the tissues are invisible. Total pulp necrosis is relatively easy to diagnose (because of the high sensitivity and specificity of pulp tests under those conditions) but partial pulp necrosis and infection pose a problem, particularly in multirooted teeth.

Diagnosis is based on taking a systematic and careful history and on clinical examination; encompassing both endodontic and periodontal components. The key elements, which should be considered together, include:

- history of dentinal, pulpal or periapical pain;
- history of periodontal symptoms (bleeding, recurrent infection, mobility);
- signs and symptoms of pulp/periapical disease (including vitality tests);
- periodontal charting including the probing profile around the tooth;
- radiographic pattern of marginal and periradicular bone loss.

History of dentinal, pulpal and periapical pain

This may give clues about the pulpal history of the tooth and the likelihood of partial pulp necrosis as the cause of the presenting findings.

History of periodontal symptoms

The duration and nature of the periodontal symptoms will help to characterize the general periodontal status and should include an assessment of risk factors such as smoking. The information will give an indication of the individual's susceptibility to periodontal breakdown and will also help differentiate and distinguish problems associated with generalized periodontal problems as opposed to those associated with local periodontal breakdown or associated with other non-periodontal causes. This aspect of the examination is also important, especially in patients with generalized periodontal breakdown, as the prognosis of the teeth can then be assessed in relation to the patient's motivation and compliance, which will affect the response to treatment.

Signs and symptoms of pulpal or periapical disease

The involved and adjacent teeth should be examined carefully for evidence of pulpal or periapical disease. This includes performing vitality tests on the teeth using cold, heat and electrical tests as each of these tests give different clues. Each root or cusp of a multirooted tooth should be tested separately to elicit unique responses from each part of the tooth. Although it may be thought that pulp-test responses on a tooth would be uniform over its surface, there are local variations which may be attributed to differences in thickness of enamel and dentine but which may also be due to partial necrosis of the pulp.

Root-filled teeth may also be associated with perio–endo lesions. The quality of the root filling, how long ago it was performed, and by whom, should be determined. The quality of the root filling (poor or good) does not necessarily correlate with the presence or absence of residual root-canal infection. This must be gauged from other clinical signs of infection.

Periodontal charting including the probing profile of the tooth

A full periodontal assessment must be performed if the patient gives a periodontal history. It should include a record of the recession, mobility and furcation involvement. The nature of the restorations should also be noted, especially on teeth designated with combined problems. Teeth suspected of having perio–endo lesions should have their periodontal probing profile recorded in detail using continuous probing (see below, **11.39–11.41**).

Clinically, attachment loss is measured by probing the pocket from a fixed reference point. Ideally this should be the cemento–enamel junction (CEJ), however, due to difficulties of ascertaining the position of the CEJ, the gingival margin is often used as the reference point. The probing depth, described as the distance between the gingival margin and the apical depth of probe penetration, is used to characterize the distribution of the attachment and bone loss. The accuracy and reproducibility of probing is dependant upon the type of probe used, the force applied to the probe and the position of the

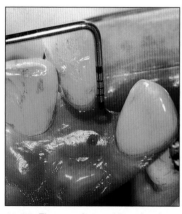

11.39 Three-point probing depths palatally – distopalatal probing

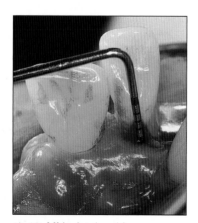

11.40 Midpalatal probing

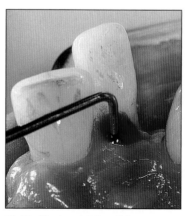

11.41 Mesiopalatal probing

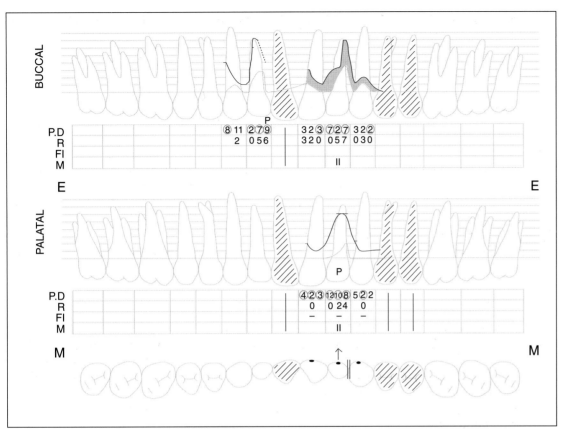

11.42 Six-point probing chart produced for the maxillary incisor in **11.39–11.41**

P = pus
PD = probing depth in millimetres (mm)
R = recession in mm
FI = furcation involvement
M = mobility (11 = grade of mobility)

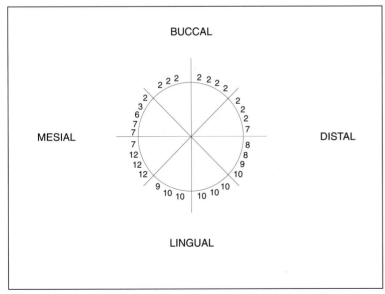

11.43 Charting continuous probing profile of the tooth

In contrast to this a *continuous probing profile* is obtained by running the probe gently along the entire circumference of the gingival sulcus of the tooth suspected to be associated with a perio–endo lesion (**11.17–11.19**). An accurate record of the continuous probing profile is maintained by dividing the tooth into sections as shown in **Figure 11.43**. The probing profile will help define the nature of the pocket, i.e. whether it is long and narrow or broad and wide, and also aid monitoring of its response to treatment.

Long, narrow pockets are classically considered to be of endodontic origin (**11.44, 11.45**). However, lateral endodontic abscesses may result in 'blow-out' lesions that exhibit extremely wide, as well as deep, probing profiles (**11.46**), yet respond favourably to endodontic treatment alone. The so-called endodontic lesions with secondary periodontal involvement should by definition have deep but narrower probing profiles and should respond favourably to endodontic treatment. They may also require adjunctive periodontal management. There are, however, few recorded cases that demonstrate such true natural progression of endodontic to periodontal disease.

Radiographic pattern of bone loss

The radiographic pattern of bone loss further helps characterize the nature and extent of the periodontal breakdown and is read in conjunction with the probing profile. The apical extent of the bone loss

probe in relation to the tooth. It is denoted with a 6-point charting (3 points buccally and 3 points palatally or lingually) (**11.39–11.42**) of the whole mouth and is used in conjunction with standardized accurate full-mouth, parallel-view periapical radiographs.

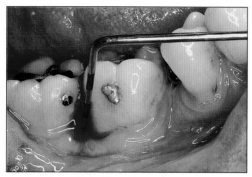

11.44 Probing on the distal aspect of an endodontically compromised molar

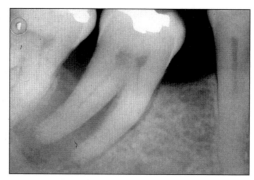

11.45 Radiograph of the same molar

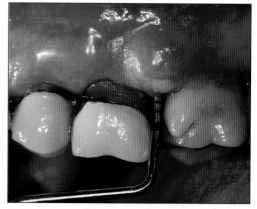

11.46 Probing lateral endodontic abscess

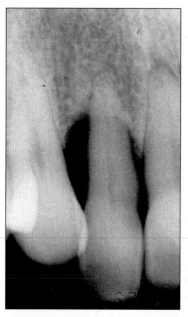

11.47 Bone loss involving the apical third

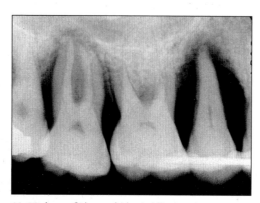

11.48 Loss of the periodontal ligament space around 15 and 17

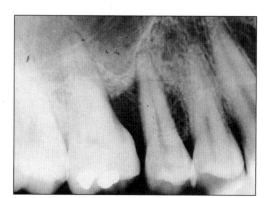

11.49 Bone loss between 15 and 16

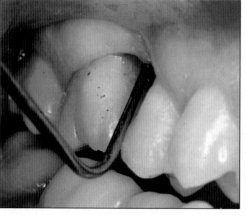

11.50 Probing the bone defect

(**11.47**), absence of definition of the periodontal ligament space around the periapex (**11.48**) and the general shape of the bone defect (angularity and presence of marginal bone) (**11.49, 11.50**),

all help to characterize the lesion. In patients with generalized periodontal disease, the following types of bone defects are more likely contributed to by pulp infection in the associated tooth:

● periodontal intrabony defect affecting more than two-thirds of the root length;
● horizontal bone loss affecting more than two-thirds of the root length;
● periodontal bone loss involving the root-end.

The chance of pulp involvement is further enhanced by the presence of;

● large restorations with marked changes in contour of the pulp chamber;
● negative or delayed vitality responses;
● technically poor root filling(s).

As a rule, acute pain is not a common presenting feature of 'perio–endo' lesions because of their 'open' nature. However, acute exacerbations do occur and are frequently mistaken for those of endodontic origin but they can arise equally commonly from either source. It has been suggested that dento-alveolar abscesses with 30–60% spirochaetes on dark-field microscopy are more likely to be of periodontal origin and those with 0–10% spirochaetes, of endodontic origin.

POSSIBLE CAUSES OF PERIO-ENDO LESIONS

In addition to the key elements used in the diagnosis, lesions with a higher chance of primary periodontal aetiology exhibit the following features:

- generalized periodontal disease;
- poor oral hygiene and presence of calculus;
- periodontal probing defects that are generally broad rather than narrow.

Relatively narrow, deep, isolated, periodontal probing depths are more likely to have a primary endodontic aetiology. There are numerous causes of lesions with such presenting features but the exact presentation depends upon the cause, history, duration and episodes of acute exacerbation. The different causes and their presenting features are described below.

Single isolated perio–endo lesion

Root canal infection

This may result in lateral areas of bone loss without involving the root apices due to the presence of lateral canal(s) as a result of partial necrosis of the pulp (**11.13, 11.14**). In some cases the periradicular area may extend around the whole of one side of the root (**11.51, 11.52**). In addition, if the lesion (**11.53**) is suppurative, then it may drain through a sinus tract in the oral mucosa (**11.54**) or the periodontal ligament (**11.55–11.57**). A lateral abscess may result in a much larger width of periodontal attachment loss. Diagnosis is straightforward when the vitality tests are negative. When they are equivocal, because of partial pulp necrosis, the diagnosis is difficult and other clues have to be sought to arrive at a definitive diagnosis. Root-canal treatment alone should result in complete resolution (**11.56–11.59**) and in doubtful cases will act as the definitive diagnosis (in retrospect). In fact, root debridement may compromise successful reattachment of periodontal tissues if it is aggressive enough to damage cells on the root surface.

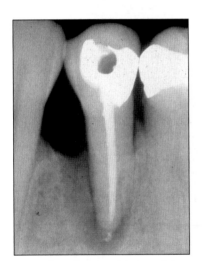
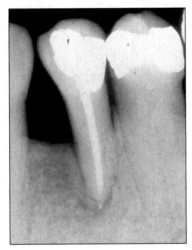

11.51 Bone loss involving mesial side of mandibular premolar

11.52 Resolution following root canal treatment

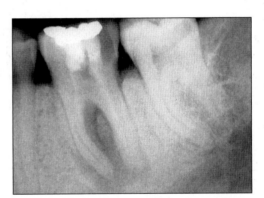

11.53 Furcal and apical bone loss associated with mandibular molar

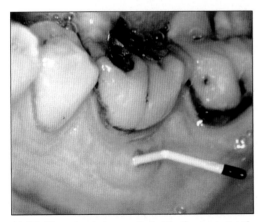

11.54 Sinus tract demonstrated in the same tooth

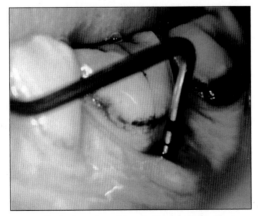

11.55 Periodontal probing before endodontic treatment

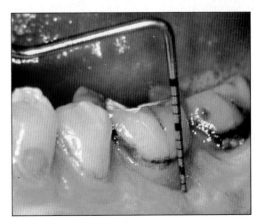

11.56 Periodontal probing after endodontic treatment

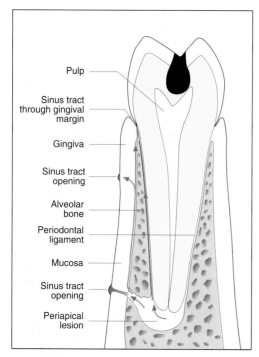

11.57 Pathways of suppuration spread

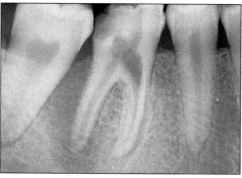

11.58 Suppurating defect associated with mandibular molar

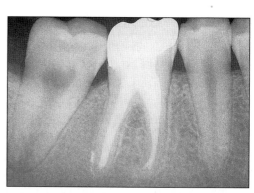

11.59 Healing following root canal treatment

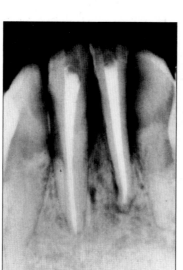

11.60

11.60–11.61 Gutta-percha points used to trace localised deep probing defects on opposite sides of premolars

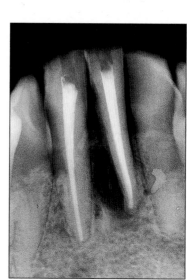

11.61

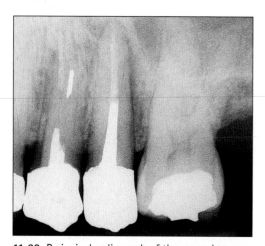

11.62 Periapical radiograph of the premolars

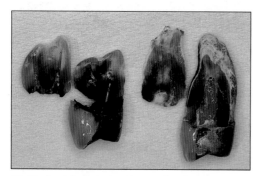

11.63 Root fragments of premolars in 11.62 following extraction

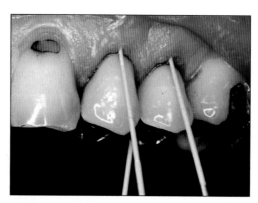

11.64 Root-filled mandibular incisors, one of which is fractured

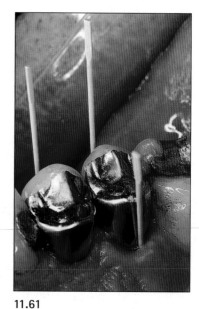

11.65 Radiograph showing the 'J' shaped pattern of bone loss around the fractured incisor

Root fractures

Surprisingly these can survive for several years without catastrophic failure. In the meantime, they produce periodontal breakdown with pathognomonic probing (**11.60–11.63**) and bone loss (**11.64, 11.65**) patterns. In **Figures 11.60–11.63**, the long-standing fracture survived with two localized, deep probing defects on opposite surfaces of the root with mild symptoms and without decementation until the extraction of the teeth. The staining inside the root fragments shows the extent and duration of the fracture (**11.63**). The 'J'-shaped radiographic lesion is the classical sign of a long-standing root fracture, usually in the mesio-distal plane (**11.65**). However, the precise presentation depends upon the direction, extent and duration of fracture. A fracture in the mesio-distal plane that is prevented from progressing further apically by a crown, may result in an associated bone defect that is limited to the coronal part of the root (**11.66**). The presence of a radicular post may mask radiographic signs of a bucco-palatal fracture (**11.67, 11.68**). In general fractures will not be visible unless they are within five degrees of the X-ray beam. Fractures can arise in the following ways:

- crown (vital or non-vital teeth);
- root (vital or non-vital teeth).

Sometimes they can only be confirmed by surgical exploration.

Fractures in teeth with vital pulps seldom reach a point of established periodontal pocketing as the tooth is extremely painful on biting (in a particular way) and the patient will seek help earlier (e.g. cracked-tooth syndrome). The fracture line is often invisible in these cases, unless the pain is less acute, when the fracture line can become stained thus becoming visible. Diagnosis is confirmed by cementing a well-fitting orthodontic band that will often prevent movement of the tooth fragments and stop the pain (**11.69**). Definitive treatment involves placement of a cusp-covered cast restoration (**11.70, 11.71**).

Fractures may arise in the roots of vital teeth (**11.72, 11.73**) and diagnosis may initially be problematic (**11.74–11.76**). In this case, pulp involvement was suspected and a fracture was only noticed later during treatment when bleeding into the canal could not be controlled. The tooth required surgical treatment.

Fractures in non-vital, infected teeth usually progress to extensive inflammation of the periodontium (**11.77**), together with matching bone loss (**11.78**). Symptoms may be mild, unless there are acute exacerbations. Patients may report a bad taste and odour in the mouth. Fractures commencing in the crown (**11.79–11.83**), may be visible with good lighting and will often respond to biting tests on individual pairs of cusps. It is important to protect such teeth from progression of the fracture by placing a band while endodontic treatment is carried out (**11.81**) and subsequently by placing a

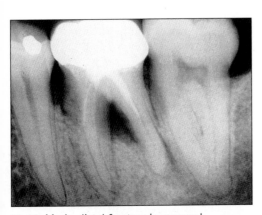

11.66 Mesio-distal fracture in crowned mandibular molar

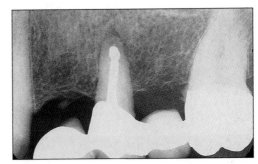

11.67 Bucco-palatal fracture in maxillary premolar

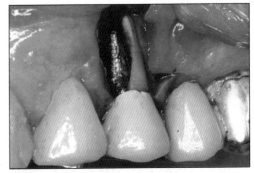

11.68 Appearance following removal of the fractured portion of root

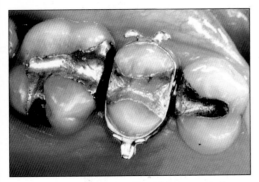

11.69 Banded vital premolar with suspected cuspal fracture

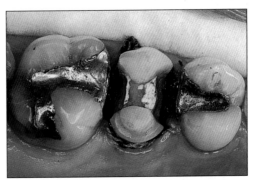

11.70 Preparation for a restoration providing occlusal protection

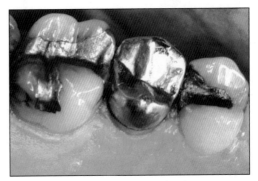

11.71 Partial veneer restoration in place

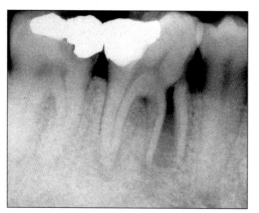

11.72 Fracture in mesial root of vital mandibular first molar

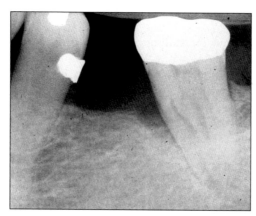

11.73 Root fracture in mandibular second molar

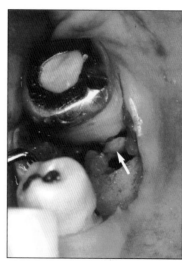

11.74 Surgical exposure of root fragment (arrowed) in mandibular second molar

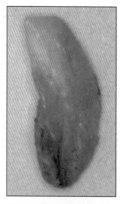

11.75 Root fragment following extraction

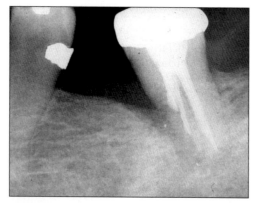

11.76 Tooth in 11.73 following endodontic and surgical treatment

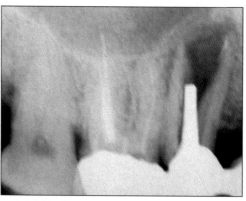

11.77 Fractured premolar with post-retained restoration

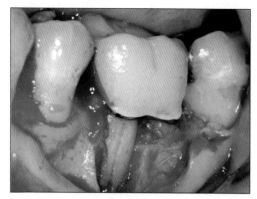

11.78 Bone loss related to fracture of the mesial root of a mandibular molar

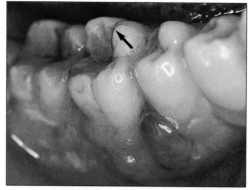

11.79 Mandibular first molar with mesio-distal fracture (arrowed)

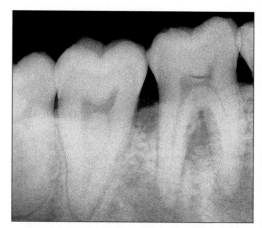

11.80 Periapical radiograph of tooth in 11.79 showing periradicular bone loss

permanent cast restoration with full cuspal coverage (**11.82, 11.83**). Fractures extending to the roots usually have poor prognosis and should be extracted.

Teeth with fractures commencing in the root may also be tender to bite on but display no differential discomfort on individual pairs of cusps. Such a fracture only results in a probing defect once the fracture line progresses to the crown. Until then, if the fracture line is superimposed on a root filling, diagnosis may be reliant upon surgical exploration (**11.84, 11.85**). The degree of pocketing and its width varies from a localized, narrow deep defect in an incipient fracture to a wider defect in a more established and long-standing fracture. The treatment will usually consist of root resection in a multirooted tooth or tooth extraction depending on the extent of the fracture.

Teeth with horizontal root fractures may exhibit increased mobility but do not require root canal treatment (**11.86**) unless pulpal or periapical symptoms intervene (**11.87**). Under these circumstances, it is usually not necessary to treat both coronal and apical fragments

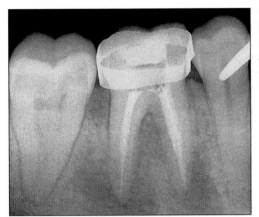

11.81 Periapical radiograph following root canal treatment and the placement of a supporting orthodontic band

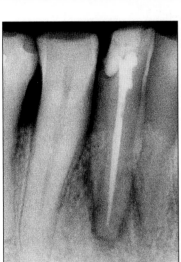

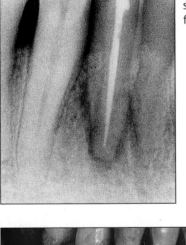

11.84 Root-filled mandibular incisor with suspected fracture

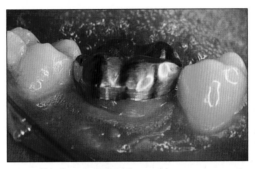

11.82 Tooth restored with a gold veneer crown to provide occlusal protection

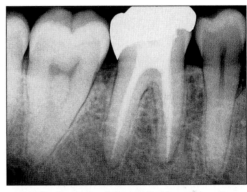

11.83 Radiograph of the tooth 15 months after commencement of treatment – there is evidence of periradicular healing

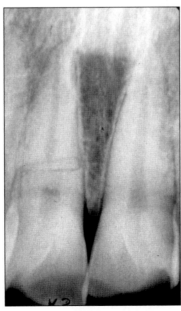

11.86 Maxillary incisor with horizontal fracture

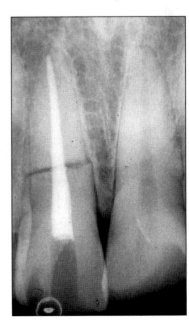

11.87 Root canal treatment of fractured incisor because of pulpal symptoms

11.85 Surgical exposure of the fracture

as the apical fragment is rarely infected (**11.88, 11.89**). The horizontal fracture line may be better revealed by an occlusal view if the fracture line is more oblique but if even this does not show it up, two radiolucent lesions on either side of a fracture line give it away (**11.90**). Horizontal fractures in the coronal third of the root are regarded as having poor prognosis but many survive the dentist's pessimism (**11.91, 11.92**) – this has lasted for 30 years!

Root perforation

During root canal treatment or restorative procedures, root perforation will expose any residual infection within the root canal system to the periodontium and consequently lay the tooth open to the development of a perio–endo lesion in the same way as for root-canal infection (**11.93**). Coronal root perforations that traumatize the marginal attachment may present with wider probing defects and are difficult to manage without crown lengthening procedures (**11.94, 11.95**). Perforations that are more apical have better prognosis as they can be treated as 'iatrogenic canals' (**11.96, 11.97**). Immediate repair of the perforation without allowing it to become infected gives the best outcome. Furcation perforations stand the best chance of success in the absence of a periodontal communication (**11.98, 11.99**). The use of amalgam for repair of perforations has been superseded by MTA (ProRoot®). Used in combination with regenerative techniques in the appropriate situation it may enhance the prognosis. Exposure of the perforation to the oral environment (coronally or through a periodontal communication) decreases chances of success (**11.100**). In the case shown (**11.100–11.107**), a highly motivated patient was nevertheless treated at his insistence with informed consent. Following root-canal treatment, a flap was raised and tin foil placed as a matrix (**11.103**) to repair the perforation surgically (**11.104**). As the teeth appeared to have poor long-term prognosis, they were restored with amalgam coronal restorations (**11.106**). The furcation defect never healed and a through and through furcation morphology became established following surgery but the patient was able to maintain it with 'bottle' brushes and the tooth was functional three years later (**11.107**). Today, regenerative techniques may offer better hope for such teeth.

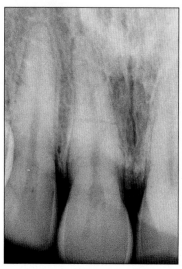

11.88 Maxillary incisor with middle-third horizontal fracture

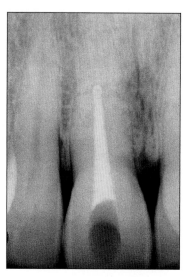

11.89 Fractured incisor following root canal treatment to the fracture line

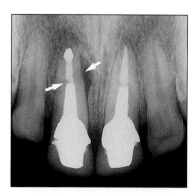

11.90 Bilateral periradicular bone loss (arrowed) associated with a fractured maxillary incisor

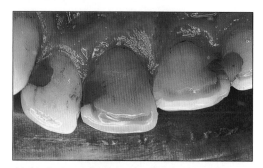

11.91 Incisor with longstanding horizontal fracture

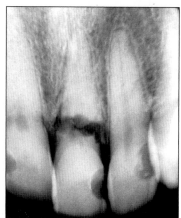

11.92 Radiograph of the tooth in **11.91** indicating an absence of interventive treatment

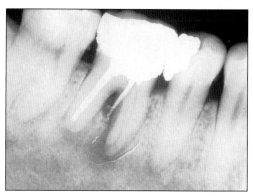

11.93 Mandibular molar with a perforation and furcal and periradicular bone loss

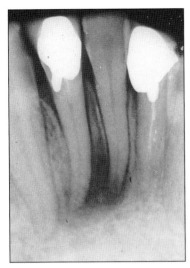

11.94 Mandibular incisors with radiographic evidence of coronal-third root perforations and a need for root canal treatment

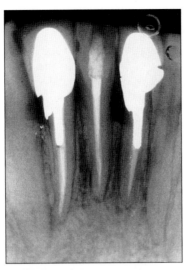

11.95 Mandibular incisors in 11.94 following crown-lengthening procedures, endodontic treatment and new post-retained restorations

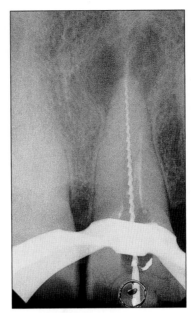

11.96 Maxillary incisor with established lateral perforation

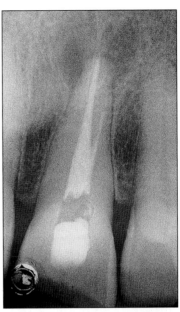

11.97 Radiographic appearance of the maxillary incisor following root canal retreatment

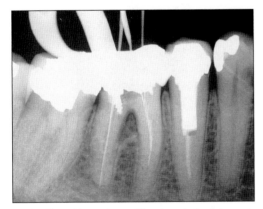

11.98 Furcal bone loss without periodontal communication in a mandibular molar with long-standing perforation

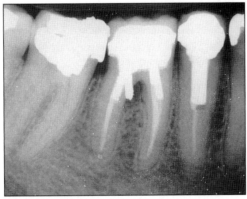

11.99 Tooth with evidence of some healing following root canal treatment and new post-retained restoration

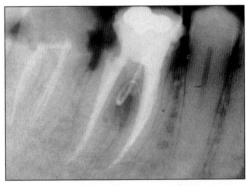

11.100 Furcal bone loss with periodontal communication in a root-treated mandibular molar

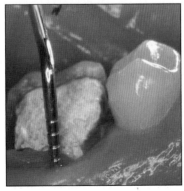

11.101 Periodontal probing of the furcal bone defect of tooth in 11.100

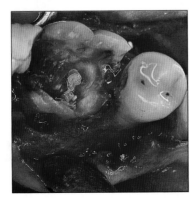

11.102 Surgical exposure of the furcal perforation

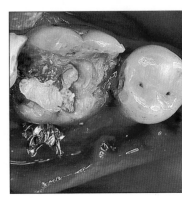

11.103 Tinfoil placed below perforation to act as a matrix

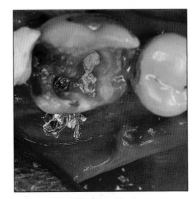

11.104 Placement of EBA cement

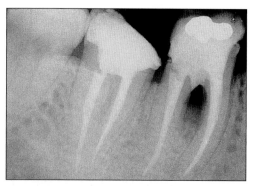

11.105 Radiograph following the sealing of the perforation

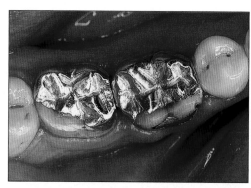

11.106 The restored mandibular molars

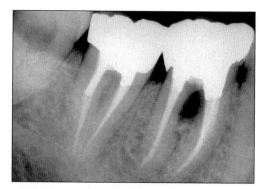

11.107 Radiograph of the mandibular molars three years later

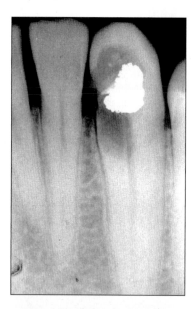

11.108 Radiograph of mandibular canine with external root resorption

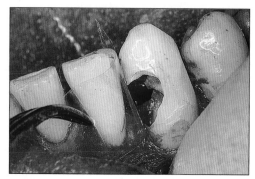

11.109 Surgical exposure and removal of the granulomatous resorbing tissue

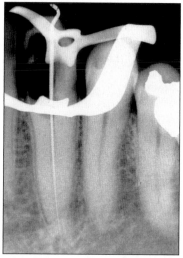

11.110 Radiograph taken during endodontic treatment

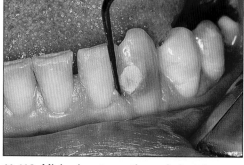

11.112 Minimal postoperative periodontal probing of the restored defect

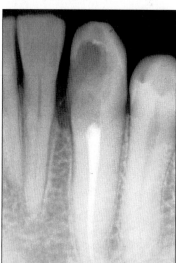

11.111 Radiograph of completed root treatment and coronal restoration

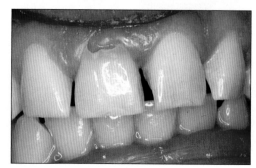

11.113 Central incisor with broad shallow cervical defect

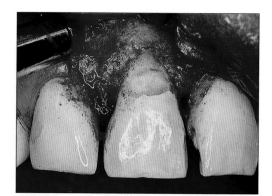

11.114 Surgical exposure and removal of granulomatous resorbing tissue. The pulp is not exposed in this case and the tooth does not require root canal treatment

Root resporption

External root resorption at the cervical margin can arise as a result of various insults to the periodontium (periodontal disease, trauma, tooth bleaching, orthodontic treatment, surgery). The pattern of resorption may vary according to the aetiology, type and severity. The entry point of resorption may be confined and deep (**11.108–11.112**) or broad and shallow (**11.113, 11.114**). It can lead to a localized periodontal probing defect though it is likely to be broader than those originating from root-canal infections or root fractures. Management requires flap surgery to expose and repair the defect but root canal treatment may also be required. The sequence of endodontic and periodontal treatment depends on the nature of the problem. Sometimes both have to be performed at the same operation for optimal outcome (**11.108–11.112**).

Internal root resorption may also create a communication between the pulp and the periodontium and, if infected, may result in a perio–endo communication in the same way as an iatrogenic perforation (**11.115, 11.116**). Treatment involves root canal therapy and, if necessary, surgery (**11.117**). For differential diagnosis of these lesions see Chapter 14.

Anatomical anomalies

These can present in a variety of ways and again the presentation is entirely dependent upon the nature of the defect. The commonest perio–endo defect associated with such anomalies is caused by developmental grooves on the palatal aspects of maxillary central or lateral incisors (**11.118–11.121**). They give the classical narrow, deep,

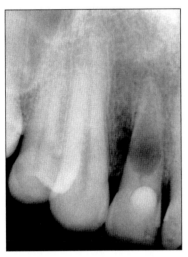

11.115 Large defect in maxillary incisor due to internal resorption

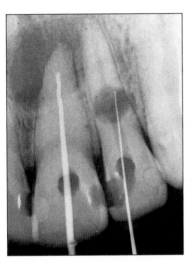

11.116 Lateral incisor with large resorptive defect involving the periodontal tissues. The central incisor also requires endodontic treatment

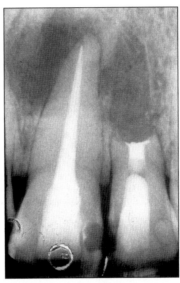

11.117 Central and lateral incisors following endodontic treatment and surgical removal of the apical portion of the lateral incisor root

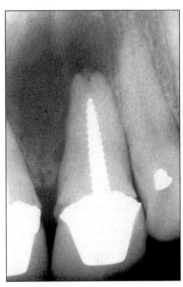

11.118 Radiograph of non-vital central incisor with periradicular bone loss

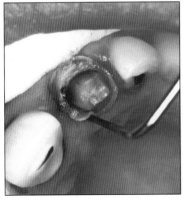

11.119 Probing the developmental groove present in the central incisor in 11.118

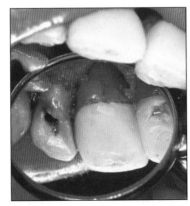

11.120 Exposure of the groove prior to debriding and flattening the groove

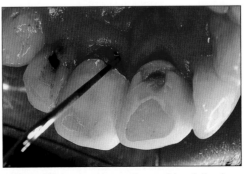

11.121 Minimal postoperative probing following surgery

localized probing defect associated with periradicular bone loss (**11.119, 11.121**). Identification of the aetiology is generally easy as the groove often extends across the palatal marginal ridge and into the cingulum pit (**11.122–11.127**). The groove may also occur bilaterally, though curiously, both teeth seldom develop perio–endo lesions.

Sometimes the groove may be deep enough to communicate with the pulp and so the tooth may become non-vital (**11.24–11.27**). Frequently though, the tooth presents with a root filling. It may be that the pulp had indeed become non-vital or that the previous operator had missed the localized periodontal pocket and had assumed the problem to be of endodontic origin. These teeth respond surprisingly well to surgical correction involving widening or flattening of the groove by judicious drilling (**11.121, 11.125–11.127**). The adjunctive use of glass ionomer cement to fill the groove if it is very

deep and guided tissue regeneration in the management of these lesions can be successful and is described later.

Other anatomical anomalies include root divisions (**11.128, 11.129**), fused teeth (**11.130–11.132**) and invaginations that communicate directly with the periodontium rather than the pulp (**11.133–11.135**) Consequently, the pulp may remain vital and normal while the tooth is associated with a periradicular radiolucency (**11.136**).

Another developmental anomaly that may lead to localized periodontal breakdown is the presence of enamel 'pearl(s)' in the furcation or proximal areas (**11.137, 11.138**).

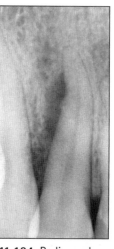

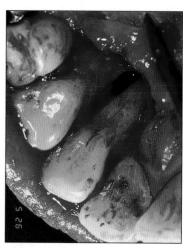

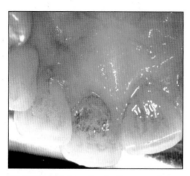

11.122 Palato-gingival groove in maxillary lateral incisor

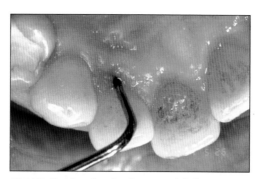

11.123 Probing the developmental defect

11.124 Radiograph of the lateral incisor prior to treatment

11.125 Surgical exposure of the defect

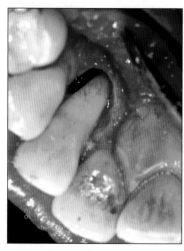

11.126 Groove flattened and debrided

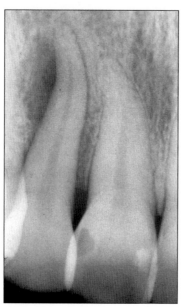

11.127 Postoperative radiograph of the lateral incisor

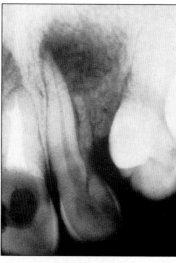

11.128 Radiograph of maxillary lateral incisor with two roots and a palato-gingival groove

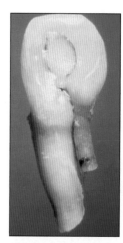

11.129 Extracted specimen of maxillary lateral incisor with root division and grooving

Orthodontic treatment

Rarely, orthodontic treatment may result in localized periodontal breakdown due to an adverse combination of factors such as poor plaque control, unfavourable soft tissue anatomy (thin quality tissues), tooth spacing and bone morphology. Such a situation may arise for example when an impacted maxillary canine is orthodontically moved into position (**11.139**).

Tooth transplantation and replantation

These have traumatic impact on the periodontal attachment whether the procedure is elective or accidental. Both can result in localized permanent damage to the attachment apparatus leading to a periodontal probing profile that varies according to the extent of injury.

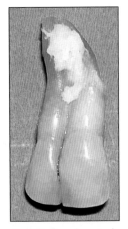

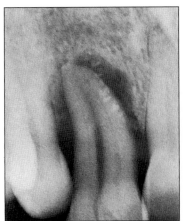

11.131 Radiograph of the fused teeth prior to extraction

11.130 Fused central and lateral maxillary incisors (buccal view)

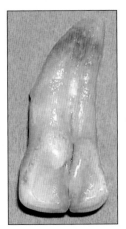

11.132 Extracted fused teeth (palatal view)

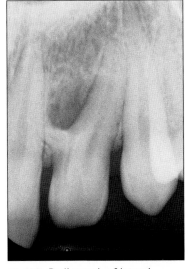

11.133 Radiograph of lateral incisor with anatomical defect and bone loss

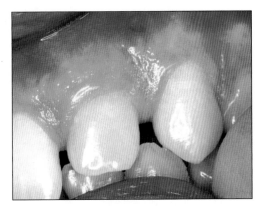

11.134 Clinical appearance of the lateral incisor

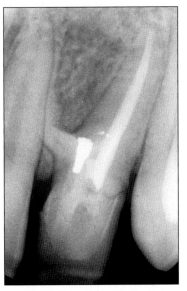

11.135 Radiograph of the lateral incisor following root canal treatment, debridement and sealing of the defect

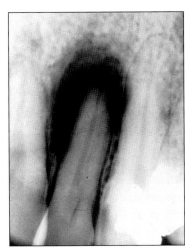

11.136 Vital lateral incisor with large periradicular radiolucency

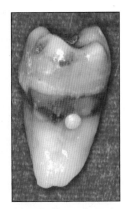

11.137 Enamel pearl on the root surface of a maxillary molar

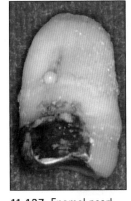

11.138 Enamel pearl on the root surface of a mandibular molar

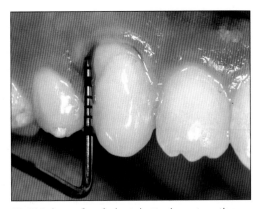

11.139 Loss of periodontal attachment on the distal side of a maxillary canine following orthodontic treatment

Poorly designed restorations

These may result in localized breakdown of the periodontal attachment (**11.140**) by compromising the patient's ability to maintain the plaque levels in these sites. Overhanging restorations, over-contoured crowns and poor embrasure contours all contribute to periodontal breakdown either by compromising the oral hygiene or encroaching on the biologic width. The linking of adjacent crowns to provide splinting is occasionally employed but the design must ensure adequate access for cleaning (**11.141**). In addition to design, compliance from the patient in maintaining cleanliness is essential to avoid secondary periodontal problems (**11.142**). The probing profile in these situations is localized to the site of restorations but is

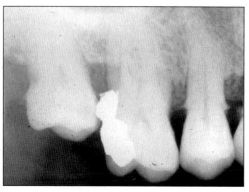

11.140 Localized periodontal breakdown related to a poorly placed restoration

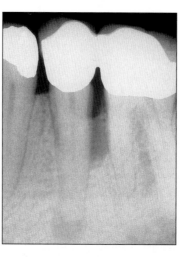

11.141 Localized periodontal breakdown related to splinted restorations

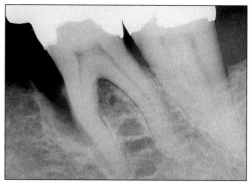

11.142 Failure to maintain the cleanliness of a fixed prosthesis has led to localized periodontal destruction

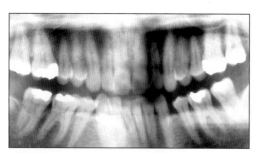

11.143 OPG showing localized periodontal disease in quadrant three

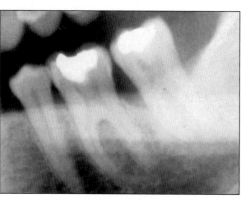

11.144 Close up radiograph of the area affected

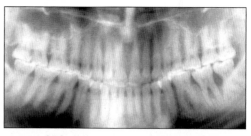

11.145 OPG showing localized periodontal disease in quadrant three

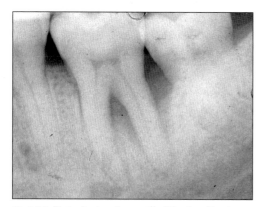

11.146 Periapical radiograph of the localized destruction

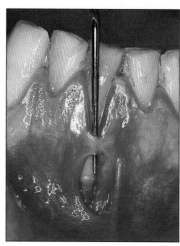

11.147 Localized periodontal breakdown related to a mandibular incisor

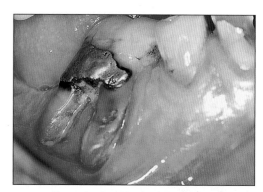

11.148 Extensive localized recession related to a mandibular molar

usually of the broad type. Replacing the restorations with those of acceptable contours and improvement of oral hygiene usually stabilizes the situation.

Localized periodontal disease

This is a rare phenomenon but can occur around a single tooth in an otherwise periodontally intact dentition (**11.143–11.146**). In the cases shown only one tooth was involved, and each had a unique probing profile that was deep although not strictly narrow. The profiles were broad but, at least initially, restricted to one surface. Presentation of similar localized breakdown on the buccal surface usually leads to extensive localized recession (**11.147, 11.148**).

Multiple perio–endo lesions

Isolated lesion(s) superimposed upon a generalized periodontitis

Any of the above isolated lesions can be found superimposed upon generalized periodontitis. The identification of some of these lesions becomes more challenging because of their occurrence together with multiple localized sites of periodontal breakdown (**11.9**). However, careful evaluation of the presenting features along with the clinical examination may help locate those lesions with a pure endodontic aetiology which have a better outlook as opposed to those with a primary periodontal aetiology (**11.149–11.151**), which do not respond to root canal treatment (**11.152**).

Chronic periodontitis

Previously termed adult periodontitis this group embraces the constellation of destructive periodontal diseases which are slowly progressive. Individuals in this group will usually have poor levels of plaque control and multiple deposits of calculus, both supra- and subgingival. The role of general and local modifying factors should be considered and both smoking and diabetes (uncontrolled) are positive risk factors for periodontitis. Within this group, bone loss can be characterized as either irregular or horizontal. The involved teeth normally give positive responses to vitality testing, indicating vital but not undiseased pulp status. Teeth with extensive attachment loss of periodontal origin have poor prognosis and should be extracted (**11.153, 11.154**). If such teeth give a negative response

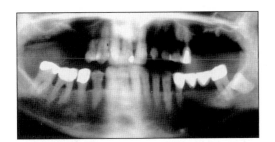

11.149 OPG of patient with a long-span mandibular fixed prosthesis

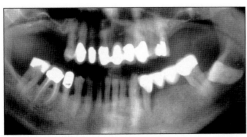

11.150 OPG taken 5 years later with a developing primary periodontal lesion related to the mesial abutment

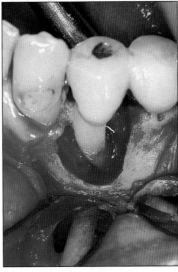

11.151 Surgical exposure of the periodontal defect demonstrating the extent of bone loss

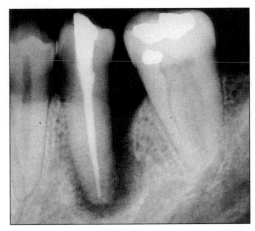

11.152 Bone loss around a non-vital mandibular premolar which has not responded to endodontic treatment – lesion of primary periodontal origin

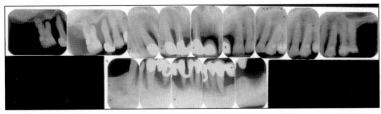

11.153 Radiographs of patient with teeth of poor prognosis

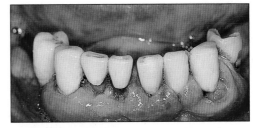

11.154 Clinical view of the same patient as in **11.153**

to vitality testing, it will not be clear without good insight into the clinical and radiographic history whether pulp necrosis is primary or secondary to periodontal disease. In cases of uncertainty, performance of first stage endodontics followed by review of response will indicate endodontic origin if there is a good response (**11.155, 11.156**).

Aggressive periodontitis (JP; RPP)

This category comprises a group of severe, rapidly destructive and progressive form of periodontitis. It includes categories previously embracing diseases affecting the young such as prepubertal periodontitis (**11.157**) and juvenile periodontitis (JP) (**11.158**) and rapidly progressive periodontitis (RPP) (**11.159, 11.160**). The time of onset of the diseases is usually not known at presentation and a number of them have an underlying genetic predisposition. Although host susceptibility in these groups has been identified to play a more significant role in disease progression, high proportions of specific bacteria e.g. *Actinomyces actinomycetemcomitans* (AA) have also been associated with these diseases. Clinical features

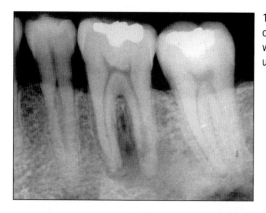

11.155 Radiograph of mandibular molar with bone loss of uncertain aetiology

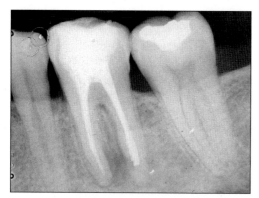

11.156 Radiograph of mandibular molar indicating the response to root canal treatment

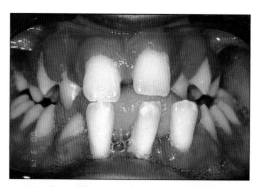

11.157 Case of prepubertal periodontitis

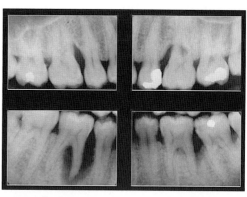

11.158 Radiographs of patient with juvenile periodontitis

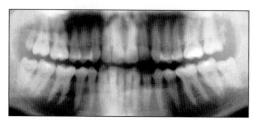

11.159 Rapidly progressive periodontitis (29 years of age)

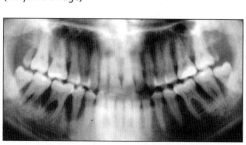

11.160 Rapidly progressive periodontitis (34 years of age)

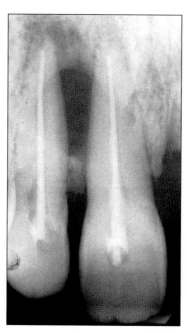

11.161 Radiograph of infected lateral periodontal cyst

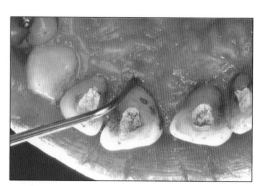

11.162 Confirmation of communication with the mouth

normally include good oral hygiene with extensive inflammation and severe periodontal breakdown (attachment and bone loss) that is not consistent with the low level of plaque accumulation. Within this group isolated vertical bone-loss patterns may be superimposed upon the generalized horizontal bone-loss pattern affecting more than two-thirds of the root length. In patients with localized aggressive disease (localized juvenile periodontitis), bone loss to the root end of the first molars is common. Given the rapid nature of periodontal destruction, there is usually insufficient time for irreversible pulp damage to occur consequently such periodontal lesions rarely have an endodontic component. Therefore, although the lesions may resemble perio–endo lesions and are often categorized as such, they rarely benefit from root canal treatment. Such extensive lesions require more radical management by extraction.

MANAGEMENT OF PERIO–ENDO LESIONS

Estimation of prognosis

In common with other endodontic or periodontal problems, the management of these lesions depends upon a correct diagnosis. Perio–endo lesions by definition imply a lack of definitive diagnosis at the outset. In many cases the true origin is not confirmed until either endodontic or periodontal treatment or sometimes both treatments have been completed. Progress in management is, therefore, based on an initial provisional diagnosis derived on the basis of an educated guess about the endodontic contribution to the problem.

The decision to embark on a course of treatment is usually based on estimating the prognosis of the teeth and the strategic value of the tooth. In perio–endo cases, it is unique that the prognosis cannot be ascertained until the origin is known, that is until either endodontic or periodontal intervention has been completed. In some cases both types of intervention may fail to resolve the problem. This is classically the difficulty in the case of infected lateral periodontal cysts that communicate with the mouth (**11.161, 11.162**).

Treatment of perio–endo cases

Any acute problems (pain and infection) should be dealt with first. Primarily debridement of the pocket is the main form of treatment when present and only used in conjunction with antibiotics if there is spreading infection and fever. The issue usually centres on whether the primary therapy should be periodontal or endodontic. In cases of doubt (where there may be partially necrotic and infected pulp tissue but this cannot be confirmed) the simplest and least damaging therapy should be undertaken first; that is periodontal debridement. In such a case, caution should be exercised in root debridement lest the lesion is of endodontic origin and viable cells on the root surface are destroyed. In the absence of any sign of resolution after a short review period following the initial periodontal debridement, the decision to intervene endodontically may be taken. The first stage of root canal treatment may be carried out (noting the contents of the canal as healthy or necrotic pulp) and the tooth dressed with non-setting calcium hydroxide to gauge the response. By this stage a definitive diagnosis will be possible but some cases will fail to respond after both measures and may need either further evaluation to determine the causative factor or extraction.

Only when the tooth is clearly non-vital and infected should root canal treatment be initiated first and the tooth dressed with calcium hydroxide. Periodontal treatment should follow in quick succession in the absence of a lack of immediate healing after root-canal treatment.

Where the patient motivation is poor or extensive primary dental disease prevails, the alternative of extraction should be considered as a first option. **Figure 11.163** shows a decision-tree for aiding the planning of treatment of isolated perio–endo lesions.

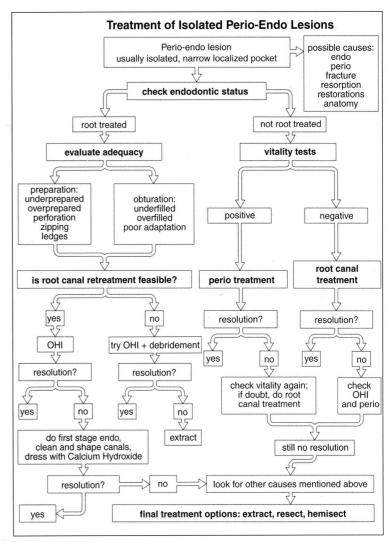

11.163 Flow chart for management of perio–endo lesions

ROOT RESECTION

Root resection is the sectioning and removal of one or two roots of multirooted teeth. This option may be considered for molar teeth where loss of periodontal attachment has involved the furcation. A detailed understanding of the anatomy and morphology of molar teeth is critical and the differences between the root shape and size in relation to the different molars must be appreciated (**11.164**). The degree of furcation involvement is classified on the basis of the amount of periodontal tissue destruction in the interradicular area:

- Degree I horizontal loss of periodontal support < one-third of the width of the tooth;
- Degree II horizontal loss of periodontal support > one-third but not encompassing the total width of the tooth; and
- Degree III horizontal through and through destruction of the periodontal tissues in the furcal area.

Classifications based on vertical loss of bone are not in common use. In maxillary teeth furcation involvement is evaluated from mid-buccal, mesio-palatal and disto-palatal aspects. While in mandibular teeth, they are evaluated from the mid-buccal and mid-lingual aspects. Furcation probing is performed with special probes, such as the Naber's probe which is curved to allow access into the furcation (**11.165**). These clinical findings are used in conjunction with radiographic findings.

Root resections are considered when the furcation is compromised by endodontic complications or Degree II or III involvement. Factors to be considered when deciding on root resection are:

- *Tooth-related factors*:
  — restorability of the tooth;
  — strategic value of the tooth;
  — feasibility of endodontic treatment;
  — post-treatment stability.
- *Root-related factors*:
  — *length of the root trunk* – ideally a tooth with a short root trunk is a better candidate for resection. Teeth with long trunks will have a low furcation entrance and once established the amount of periodontal support remaining around the roots will be poor.
  — *divergence between the roots* – the smaller the divergence (closely proximated roots), the smaller the inter-radicular space and these teeth are poor candidates for resection.
  — *length and shape of roots*. – short and small roots may show increased mobility after resection.
- *Bone-related factors*:
  — the residual bone around the remaining roots should be assessed;
  — localized deep-attachment loss at one surface of the root may compromise the long-term prognosis of an otherwise ideal abutment.

If the tooth has poor restorability or endodontic prognosis then extraction is the treatment of choice. The coronal and radicular access cavities for endodontic treatment should be conservative and

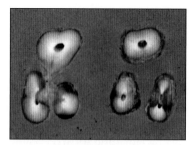

11.164 The shapes of the roots of maxillary first and second molars

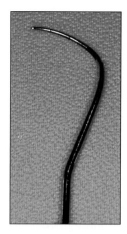

11.165
Naber's probe

compatible with the requirement of debridement to achieve the goals of infection elimination as well as maintaining restorability. The roots to be retained should exhibit both good endodontic and restorative prognoses. The root(s) to be sacrificed do not require root canal treatment unless it is suspected that pulp necrosis is contributing to the periodontal lesion. The canals in the root to be resected should be dressed and sealed with amalgam. Some operators prefer glass ionomer cement but this can disintegrate in the mouth and, therefore, is not the preferred choice. It is preferred practice to complete root canal treatment first followed by the resective surgery. The flap design is dictated by the extent of periodontal breakdown. Although some operators use 'buccal' flaps only, it is important that both a buccal and palatal (or lingual) flap is raised to allow access to all the furcal entrances. Relieving incisions are only used when visibility into the furcation and periodontal defect is poor. Intracrevicular incisions are normally used and it is important that a full thickness flap is elevated to allow access to both the furcal entrances from a buccal and palatal aspect (**11.166–11.171**). Following resection, the undersurface of the crown should be bevelled to eliminate the natural concave curvature in the apico-coronal direction. The root resection in **11.172** shows poor contouring.

On rare occasions where a vital resection becomes necessary, it is important that endodontic treatment is initiated within two weeks of the surgery to reduce the risk of any postsurgical infection. Such cases are difficult to manage endodontically because of the potential for microbial leakage into the root canal system that may compromise outcome – a fact that should be pointed out to patient and periodontist alike.

ROLE OF REGENERATIVE TECHNIQUES IN TREATMENT OF PERIO–ENDO LESIONS

Guided tissue regeneration refers to procedures that are used to regenerate the lost periodontal structures through differential tissue development. A number of methods have been adopted to achieve this and can be classified into:

- barriers;
- enamel matrix derived proteins.

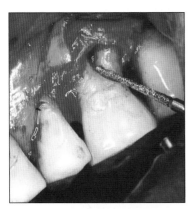

11.166 Surgical exposure of furcation prior to sectioning the disto-buccal root

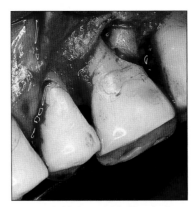

11.167 Initial cut with diamond instrument

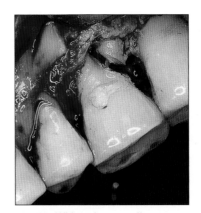

11.168 Widened cut to allow instrumentation

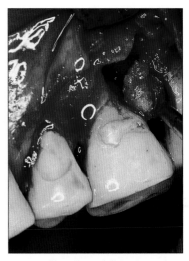

11.169 Elevation of disto-buccal root

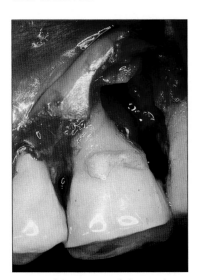

11.170 Appearance of the tooth following removal of the distobuccal root

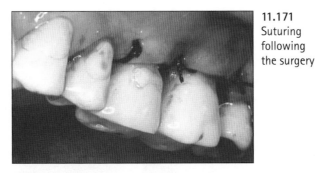

11.171 Suturing following the surgery

11.172 Poor contouring associated with root resection

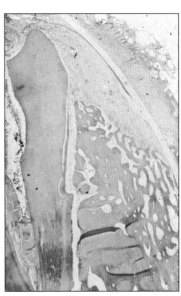

11.173 Histological section showing new attachment formation using a barrier

In the management of perio–endo lesions, barriers have been used with a degree of success. Barriers function on the principle of selective exclusion of cells to enable the desired cells (in this case the periodontal ligament cells) to repopulate the wound thus enabling new attachment formation to the root surface (**11.173**). The first barriers used were non-resorbable, however due to problems with their exposure, infection and the need for resurgery to remove the barrier six weeks later these have been superseded by bio-absorbable barriers. The latter group fall into two types:

- collagen-based (usually derived from bovine or porcine source); and
- synthetic-based (copolymers of polylactic and polyglycolic acid).

A successful outcome requires that the barrier is stiff enough to preserve the space into which cells can proliferate, but also allow the wound to remain stable. After surgery it is important to obtain primary closure, although exposure of the barrier a few weeks later is a common complication. This does not appear to cause significant problems as the barrier does not become infected but instead begins to absorb sooner.

The following case shows the use of a barrier in the management of localized perio–endo lesion associated with a deep palato-gingival groove.

The patient in **11.174** presented with a localized palatal breakdown associated with the upper left 2. The tooth had been root treated twice before, however there was no resolution of the residual probing defect, which tracked along the line of the palato-gingival groove (originally undiagnosed). Following referral, careful assessment and planning, the patient underwent root canal retreatment and regenerative surgery **11.174**. At surgery it was noted that the

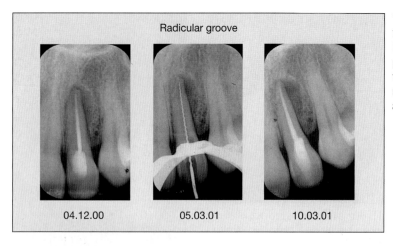

Radicular groove

04.12.00   05.03.01   10.03.01

11.174 The three radiographs show the retreatment of the left maxillary lateral incisor with a radiolucency and palatal periodontal breakdown related to a palato-gingival groove. The three radiographs cover the period during and after the regenerative surgery

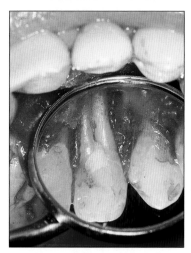

11.175 Surgical exposure of the developmental groove

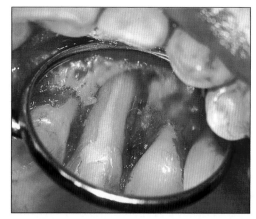

11.176 Groove sealed with glass ionomer

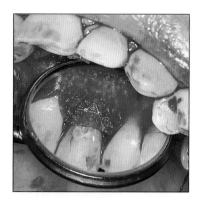

11.177 Resorbable barrier placed

groove which was deep, gave the root a bifid appearance, tracked along the palatal aspect and terminated in the apical third (**11.175**). The groove was cleaned and opened slightly with a narrow ultrasonic tip. The residual bone defect, which had a narrow three-walled morphology, was debrided and all the granulation tissue removed. The palato-gingival groove was filled with glass ionomer cement (**11.176**) and a resorbable barrier was placed (**11.177**). At follow-up

healing had been uneventful with no persistent probing depths and complete resolution of the bone defect as shown in **11.174**.

Successful outcomes with barriers require good case and site selection (including the soft tissue assessment and the defect anatomy) as well as close postoperative follow-up. Early follow-up helps to identify complications such as infection, which should be managed promptly. Although enamel matrix derived proteins have been extensively used in periodontal regeneration for periodontitis patients, they have not yet been applied to the combined perio–endo lesion.

References

Kirkham DB (1975) The location and incidence of accessory pulpal canals in periodontal pockets. *J Am Dent Assoc* **91**, 353–6

Lowman JV, Burke RS, Pellu GB (1973) Patent accessory canals: incidence in molar furcation region. *Oral Surg, Oral Med, Oral Pathol* **36**, 580–4.

Rubach WC, Mitchell DF (1965) Periodontal disease, age, and pulp status. *Oral Surg, Oral Med, Oral Pathol* **19**, 483–93.

Vertucci FJ, Gegauff A (1979) Root canal morphology of the maxillary first premolar. *J Am Dent Assoc* **99**, 194.

Vertucci FJ, Williams R (1974) Furcation canals in the mandibular first molar. *Oral Surg, Oral Med, Oral Pathol* **38**, 308–14.

Chapter 12

Surgical endodontics

J D Regan and S Rahbaran

INTRODUCTION

Endodontic surgery has been performed for many hundreds of years. For most of this time little attention was paid to addressing the elimination of the aetiological factors necessitating the surgical treatment in the first place. It is only in recent decades that it has been widely understood that microorganisms play a central role in the development and progression of periradicular disease. Armed with this new-found knowledge clinicians began to consider the nature of the aetiological factors and how these factors could be eliminated rather than focusing on removal of the reactive tissue surrounding the root apex.

RATIONALE FOR SURGICAL ROOT CANAL TREATMENT

Most pulpal and periradicular conditions are best managed by non-surgical root canal treatment (NSRCT) which has been shown to be predictable and reliable in the great majority of cases, whether previously untreated (**12.1, 12.2**), or previously treated with evidence of failure (**12.3, 12.4**). Even cases, which at first appear to lend themselves to surgical management can be dealt with in a non-surgical manner (**12.5–12.7**).

The rationale for performing surgical endodontics is the elimination of periradicular disease where this cannot be achieved by non-surgical means. The objectives of a surgical approach are to remove diseased tissue, debride the canal system as far as possible and to 'seal' the cavity or defect to prevent or reduce the egress of microorganisms into the periradicular tissues, thereby providing an environment conducive to regeneration of a histologically normal periodontal apparatus (**12.8**).

12.1–12.4 NSRCT is usually associated with a high degree of success.

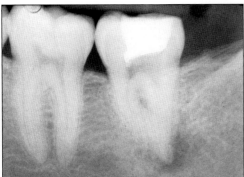

12.1 Preoperative radiograph

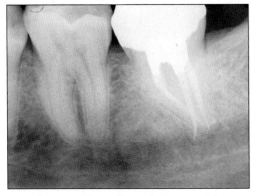

12.2 Postoperative radiograph demonstrating evidence of regeneration of periradicular structures

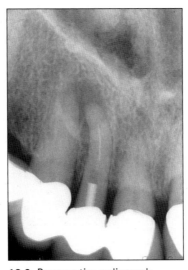

12.3 Preoperative radiograph

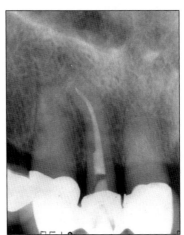

12.4 Postoperative radiograph demonstrating evidence of regeneration of periradicular structures

Historically, a plethora of indications have been listed for surgical root canal treatment. However, as our understanding and knowledge of endodontology increases, the indications for surgery can be greatly simplified. The two main indications for surgical root canal treatment are:

- to obtain a biopsy;
- to achieve what could not be done by non-surgical root canal treatment (NSRCT) alone.

When treatment planning a case, it is important to see beyond the obvious impediments to non-surgical root canal retreatment such as presence of posts or fractured instruments (**12.5–12.7**). Surgical root canal treatment (SRCT) should not be considered in isolation but rather as an extension of root canal treatment necessary to prevent the loss of a natural tooth. The surgical option may be tempting for its expediency when faced with the temporal and financial implications of dismantling crown and bridgework. However, there is a strong likelihood that periradicular surgery will ultimately fail if the infection in the root canal system is not addressed in the first instance.

In recent years two main factors have influenced the change in the nature and number of the cases being treated surgically. On the one hand, more endodontic treatment is being carried out as the general population has become more dentally aware and is undergoing more extensive restorative treatment in order to retain their natural teeth. Frequently, surgery is the only option available. On the other hand, as our understanding of endodontology increases coupled with an increased awareness of the complexity of the root canal systems and improvements in instrumentation design the success of non-surgical treatment and retreatment is improving thereby reducing the necessity for surgical intervention. In addition there continues to be instances where the clinician may need to consider other factors such as the extra temporal and financial costs involved in dismantling extensive crown and bridgework or the patient's inability to attend for follow-up appointments.

PROGNOSIS FOR SURGICAL ROOT CANAL TREATMENT

The reported success rates for periapical surgery range from 28 to 95% (**Table 12.1**). The outcome studies differ in design, case selection, treatment procedures, evaluation period, statistical analysis and criteria for evaluation of success. These differences may account for the wide range of success rates quoted.

The parameters used to assess the outcome following endodontic surgery are limited to clinical, radiographic and histological evaluation. Even though the clinical and radiographic evaluations are the only practical ways in which the clinician can assess success or failure it must be remembered that the only truly accurate assessment of the treatment outcome involves histological examination. As this is invariably impractical in the clinical setting periapical surgery is usually considered successful where no clinical signs or symptoms are present and there is radiographic evidence of bony repair.

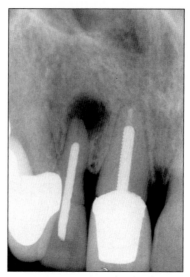

12.5 Preoperative radiograph of lateral incisor restored with porcelain crown with post-retained core.

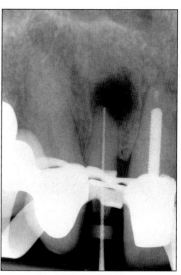

12.6 Working-length determination radiograph following dismantling of the restoration

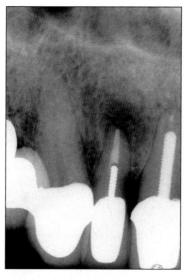

12.7 Postoperative radiograph of completed case

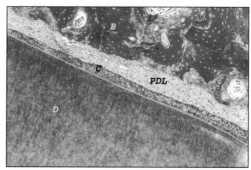

12.8 Masson's Trichrome histological section of normal periodontal architecture: B = bone; PDL = periodontal ligament; C = cementum; D = dentine

12.5–12.8 NSRCT should always be considered first, even if factors such as restorations complicate the treatment

Table 12.1 Surgical root canal treatment outcome studies

Authors	Year	Teeth (No.)	Tooth position	Recall period (years)	Recall rate (%)	Success rate (%)	Uncertain healing (%)	Failure rate (%)
Nordenram & Svärdström	1970	697	All teeth	0.5–6	87.5	49.5	30	20.5
Harty et al.	1970	1016	All teeth	0.5–6	74	90	–	10
Rud et al.	1972	1000	All teeth	1–15	61	66–81	32–15	2–4
Persson	1973	129	No molars	0.5–3	98.2	36.4	25.6	38
Ericson et al.	1974	314	No incisors	0.5–12	94	53.5	25.2	21.3
Altonen & Mattila	1976	93	Molars	1–6	80	72	11	17
Finne et al.	1977	218	Not known	3	–	49.5	18.8	31.7
Hirsch et al.	1979	572	All teeth	0.5–2	42.5	46.7	26.2	27.1
Ioannides & Borstlap	1983	182	Molars	0.5–5	81.4	72.8	21.4	5.7
Mikkonen et al.	1983	174	All teeth	1–2	–	56.9	27	16.1
Reit & Hirsch	1986	35	No molars	1–4	–	71	23	6
Allen et al.	1989	311	All teeth	> 0.5	44.7	58.8	24.8	16.4
Amagasa et al.	1989	64	No molars	1–7	–	95.3	–	4.7
Crosher et al.	1989	85	No molars	> 2	92.6	80	15.3	4.7
Dorn & Gartner	1990	488	Not known	> 0.5	–	65	17	18
Grung et al.	1990	477	All teeth	1–8	87.5	78	15	7
Molven et al.	1991	224	All teeth	1–8	–	76.6	16.6	6.8
Friedman et al.	1991	136	No incisors	0.5–8	–	44.1	22.8	33.1
Rapp et al.	1991	428	All teeth	0.5–>2	60	65	29.4	5.6
Zetterqvist et al.	1991	105	Not known	1	–	62	28.5	9.5
Rud et al.	1991	338	All teeth	0.5–1	67.5	74	19	7
Frank et al.	1992	104	All teeth	> 10	–	57.7	–	42.3
Pantschev et al.	1994	103	Not known	3	79	54.4	21.3	24.3
Lyons et al.	1995	86	All teeth	5	27 (54)	89	–	11
Jesslén et al.	1995	82	Not known	5	79	58.5	26.9	14.6
August	1996	39	All teeth	10.9–23.5	19	74.4	15	10.6
Jansson et al.	1997	69	No molars	0.9–1.3	85.5	30.6	54.9	14.5
Rubenstein & Kim	1999	94	All teeth	1	–	90.4	6.4	3.2
Kvist & Reit	1999	47	Incisors and canines	4	95	57	–	–
Rahbaran et al.	2001	176	All teeth	> 4	41	27.8	34.1	38.1
Rubenstein & Kim	2002	59	All teeth	> 5	63	83	8.5	8.5

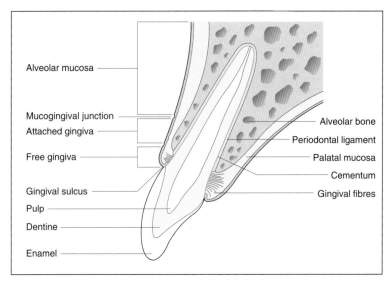

12.9 Diagramatic section of periodontium

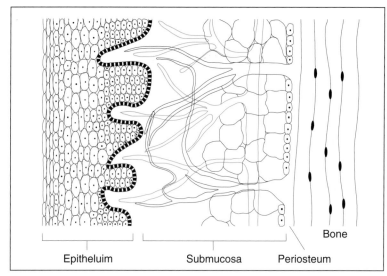

12.10 Diagrammatic section through mucoperiosteum

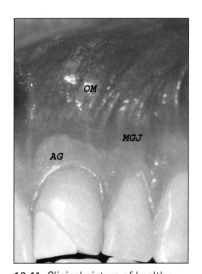

12.11 Clinical picture of healthy oral tissues: AG = attached gingivae; MGJ = mucogingival junction; OM = alveolar mucosa

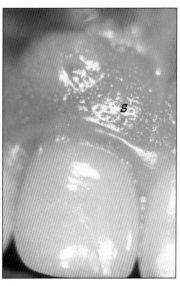

12.12 Stippled appearance of attached gingivae

The effect of individual variables on the outcome of periapical surgery have been analysed by numerous authors and the findings are contradictory. There is a consensus that age, gender, tooth type and preoperative signs and symptoms do not significantly affect postsurgical healing (Hirsch *et al.* 1979; Mikkonen *et al.* 1983; Grung *et al.* 1990; Lyons *et al.* 1995). The majority of studies have reported that the quality of the pre-existing root canal filling (Hirsch *et al.* 1979; Friedman *et al.* 1991), presence and size of preoperative periapical radiolucency (Harty *et al.* 1970; Persson 1973), loss of cortical plate (Grung *et al.* 1990), placement of root-end filling (Rud *et al.* 1972, Hirsch *et al.* 1979, Lustmann *et al.* 1991) and

presence of an adequate coronal seal (Rapp *et al.* 1991; Rahbaran *et al.* 2001) can significantly influence postsurgical healing. Again, it must be emphasized that the primary cause of surgical and non-surgical root canal treatment failure is the persistence or recontamination of the root canal system by microorganisms and their by-products.

ANATOMY AND PHYSIOLOGY OF PERIRADICULAR TISSUES

It is essential for all surgeons to have an intimate knowledge of the tissues that they are operating on. In endodontic surgery, the tissues are collectively known as the periodontium (**12.9, 12.10**). The tissues of the periodontal apparatus include dentine, cementum, bone, periodontal ligament and alveolar mucosa. Understanding the strengths and weaknesses of each of these tissues will allow the operator to manipulate the tissues to ensure the greatest chance of complete healing. The clinical appearance of these tissues in health (**12.11, 12.12**) should be appreciated.

A complete examination of the surgical site allows the surgeon to become familiar with the more local anatomical features as well as the broader aspects of the orofacial anatomical structures (**12.13, 12.14**). Some major anatomical structures of interest include the maxillary sinus, the greater palatine vessels and the inferior alveolar and mental nerves (**12.15**). In addition, local structures such as the root anatomy and the relationship of the tooth to the periodontal apparatus and adjacent teeth must be considered. The design of the flap will be determined, in the main, by these anatomical considerations and by the demands of surgical access.

In addition, a thorough understanding of the radicular anatomy will enable the operator to anticipate the presence of isthmi, anastamoses, and other anatomical complexities that could harbour bacteria or their products. This in turn will facilitate the design of the root-end preparation.

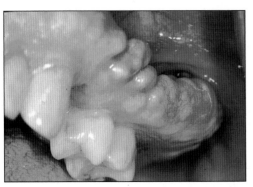

12.13 Maxillary tori

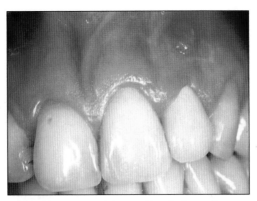

12.14 Frenae – position and level of attachment

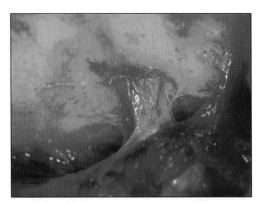

12.15 Mental nerve location

12.13–12.15 Local anatomical features must be considered prior to surgery

SYSTEMIC AND PHARMACOLOGICAL CONSIDERATIONS

As in all areas of dentistry the necessity for collection and analysis of all relevant medical information prior to treatment is obvious. The basis for this has been established elsewhere in this book. However, a number of issues requiring emphasis will now be discussed briefly.

A review of the main systems will provide a framework for establishing the health status of the patient. A written medical questionnaire completed by the patient prior to treatment is essential. However, studies have indicated that the most effective means of gathering medical history details are for the practitioner to interview the patient directly. A combined approach will undoubtedly provide the most accurate assessment overall.

As demographic studies indicate, the population of the western world is an aging one. Edentulousness is no longer accepted as an integral part of growing old. Consequently, an increasing number of medically compromised patients will be presenting for both surgical and non-surgical endodontic treatments. Generally, few special considerations need to be taken for surgical patients that do not apply equally to non-surgical patients. The main areas where exceptions occur are related to haemostasis during and subsequent to the surgical procedure.

In dentistry local analgesic agents are usually combined in a single carpule with vasopressors. The function of the vasopressor is to provide local haemostasis and to delay the absorption of the analgesic agent. This, in turn, prolongs the duration of action of the analgesic. In surgical endodontic procedures good haemostasis is an absolute requirement especially during root-end preparation and root-end filling and in corrective procedures. Good haemostasis allows for clear inspection of the resected root surface and facilitates placement of a root filling by providing a blood-free environment (**12.16, 12.17**).

Vasopressors such as adrenaline (epinephrine) exert their influence on blood flow by stimulating α-adrenergic receptors found on the smooth muscle cells of the microcirculation in the alveolar submucosa. It is important to avoid injection into skeletal muscle, as the

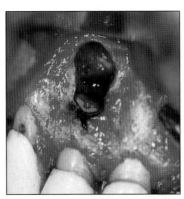

12.16 Good haemostasis permits clear inspection of the root and surrounding tissues

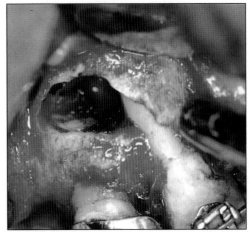

12.17 Good haemostasis permits clear inspection of the root and surrounding tissues

predominant receptor type here is β-adrenergic, stimulation of which results in vasodilation. This would cause an increase in local blood flow, more rapid removal of the analgesic agent with concomitant loss of profound analgesia, and a loss of haemostasis control.

Adrenaline (epinephrine) is the most effective, potent and frequently used vasopressor. In healthy patients, the influence of the adrenaline (epinephrine) injected with the local anaesthetic tends to be minor in most patients provided the injection is administered slowly and avoids a direct intravascular bolus of adrenaline. This is true of all concentrations of adrenaline (epinephrine) available in combination with local analgesic. Absolute contraindications to the use of adrenaline (epinephrine) include cases where the patient has uncontrolled hyperthyroidism. Administration of exogenous adrenaline (epinephrine) could provoke a 'thyroid storm' or 'crisis'. Other conditions that require special consideration prior to administration of vasopressor agents include unstable angina, cardiac arrythmias, history of myocardial infarction, hypertension and uncontrolled diabetes. Although not absolutely contraindicated, caution should also be exercised in patients on tricyclic antidepressants.

Problems arising during and after surgery are frequently encountered with patients with bleeding disorders. It is therefore imperative that any patient with a history of bleeding disorder or those taking anticoagulant medications should be referred to their medical practitioners for further assessment and adjustment of their medications. If necessary, a number of haematological tests can be used to assess the patients status, and these are readily available in many centres in most communities. These screening tests include platelet count and function tests, activated partial thromboplastin time (APTT) and international normalized ratio (INR) formerly known as the prothrombin time (PT). The INR allows for the interpretation of PT with respect to variations among laboratories.

BASIC 'REQUIREMENTS' PRIOR TO SURGERY

Before any surgical endodontic procedure is embarked on, a number of fundamental requirements need to be assured. These are:

- indication(s) for the surgical procedure;
- complete general medical history including administration of prophylactic antibiotics if necessary;
- comprehensive dental history;
- understanding of general and local anatomical relationships;
- understanding of the physiological and pharmacological factors affecting treatment;

- diagnostically excellent radiographs from different angles;
- complete surgical armamentarium;
- full clinical nursing and assistant support;
- the patient's informed consent.

Surgical armamentarium

A complete armamentarium should be available for surgical endodontic procedures to include those items required for all surgical procedures including:

- sterile towels;
- gauze swabs and ribbon;
- bowl for saline irrigant;
- irrigating syringe;
- college tweezers;
- surgical round and tapered burs;
- tear-venting surgical handpiece;
- ultrasonic unit and root-end preparation tips;
- tissue forceps;
- needles and suitable suture material;
- local analgesic equipment;
- aspiration equipment;
- an endodontic surgical tray (**12.18**), which should include:
  — front-surface mirror and small microsurgical mirrors
  — lesions and root apices;
  — hooked, curved and angled probes;
  — a range of surgical scalpels (**12.19**);
  — periosteal elevators (**12.20**);
  — periosteal retractors (**12.21**);
  — lip and flap retractors with fibre-optic attachments (**12.22**);
  — bone curettes;
  — periodontal curettes;
  — surgical scissors;
  — needle holder;
- Endodontic instruments for canal preparation and obturation may also be required.

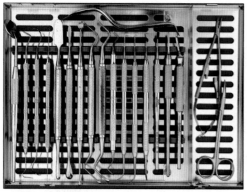

12.18 Surgical tray

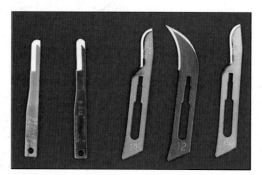

12.19 Scalpel blades

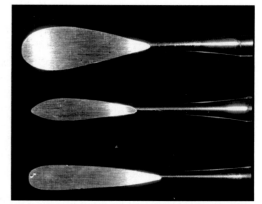

12.20 Elevators

CLASSIFICATION OF ENDODONTIC SURGICAL PROCEDURES

It is frequently useful for the purpose of discussion to classify endodontic surgical procedures under the following headings:

- *emergency surgery*;
  - incision and drainage;
  - trephination;
- *biopsy*;
- *periradicular surgery*;
- *corrective surgery*;
  - perforation repair;
  - root resection;
  - hemisection;
  - intentional replantation;
- *regenerative procedures*;
- *decompression*.

Emergency surgery

- incision and drainage
- trephination

Incision and drainage

A surgical opening in soft tissue created for the purpose of releasing exudate, this procedure may be performed to release a localized intraoral collection of pus and exudate (**12.23**) and is a relatively minor procedure. However, when the swelling extends to the tissue spaces with an extraoral component this may result in life-threatening situations such as occlusion of the airway. Cellulitis (**12.24**) is a symptomatic oedematous inflammatory process that spreads diffusely through the fascial planes. This infection demands immediate treatment with both antibiotic and analgesic medication and establishment of drainage if at all possible.

Trephination

This is the surgical perforation of the alveolar cortical plate to release accumulated periradicular tissue exudate. In these cases the absence of any obvious intra- or extraoral swelling prevents drainage and indicates that the inflammatory exudates have not perforated the cortical plate of the alveolar process. Mishaps can occur with this technique (**12.25**) and damage to the tooth may require surgical correction (**12.26**).

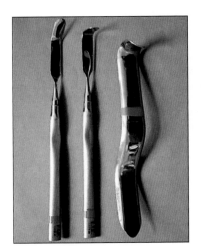

12.21 Retractors

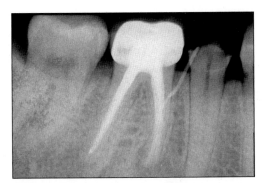

12.22 Retractors and elevators with fibre-optic light attachments

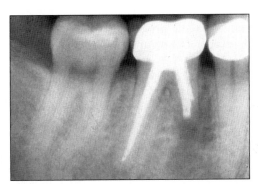

12.23 Incision and drainage

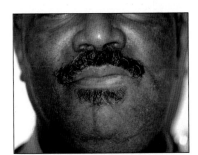

12.24 Cellulitis is a symptomatic oedematous inflammatory process that spreads diffusely through fascial planes

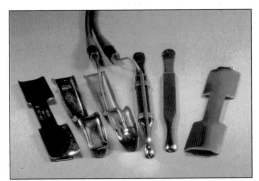

12.25 Radiograph of lower molar: mishap involving perforation of the mesial root during a trephination procedure. GP cone placed in sinus tract originating at mid-root level

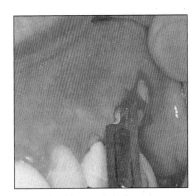

12.26 Postoperative radiograph two months following resection of the mesial root to the level of a clearly outlined bur hole formed by the misdirected trephine

In general, the aim of these procedures is to establish a communication between the oral cavity and the underlying soft or hard tissues that can reasonably be expected to provide necessary drainage. These procedures are performed when drainage through the root canal is not possible. The main objectives are to prevent adverse clinical signs or symptoms and to relieve acute symptoms. Antibiotics are required only when there is systemic involvement.

Biopsy

The aim of taking a biopsy is to establish a definitive diagnosis by histologic examination. It involves the surgical removal of a soft and/or hard tissue specimen for histological evaluation (**12.27**). The value of routine histopathological examination during endodontic surgical procedures must not be underestimated. The taking of a biopsy during periradicular surgical procedures has come to be accepted as the standard of care. Correct handling of the removed tissue is central to the formation of an accurate histological diagnosis. Recovered tissue must be placed immediately in a 10% formalin solution and sent with complete relevant details to the pathology laboratory (**12.28**). A biopsy request should include:

- a history of the case, including patient details;
- a clinical description of the lesion;
- a gross description of the biopsied tissue including size, location, duration, colour, texture, consistency and radiographic appearance;
- a provisional diagnosis.

Biopsies are usually excisional or incisional. Excisional biopsy is used to remove the lesion in its entirety and is, therefore, therapeutic. An incisional biopsy is only used to establish a diagnosis.

Periradicular surgery

The most common endodontic surgical procedures involve periradicular surgery and include curettage, root-end resection, root-end cavity preparation and root-end filling.

As a preliminary procedure for all periradicular procedures a tissue flap must be reflected. Careful and considered soft tissue management greatly enhances the prognosis of the surgical procedure and improves the postoperative wound healing.

Flap design

The main considerations governing flap design are access and vision. In addition it is important to aim to minimize trauma to the soft tissues, to maintain a good blood supply to the flap tissue, to avoid damage to the surrounding structures and to facilitate wound closure. The flap design should include the tooth to be treated and one or more teeth on either side. It is always preferable to extend the flap further than to attempt to work in a restricted field. Factors which influence the extent of the flap include position of the mental nerve, muscle and fraenal attachments, root and bony eminences and large bony defects. Full and limited mucoperiosteal flaps are used in endodontic surgery. Mucoperiosteal flaps consist of the periosteum along with the overlying alveolar mucosa and gingival tissues. Flaps are described according to their shape and include triangular (**12.29**), rectangular (**12.30**), semilunar (**12.31**), submarginal (**12.32**), and palatal (**12.33**). Flaps with vertical relieving incisions are less likely to produce excessive bleeding because of the orientation of the submucosal vasculature (**12.34**). Incision lines should always be placed so that wound closure is on sound bone. Buccal flaps are most commonly used to gain access to the periradicular tissues, however a palatal approach may be indicated for gaining access to palatal roots or defects (**12.33, 12.35**). The only indications for lingual flap reflection are crown lengthening procedures or repair of a coronal, lingually located defect is planned.

Full mucoperiosteal flaps These may be triangular (**12.29, 12.36**), rectangular (**12.30, 12.37**), or trapezoid. The vertical component of the trapezoid flap is angulated, cutting across the vasculature (**12.34**) and generally its use is not recommended. Therefore the rectangular and triangular flaps are the types most commonly used. The triangular flap has the advantage of flexibility as the flap may either be extended or converted into a rectangular

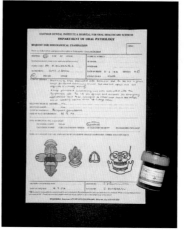

12.27 Taking an excisional biopsy for histological examination during a periradicular surgical procedure

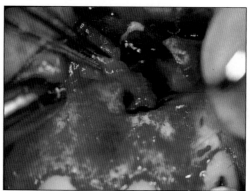

12.28 Biopsy bottle containing 10% formalin and correctly completed clinical biopsy request form

one if necessary. It is created by the use of an intrasulcular and relieving incision (**12.38**). The relieving incision is started in alveolar mucosa, passes through the attached and marginal gingivae and ends on the mesial or distal aspect of the teeth. The gingival papillae should not be incised in order to facilitate repositioning of the flap and to prevent sloughing of the papillae. Elevation of the flap should commence in the attached gingivae of the vertical incision (**12.39**). The advantages of the full flaps include provision of good access to the root tissues (**12.40**), ease of reflection and repositioning and provision for excellent healing, usually without scarring, thereby minimizing postoperative pain and swelling. The only disadvantage of these flaps is the possibility of postoperative recession. This has been shown to be minimal with the correct handling of the tissues and is more likely to occur with thin marginal tissues.

Limited mucoperiosteal flaps These flap designs eliminate the need to disturb the gingival margins especially those around restorations where recession would be most marked. They include the semilunar (**12.31**), submarginal (Leubke–Ochsenbein) (**12.32, 12.41**) and the papilla-base flaps. The semilunar flap is created by cutting a semilunar incision in the alveolar mucosa. The access provided is limited and scarring is a frequent complication (**12.42**). The submarginal flap consists of two vertical and a scalloped horizontal incision in the attached gingivae, which follows the outline of the gingival margin. It must be noted that the required width of the attached gingivae is 3–5 mm. The papilla-base flap involves vertical releasing incision(s) along with a shallow incision in the base of the papilla and a second incision directed to the crestal bone. This creates a split-thickness flap in the area of the papilla base.

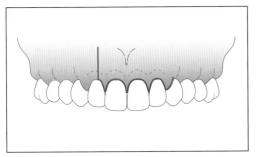

12.29 Triangular

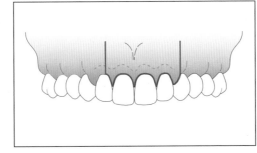

12.30 Rectangular

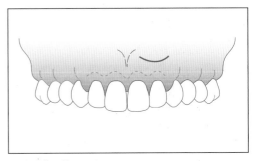

12.31 Semilunar

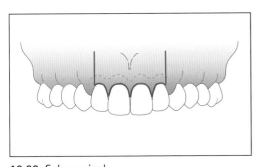

12.32 Submarginal

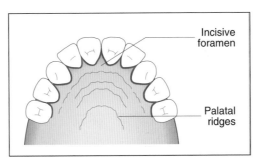

12.33 Palatal

Incisive foramen

Palatal ridges

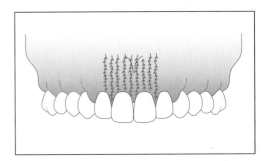

12.34 Vertical orientation of blood vessels in oral mucosa

12.29–12.34 Line drawings of the flap designs

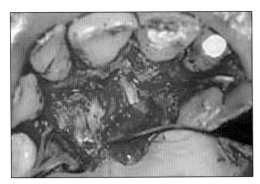

12.35 Palatal flap

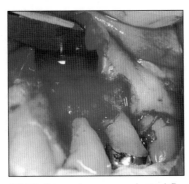

12.36 Triangular mucoperiosteal flap

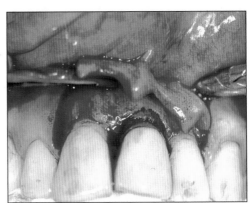

12.37 Rectangular full mucoperiosteal tissue flap

These limited flap designs may be appropriate when recession may expose the crown margins.

Incisions A variety of incisions are used during creation of mucoperiosteal flaps. These include:

- intrasulcular incision (**12.38**);
- vertical relieving incision (**12.38**);
- papilla-base incision.

Irrespective of the type, a number of basic principles apply when making incisions. These include:

- avoid crossing underlying bony defects;
- create the incision with a firm continuous stroke, which may be repeated until the tissues have been sharply incised to bone;
- plan the start and finish points of the incision;
- avoid bony eminences with vertical incisions.

Flap elevation Elevation of the flap must be performed with care in order to avoid damage to the tissues. As already indicated, elevation is commenced in the vertical incision and away from the gingival margin, in the attached gingivae (**12.39**). This minimizes damage to the delicate papillary tissues. The flap should be gently undermined (**12.36**, **12.39**). All reflective forces should be applied to the periosteum which then allows for passive reflection of the overlying alveolar mucosa and gingivae. The small tissue tags which remain attached to the cervical regions of the teeth or the underlying alveolar bone must be preserved in order to enhance reattachment (**12.43**, **12.44**). Scarring from previous surgery or the presence of a sinus tract can complicate flap elevation.

Flap retraction Care for the reflected soft tissues is essential to good postoperative wound healing. The operator must ensure that the retractor is placed firmly on the bone avoiding pinching of any soft tissue (**12.40**). Frequent irrigation of the surgical site prevents

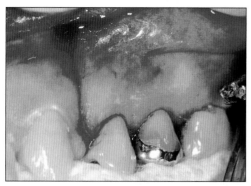

12.38 Intrasulcular and vertical relieving incision

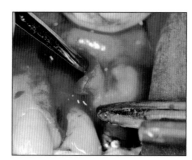

12.39 Elevation of tissue commencing in the attached gingivae of the vertical incision

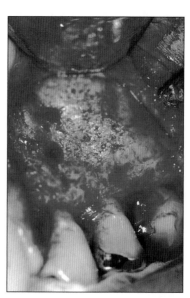

12.40 Excellent access provided by full mucoperiosteal flaps

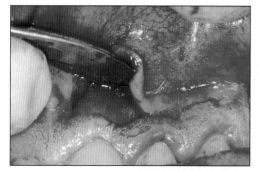

12.41 Limited mucoperiosteal flap. This flap is frequently created in cases where there is a concern about the aesthetics associated with potential recession

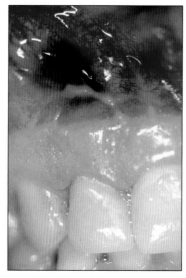

12.42 Scarring of tissues subsequent to creation of a semilunar incision in the oral mucosa

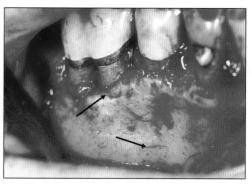

12.43 Retained tissue tags (arrows) on the cortical bone enhance reattachment and postoperative healing

dehydration of the flap and the tissue tags attached to the teeth, encouraging optimum healing. In the lower premolar region, the mental nerve should be identified and protected with a retractor.

Osteotomy Access to the periradicular tissues and root-end is gained by removing the overlying alveolar bone (**12.45**). The periradicular lesion may perforate the cortical plate. This aids location of the root apex (**12.46, 12.47**). If the cortical plate is intact, measurements from radiographs or from working lengths obtained during a non-surgical treatment must be used to estimate the position of the root apices. In conjunction with copious sterile irrigation a rearventing surgical handpiece (**12.45, 12.48**) is used to remove the bone with gentle brushing motion. Large round tungsten–carbide burs (**12.49–12.50**) have been shown to be most suitable for safe bone removal. Excessive heating of the bone by the use of excessive pressure on the rotating instrument, excessive depth of cutting, inadequate cooling or the use of the wrong cutting instrument can result in stagnation of the local bone circulation and eventual tissue necrosis. Caution must be exercised at all times not to damage adjacent teeth and soft tissues.

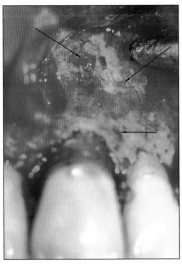

12.44 Retained tissue tags (arrowed) wound repair following repositioning of the tissue flap

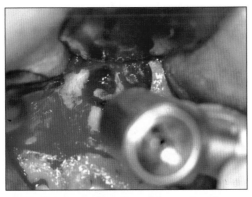

12.45 Osteotomy. Location of the root surface during periradicular surgery usually involves removal of overlying bone unless the lesion has already perforated the cortical plate (**12.47**) or a natural dehiscence or fenestration exists

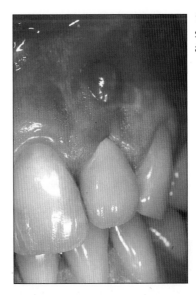

12.46 Preoperative view showing existing sinus associated with tooth 22

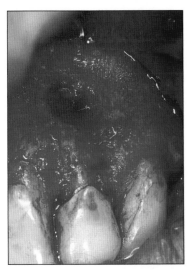

12.47 Perforation of the cortical plate of bone over tooth 22 by the periradicular lesion

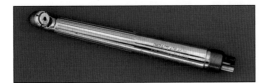

12.48 A high-speed surgical handpiece must have a rear-venting exhaust in order to avoid development of surgical emphysema

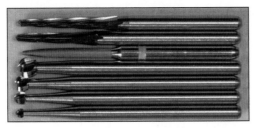

12.49 Burs used during periradicular surgery

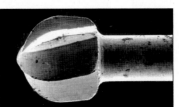

12.50 SEM of a large round surgical tungsten–carbide which generates the least frictional heat

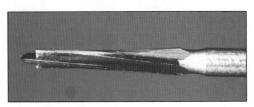

12.51 A Lindeman bone-cutting bur used for root-end resection

Curettage This has been defined as a surgical procedure to remove diseased or reactive tissue and/or foreign material from the periradicular bone surrounding the root of an endodontically treated tooth (American Association of Endodontics 1998). Resection of the root-end can facilitate curettage as access to the palatal/lingual surfaces is improved. All curetted tissue must be sent for histopathological examination as sinister lesions have been identified in the past. The histology of the lesion may give the clinician an insight into the aetiology of the periradicular disease.

Ideally, all the soft tissue in the lesion should be removed in case of a sinister lesion. According to Fish (1939) the outer layers of a lesion (**2.26**) are reparative in nature and demonstrate angiogenic tissue along with fibroblasts and newly formed granulation tissue.

Root-end resection The level at which the root-end is resected and the angle of resection are important considerations. It is recommended that the apical 3 mm of the root-end be removed. The majority of the anatomical aberrations are found in the apical region and resection at this level would eliminate a large proportion of root-canal ramifications. In certain circumstances, it is not possible to remove the recommended 3 mm. For instance a long-post or reduced-bone support limit the amount of root-end removal, and close proximity of the apex to neurovascular bundles may demand a high level of resection.

Ideally the root should be resected with a bevel as close to zero degrees from horizontal as possible. Such a resection angle reduces the number of dentinal tubules exposed, decreasing the communication pathways between the canal system and periradicular tissues. The forty-five degree resection angle was previously recommended to improve access and visibility, however, with the introduction of microsurgical instruments, this problem has largely been overcome.

Visualization of the root-end outline is frequently enhanced by staining it with a 1% solution of methylene blue dye (**12.52–12.54**). The root-end should be carefully inspected for anatomical details, fractures and incomplete resection. Identification of the canal anatomy and in particular isthmi facilitates the correct extension of the root-end preparation.

Root-end cavity preparation The rationale for preparation and filling of the root-end is to debride the canal system and seal off any residual intracanal infection. The rationale for placement of a root-end filling is to prevent egress of any intracanal microorganisms and/or their products into the periradicular tissues. A '*double seal*' (Regan et al, 2002) consisting of the physical barrier provided by the root-end filling material as well as a biological seal formed by regeneration of the periodontal apparatus over the resected root face is the ideal outcome. This has been shown to be achievable with the root-end filling materials available today, such as Diaket (**12.55**) and Mineral Trioxide Aggregate (MTA) (**12.56**).

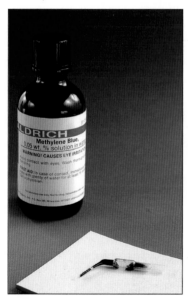

12.52 A 1% solution of methylene blue dye is used to stain the root to facilitate visualization of vertical root fractures or to outline the resected root face

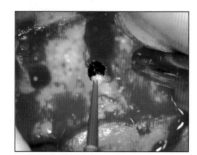

12.53 Application of dye with sterile sponge applicator

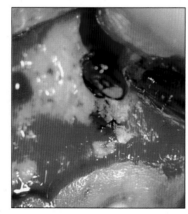

12.54 Resected root face outlined with methylene blue

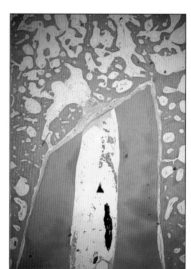

12.55–12.56 Histological sections demonstrating the formation of a 'double seal' at the root-end

12.55 H&E of a Diaket section

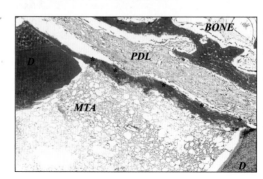

12.56 Masson's Trichrome stained section showing MTA as a root-end filling associated with regeneration of the periodontal apparatus

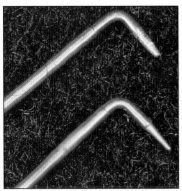

12.57 EMS® root-end preparation tips (Electro Medical Systems, Switzerland)

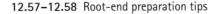

12.57–12.58 Root-end preparation tips

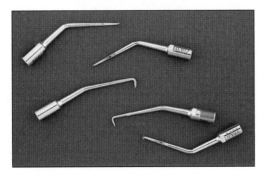

12.58 Dentsply Tulsa Dental ProUltra™ tips

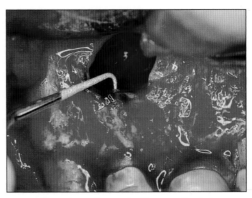

12.59 Use of an ultrasonically energized tip to create a root-end preparation

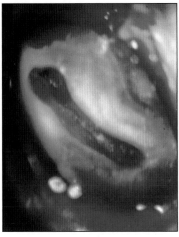

12.60 Root-end preparation created with ultrasonically energized tips (courtsey Dr David Dickey)

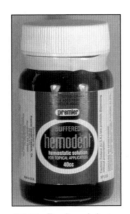

12.61 Ferric sulphate haemostatic agent

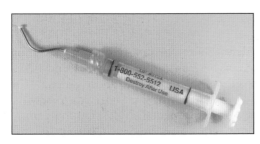

12.62 Ferric sulphate applicator

The ideal root-end cavity should be prepared along the long axis of the root, have near parallel walls, be 3 mm deep and encompass the root-canal anatomy. The introduction of ultrasonic root-end tips (**12.57, 12.58**) have revolutionized root-end preparation (**12.59, 12.60**). The smaller size of the ultrasonic handpiece and the angulation of the root-end tips, allow for less bone removal and better access. A recognized complication of root-end preparation is perforation of the lingual aspect of the root irrespective of the instrument used to create the preparation. However, this iatrogenic complication is less likely when ultrasonically energized root-end preparation tips are used instead of conventional burs in a handpiece.

It is possible to instrument the root-canal system from a retrograde approach. Bent hand files matching the canal length and held in a pair of haemostat forceps may also be used during debridement of the canal. The closer the retrograde root filling can be placed to the post or the fractured instrument, the more successful is the treatment outcome (Reit & Hirsch 1986).

Haemostasis Adequate haemostasis is central to the periradicular surgical procedures. This is especially true for root-end preparation and root-end filling. Administration of adequate amounts of vasopressor agents contained in the local analgesic carpules will usually ensure good haemostasis which will be maintained throughout the procedure provided that the procedure is completed within a reasonable time frame. After this 'window of opportunity' control of the blood flow is lost and a massive increase in bleeding occurs due to the 'rebound phenomenon'.

A number of locally applied haemostatic agents are available for use during the surgical procedure. These include Racellets® (adrenaline (norepinephrine) impregnated cotton pellets), ferric sulphate (**12.61, 12.62**) (e.g. Cutrol), bone wax, oxidized cellulose (Surgicel®), gelatine-based foam (Gelfoam) and bovine-derived collagen (Collacote® or Collaplug®) (**12.63, 12.64**). Application of pressure on plain cotton pellets placed into the bony defect may also arrest bleeding. Complete removal of the haemostatic agents is usually recommended especially when using bone wax or ferric sulphate. Any of these materials remaining in the bony crypt will usually evoke an inflammatory foreign-body reaction which may prevent or delay healing.

Root-end filling Following root-end resection it is usually recommended that a root-end preparation and root-end filling be placed. However, this is not always the case and there is some debate as to whether a better seal can be achieved by placement of a root-end filling where the canal has recently been well obturated (Harrison & Todd 1986, Tanzilli *et al.* 1980). In all other cases root-end filling is recommended.

The ideal root-end filling material should be biocompatible, antibacterial, easy to place and remove, radiopaque, dimensionally stable,

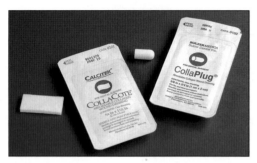

12.63 Collagen agents Collaplug and Collacote can be used to stem blood flow in the crypt both physically and by contributing to the clotting cascade

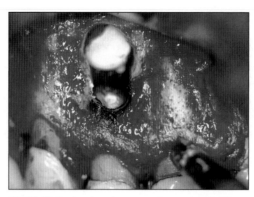

12.64 Collaplug in a bone crypt over tooth 22

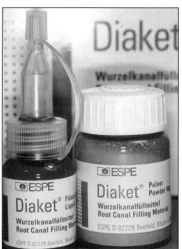

12.65 Diaket (ESPE, Germany)

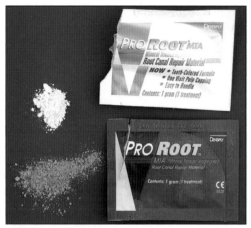

12.66 ProRoot® material (MTA) both original grey and the new white material (Dentsply, Tulsa)

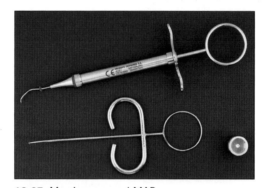

12.67 Messing gun and MAP gun

12.67–12.70 Root-end filling carriers

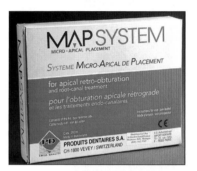

12.68 The MAP system (Micro Apical Placement system, Produits Dentaires SA, Vevey, Switzerland)

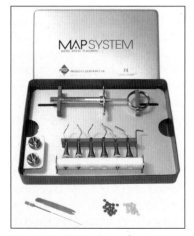

12.69 The MAP system (Produits Dentaires SA, Vevey, Switzerland)

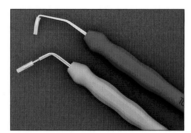

12.70 ProRoot MTA carriers (Dentsply, Tulsa)

adhere to the root canal wall, insoluble and induce regeneration of the periradicular tissues. There are a variety of root-end filling materials available, none of which fulfil all the above criteria. The materials most commonly used are amalgam, Super ethoxybenzoic acid (EBA), intermediate restorative material (IRM), gutta-percha, Diaket (**12.65**), composite resin, glass ionomer cement and the recently introduced mineral trioxide aggregate (MTA) (**12.66**). Amalgam can no longer be recommended as a root-end filling material due to new evidence demonstrating the superiority of other materials and due to the long-term failure of cases where amalgam was used (Frank et al. 1992). This failure may be due to initial leakage, formation of corrosion products and possible electrochemical reactions when in contact with a metal post. At present the most suitable materials for use in root-end cavities appear to be MTA (**12.66**), Diaket (**12.65**) or Super EBA.

Following its creation, the root-end cavity should be dried before the root-end filling is placed. This can be done with cut sterile paper

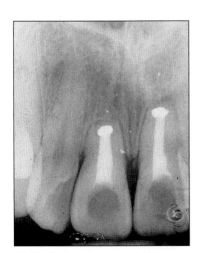

12.71 Amalgam root-end fillings

12.71–12.74 Radiographs of root-end filling

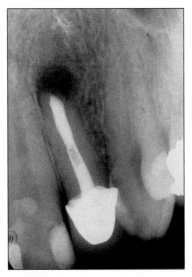

12.72 Diaket root-end filling in tooth #22

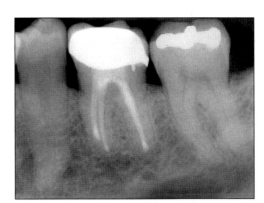

12.73 MTA root-end filling in tooth #36

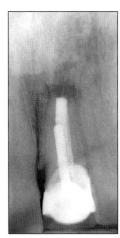

12.74 Composite root-end filling in tooth #21

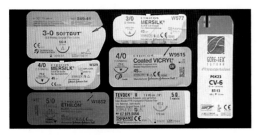

12.75 A variety of suture material is available for use for wound closure following endodontic surgery

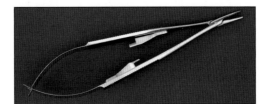

12.76 Suture needle holder

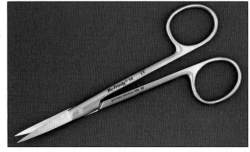

12.77 Suture scissors

points or with a short needle attached to a suction device such as the Stropko device. The surgical crypt should be packed with a collagen material such as Collaplug (**12.64**) during the placement of the root-end filling. This will help maintain a dry field and, in addition, will facilitate removal of any excess filling material at the end of the procedure. There are a number of instruments, devices and systems available to facilitate root-end filling placement (**12.67–12.70**). Surgical root-end pluggers, available in different sizes and angulations, allow good condensation and adaptation of the filling material to the canal walls. The root-end filling should be routinely burnished or polished except when MTA is used. This finish is not possible with MTA as it does not set for approximately four hours. The bony crypt should be cleared of all foreign materials such as root-end filling, haemostatic agents or cotton pellets. The surgical site is then irrigated with sterile saline. Prior to wound closure, a periapical radiograph should be exposed to confirm adequate placement and condensation of the root-end filling, as well as the absence of extraneous material in the periradicular tissues (**12.71–12.74**).

Wound closure   Optimal wound healing is dependent on correct flap replacement and suturing. The flap should be repositioned and held in place under gentle compression for a few minutes with a damp gauze. Once all the sutures have been placed, the flap should be compressed again with digital pressure for approximately 10 minutes. The rationale for this procedure is to encourage formation of as thin a clot as possible. If this is not achieved complications include infection, scar tissue formation, swelling and bruising may occur. The importance of good oral hygiene must be emphasized to the patient.

The choice of suture material used for wound closure depends on the clinician who should be aware of the advantages and disadvantages of each material (**12.75**). Black silk and catgut sutures have been widely used in oral surgery in the past and continue to be the suture of choice for many surgeons. Good quality needle holders and scissors are recommended (**12.76, 12.77**). Black silk is strong, easy to use and is relatively cheap. However, it is a braided suture and hence it encourages wicking – an undesirable property which allows microorganisms to track along the length of the suture into the wound. This in turn delays healing. In addition, black silk is non-absorbable and needs to be removed. Catgut, on the other hand is absorbable and is a monofilament. Unfortunately it is more difficult to handle. Monofilamentous sutures such as nylon, polyester and expanded polytetrafluoroethylene have many advantages. They tend to be strong, easy to handle and see, non-allergenic and available in a number of sizes. As the wound has established the greatest part of its strength after 24–36 hours, sutures can be removed much earlier than previously recommended. It has been shown that after two to three days, sutures have performed their useful function (**12.78**) and if left in place any longer they will retard healing.

When suturing the tissues it is important to ensure that the flap is not under tension. The horizontal incision is usually sutured first. The technique most commonly used in endodontic surgery involves the use of interrupted sutures. The single sling suture, vertical mattress suture and the anchor suture may also be used. Postoperative wound healing is demonstrated (**12.79–12.81**).

Wound healing   Various tissues are wounded during periradicular surgery. These are mucoperiosteal tissues (gingivae, alveolar mucosa and periosteum), periradicular tissues (bone and periodontal ligament) and radicular tissues (dentine and cementum). Harrison and Jurosky (1991a,b; 1992) give a detailed account of the three different types of wound healing: incisional; dissectional; and excisional. To promote optimum healing, the operator must ensure close approximation of the wound edges, encouraging healing by primary intention. Appropriate oral hygiene measures must be established to prevent infection of the surgical site, which may lead to wound breakdown and healing by secondary intention (scarring).

The first event in wound healing is clot formation. The function of the clot is to provide an initial seal and strength, attach the opposing wound edges and thereby provide a pathway for the migration of inflammatory and repair cells. Inflammatory cells such as polymorphonuclear leucocytes migrate to the wound site (chemotaxis) and are responsible for removal of bacteria and cellular debris (phagocytosis).

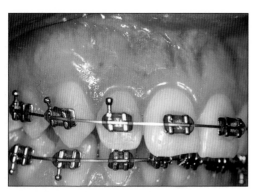

12.78 Postoperative closure of submarginal flap with gut suture material

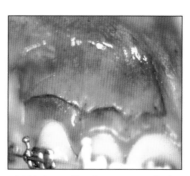

12.79 Immediately postoperatively

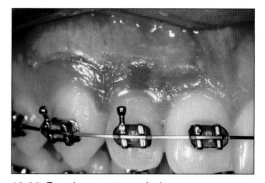

12.80 Two days postoperatively

12.79–12.81 Postoperative wound healing of submarginal flap

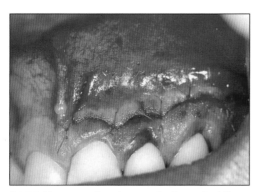

12.81 Two weeks postoperatively

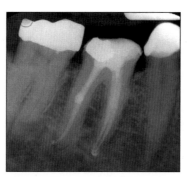

12.82 Internal resorption in tooth arrested by NSRCT

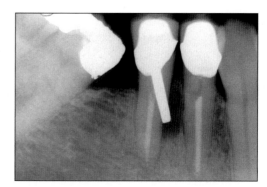

12.83 Perforation on the mesio-lingual of tooth 35 following a procedural error

Activated macrophages then invade and stimulate fibroblasts to form new collagen and small blood vessels (angiogenesis). Once an epithelial barrier has been formed, connective-tissue healing commences. With time, the connective tissue remodels and matures.

Corrective surgery

Perforation repair

A radicular perforation is an artificially created communication between the root canal system and the supporting periodontal apparatus of the tooth. Perforations compromise the health of the periradicular tissues and threaten the viability of the tooth. Perforations pose a number of diagnostic and management problems. They occur primarily through three possible mechanisms: resorptive processes (**12.82**); caries; and procedural errors (**12.83, 12.84**).

Resorptive processes, given sufficient time, will perforate the root structure. The resorptive process may be internal or external in origin and it is important to distinguish between them so that appropriate treatment can be rendered.

Caries involves destruction of dental tissues as a result of microbial action. An untreated carious lesion may invade the floor of the pulp chamber or extend along the root resulting in perforation of the root. Treatment of these perforations may require a combination of crown lengthening, root extrusion or root resection in order to retain valuable radicular segments.

Perforations resulting from procedural errors are probably the second most common cause of endodontic failure and account for close to 10% of all endodontic failures (Ingle 1994).

Irrespective of the factors involved in the creation of the perforation, the management and repair will depend on three factors: (1) the location of the perforation; (2) the length of time since the perforation was created; and (3) the size of the perforation. The most important of these is the location of the perforation. Perforations close to the height of the alveolar crest are the most difficult to repair and generally have the least favourable prognosis due to their communication with the gingival sulcus and the microorganisms contained within it. This location has been described as the 'critical crestal zone'. Coronal to this a perforation can be repaired with restorative material with or without crown lengthening. Apically, a perforation can be viewed as a secondary foramen.

The treatment of a perforation affecting the mesial root of a mandibular molar is illustrated (**12.85–12.87**).

Root resection

A root resection or root amputation is defined as the removal of an entire root leaving the crown of the tooth intact (**12.88, 12.89**). Root resections have been performed for a multitude of reasons for many decades. Today the main indications for root resection include:

- treatment of a class III periodontal defect;
- vertical root fracture of one root of a multirooted tooth;
- caries, or a resorptive defect of one root of a multirooted tooth that cannot be managed in other ways;
- removal of a root that has undergone an irreparable perforation;
- treatment of one root of a multirooted tooth that is not amenable to non-surgical or surgical treatment.

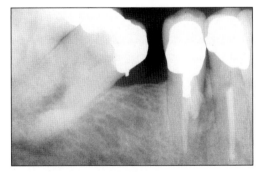

12.84 Two-year follow-up of non-surgical repair of the perforation

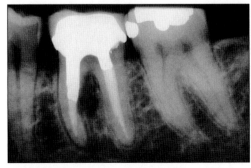

12.85 Perforation of the distal aspect of the mesial root of tooth 36

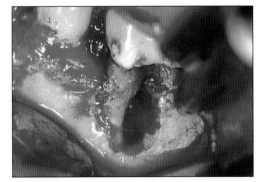

12.86 Reflected tissue flap revealing extent of the bone loss associated with the perforation

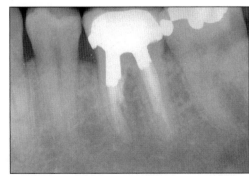

12.87 Surgical repair of the perforation with MTA

Contraindications to root resection include:

- fused roots;
- unrestorable tooth;
- paucity of support for or attachment to remaining root(s).

A case of root resection of the mesial root of a mandibular first molar is presented to emphasize procedural aspects. Where possible endodontic treatment should be completed prior to root resection (**12.90**). Amalgam has been placed in the root with the perforation that is due to be resected. This will facilitate orientation during the surgical procedure and will, more importantly, seal the remaining root canal systems from the oral cavity. Preservation of alveolar bone is important but in many cases removal of some bone around the root to be resected will be necessary. Following reflection of a soft-tissue flap, root resection is done with a high-speed, tapered tungsten carbide bur starting at the most accessible coronal aspect of the root. The instrument is directed apically towards the furcation, stopping just short of the furcation in order to avoid damage to the adjacent root surface. The root can then be completely sectioned gently fracturing the remaining root material with a fine elevator placed in the resection line. Having removed the resected root (**12.91**), the placement of a bone substitute and membrane covering further enhance healing and resolution (**12.92–12.94**). A five-year follow-up radiograph shows a favourable outcome (**12.95**). Root resection should be avoided prior to non-surgical root canal treatment (**12.96**) and it is important to confirm that no residual root spurs remain as they can lead to localized periodontal breakdown (**12.97**).

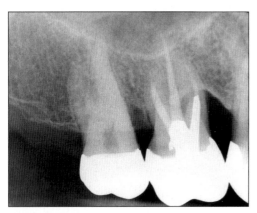

12.88 Preoperative radiograph of tooth 16 prior to resection of the mesio-buccal root which was associated with extensive bone loss. Note the use of amalgam compacted into the orifice. The amalgam acts as a permanent restoration and is easily visualized during the surgical procedure

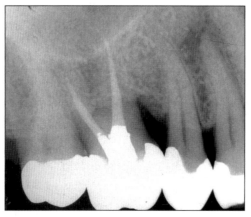

12.89 One-year postoperative radiograph of the tooth

12.88–12.89 Root resection or root amputation

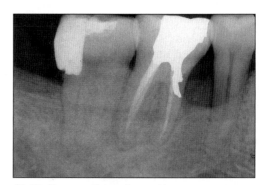

12.90 Preoperative radiograph

12.90–12.95 Root resection of the mesial root of tooth 36

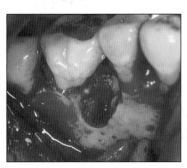

12.91 Clinical view following root resection

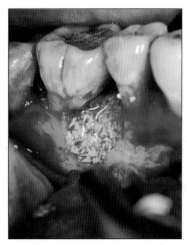

12.92 Placement of bone substitute Bio-Oss

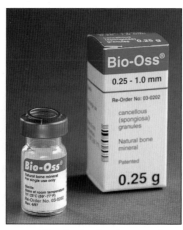

12.93 Bio-Oss bovine bone graft

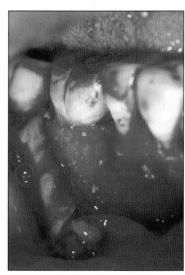

12.94 Resorbable membrane in place

Hemisection

Hemisection is defined as the surgical separation of a multirooted tooth, usually a mandibular molar, through the furcation in such a way that a root and the associated portion of the crown may be removed (American Association of Endodontics 1998) (**12.98**). The need for a mucoperiosteal flap is determined following each case evaluation. Restoration of the remaining portions of the tooth is critical to the long-term survival of the tooth (**12.99**).

When hemisection is performed prior to NSRCT (**12.100**), it is necessary to isolate the remaining tooth and complete the treatment in the normal way (**12.101, 12.102**).

Intentional replantation and transplantion

Intentional replantation is defined as the replacement of a tooth in its socket following deliberate avulsion (**12.103–12.105**). Transplantation of a tooth involves replacement of a tooth in a socket other than the one from which it had been extracted from (**12.106–12.111**). This is normally limited to procedures within the same mouth.

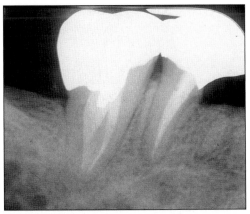

12.95 Five-year follow-up radiograph

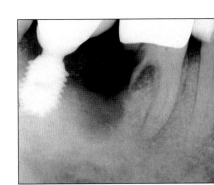

12.96 Root resection performed prior to NSRCT is not recommended – note 'spur' of dentine remaining which will complicate the periodontal management of the case

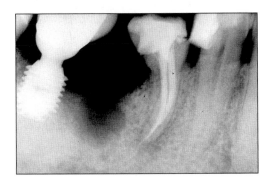

12.97 Correction of the problems by performing NSRCT and by removing the dentine spur

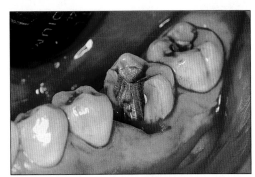

12.98 Hemisected mandibular molar

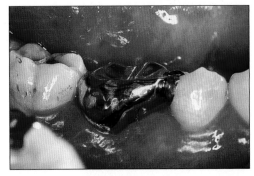

12.99 Restored distal segment

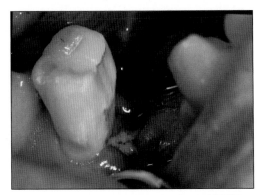

12.100 Hemisection performed prior to NSRCT – note bleeding pulpal tissue

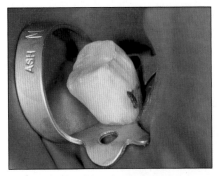

12.101 Isolated hemisected tooth

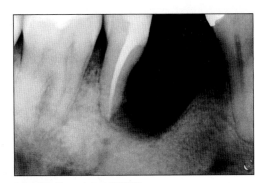

12.102 Completed NSRCT

As a general rule intentional replantation is considered a procedure of last resort although many successful cases have been reported in the literature. Much is now understood about the physiology of the periodontal ligament surrounding the root of the extracted tooth and appropriate handling of the root will enhance the chances of success following replantation.

It is desirable to perform non-surgical root canal treatment on the tooth prior to replanting or transplanting. The ligament of the

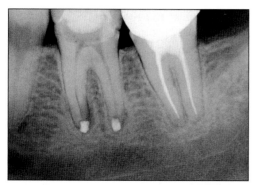

12.103 Replanted molar – note lack of NSRCT

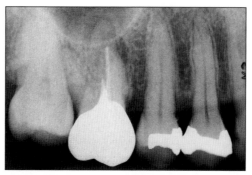

12.104 Radiograph of replantation – preoperative

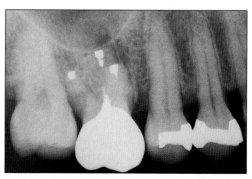

12.105 Radiograph of replantation – postoperative

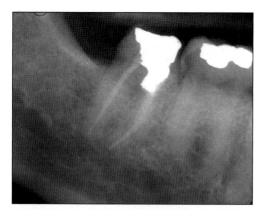

12.106 Transplantation case. Radiographic and clinical examination revealed a hopeless prognosis for the lower second molar tooth

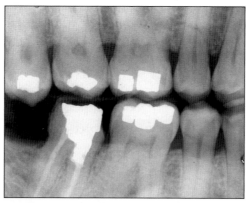

12.107 Bitewing radiograph indicating relationship of maxillary to mandibular teeth

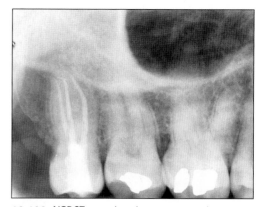

12.108 NSRCT completed on unopposed maxillary third molar

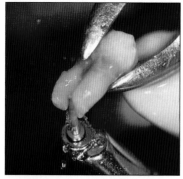

12.109 Maxillary third molar extracted gently and the root-ends resected

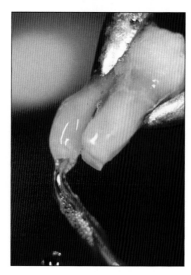

12.110 Root-end preparations prepared and obturated with Diaket root-end filling material. The palatal root had to be extensively resected in order to allow the tooth to be positioned in the recipient socket

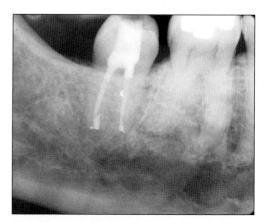

12.111 Transplanted tooth in recipient site

extracted tooth should be protected in the same way as that of an avulsed tooth. The cells of the periodontal ligament and the socket are very susceptible to damage and must be protected from trauma and from desiccation. If the tooth is out of the mouth for any time, it should be placed in a storage medium such as Hanks Balanced Salt Solution (HBSS) or Ringer's solution. These isotonic solutions provide the greatest chance of ensuring vitality of the periodontal ligament, which will in turn reduce the chance of resorption of the root at a later date. Root-end preparation and root-end filling are performed extraorally under a constant stream of isotonic saline or HBSS.

Regenerative procedures

In 1793 John Hunter said that, 'the only rational form of treatment is that which calls forth the recuperative powers of the body ...'. More recently, Melcher (1976) wrote a paper entitled 'On the repair potential of periodontal tissues', which resulted in a reappraisal of the processes involved in periodontal regeneration. The emphasis following endodontic and periodontal surgery has subsequently shifted towards regeneration of tissues as opposed to repair alone.

Regeneration of the periradicular tissues subsequent to surgery or due to the ravages of disease processes implies replacement of the various components of the tissue in their appropriate locations, amounts and relationships to each other (Aukhil 1991). Repair, on the other hand, is a biological process by which continuity of disrupted tissue is restored by new tissues that do not replicate the structure and function of the lost ones (Hammarstrom 1997).

Melcher (1976) stated that the cells that repopulate the exposed root surface determine the nature of the attachment that will form. If the rapidly growing epithelium proliferates first, a long junctional epithelium (JE) will form. If cells from the gingival connective tissue (CT) meet the root surface, root resorption might be the sequela. If bone comes in direct contact with the root, root resorption and ankylosis occurs. However, if cells from the PDL populate the root surface first, ideal new connective tissue attachment develops.

Overall, guided tissue regeneration (GTR) procedures have been shown to improve the levels of attachment. However, histometric assessment reveals that incomplete regeneration frequently occurs (Aukhil *et al.* 1986, Caffesse *et al.* 1988, Magnusson *et al.* 1990). Aukhil *et al.* (1986) described three different zones of healing after barrier therapy:

- JE;
- fibres parallel to the root surface;
- new CT attachment (new bone, PDL, cementum).

A number of commercially available membranes are currently available (**12.112–12.114**). The use of membranes in endodontic surgical cases became more widespread following the development of absorbable materials. Prior to this, the non-resorbable material such as the Gore-Tex membrane had to be removed during a second follow-up surgical procedure some six weeks after the initial procedure. Absorbable membranes include Biomend (**12.114**) and BioGide (both collagen products) and the discontinued Guidor. A new absorbable 100% synthetic membrane called Resolut Adapt has been introduced by the Gore Company. It is important to place the

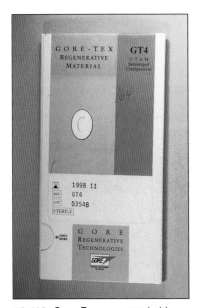

12.112 Gore-Tex non-resorbable membrane (Gore)

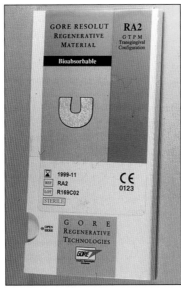

12.113 Resolut absorbable membrane (Gore)

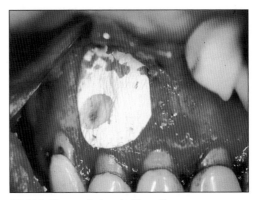

12.114 Biomend absorbable collagen membrane placed over large through and through defect with 2–3 mm extension over the osseous margins of the lesion

membrane so that its edges are fully supported by 2–3 mm of bone away from the edge of the crypt. Many clinicians prescribe antibiotics for their patients following placement of a membrane but there is no evidence to support routine use of antibiotics.

Other substitute materials are also available as supports for membranes or as regenerative materials aimed at supporting, if not inducing, bone formation. These include BioOss (**12.93**), Perioglass and calcium sulphate (**12.115, 12.116**).

Decompression

Decompression or marsupialization involves the surgical exteriorization of a large periradicular lesion in order to facilitate healing of the lesion (**5.71–5.75**). The lesion is penetrated through the periosteum and cortical plate and the patency of the opening is maintained by inserting a flanged cannula allowing for daily irrigation of the lesion by the patient. The advantages of this procedure include reduction in the risk of damaging either adjacent vital teeth or anatomical structures.

12.115

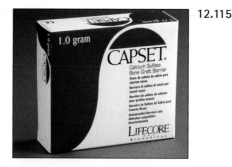

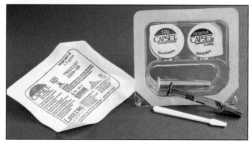

12.116

12.115–12.116 Capset calcium sulphate material

References

American Association of Endodontics (1998) *Contemporary Terminology for Endodontics*, 6th edn. Glossary, AAE, Chicago, IL.

Allen RK, Newton CW, Brown CE (1989) A statistical analysis of surgical and non-surgical endodontic retreatment cases. *J Endod* **15**, 261–6.

Altonen M, Mattila K (1976) Follow-up study of apicectomized molars. *Int J Oral Surg* **5**, 33–40.

Amagasa T, Nagase M, Shioda S (1989) Apicectomy with retrograde gutta-percha root filling. *Oral Surg, Oral Med, Oral Pathol* **68**, 339–42.

August DS (1996) Long-term, post-surgical results in teeth with periapical radiolucencies. *J Endod* **22**, 380–3.

Aukhil I (1991) Biology of tooth-cell adhesion. *Dent Clin North America* **35**, 459–67.

Aukhil I, Pettersson E, Suggs C (1986) Guided tissue regeneration. An experimental procedure in beagle dogs. *J Periodontal* **57**, 727–34.

Crosher RF, Dinsdale RCW, Holmes A (1989) A one-visit apicectomy technique using calcium hydroxide cement as the canal filling material combined with retrograde amalgam. *Int Endod J* **22**, 283–9.

Caffesse RG, Kerry GJ, Chaves ES (1988) Clinical evaluation of the use of citric acid and autologous fibronectin in periodontal surgery. *J Periodontal* **59**, 565–9.

Dorn SO, Gartner AH (1990) Retrograde filling materials: a retrospective success–failure study of amalgam, EBA and IRM. *J Endod* **16**, 391–3.

Ericson S, Finne K, Persson G (1974) Results of apicoectomy of maxillary canines, premolars and molars with special reference to oro-antral communication as a prognostic factor. *Int J Oral Surg* **3**, 386–93.

Finne K, Nord PG, Persson G, Lennartsson B (1977) Retrograde root filling with amalgam and Cavit. *Oral Surg, Oral Med, Oral Pathol* **43**, 621–6.

Fish, FW (1939) Bone infection. *J Am Dent Assoc* **26**, 691–712.

Frank AL, Glick DH, Patterson SS, Weine FS (1992) Long-term evaluation of surgically placed amalgam fillings. *J Endod* **18**, 39–8.

Friedman S, Lustmann J, Shaharabany V (1991) Treatment results of apical surgery in premolar and molar teeth. *J Endod* **7**, 30–3.

Grung B, Molven O, Halse A (1990) Periapical surgery in a Norwegian county hospital: follow-up findings of 477 teeth. *J Endod* **16**, 411–17.

Hammarstrom L (1997) The role of enamel matrix proteins in the development of cementum and periodontal tissues. In *Dental Enamel*, Ciba Foundation Symposium 205, pp. 246–53. John Wiley & Sons, Chichester.

Harrison JW, Jurosky KA (1991a) Wound healing in the tissue of the peridontium following periradicular surgery. 1. The incissional wound. *J Endod* **17**(9), 425–35.

Harrison, JW, Jurosky KA (1991b) Wound healing in the tissue of the peridontium following periradicular surgery. 2. The dissectional wound. *J Endod* **17**(11), 544–52.

Harrison JW, Jurosky KA (1992) Wound healing in the tissues of the periodontium following periradicular surgery. 3. The osseous excisional wound. *J Endod* **18**, 76–81.

Harrison JW, Todd M (1986) The effect of root resection on the sealing property of root canal obturations. *Oral Surg* **50**, 264–72.

Harty FJ, Parkins BJ, Wengraf AM (1970) The success rate of apicectomy. *Br Dent J* **129**, 407–13.

Hirsch JM, Ahlström U, Henrikson PA, Heyden G, Peterson LE (1979) Periapical surgery. *Int J Oral Surg* **8**, 173–85.

Ingle JI (1994) *Endodontics*, 4th eds. Lea & Febiger, Philadelphia.

Ioannides C, Borstlap WA (1983) Apicectomy on molars: a clinical and radiographical study. *Int J Oral Surg* **12**, 73–9.

Jesslén P, Zetterqvist L, Heimdahl A (1995) Long-term results of amalgam versus glass ionomer cement as apical sealant after apicectomy. *Oral Surg, Oral Med, Oral Pathol, Oral Radiol, Endod* **79**, 101–3.

Jansson L, Sandstedt P, Låftman AC, Skoglund A (1997) Relationship between apical and marginal healing in periradicular surgery. *Oral Surg, Oral Med, Oral Pathol, Oral Radiol, Endod* **83**, 596–601.

Kvist T, Reit C (1999) Results of endodontic retreatment: a randomized clinical study comparing surgical and nonsurgical procedures. *J Endod* **25**, 814–17.

Lustmann J, Friedman S, Shaharabany V (1991) Relation of pre- and intraoperative factors to prognosis of posterior apical surgery. *J Endod* **17**, 239–41.

Lyons AJ, Dixon EJA, Hughes CE (1995) A 5-year audit of outcome of apicectomies carried out in a district general hospital. *Ann Roy Coll Surg Engl* **77**, 273–7.

Magnusson I, Stenberg WV, Batich C, Egleberg J (1990) Connective tissue repair in circumferential periodontal defects in dogs following use of a biodegradable membrane. *J Clin Periodontal* **17**, 243–8.

Melcher AH (1976) On the repair potential of periodontal tissues. *J Periodontal* **47**, 256–60.

Mikkonen M, Kulla-Mikkonen A, Kotilainen R (1983) Clinical and radiological re-examination of apicectomized teeth. *Oral Surg, Oral Med, Oral Pathol* **55**, 302–6.

Molven O, Halse A, Grung B (1991) Surgical management of endodontic failures: indications and treatment results. *Int J Dent* **41**, 33–42.

Nordenram Å, Svärdström G (1970) Results of apicectomy. *Swedish Dent J* **63**, 593–604.

Pantschev A, Carlsson AP, Andersson L (1994) Retrograde root filling with EBA cement or amalgam: a comparative clinical study. *Oral Surg, Oral Med, Oral Pathol* **78**, 101–4.

Persson G (1973) Prognosis of reoperation after apicectomy: a clinical–radiological investigation. *Swedish Dent J* **66**, 49–67.

Rahbaran S, Gilthorpe M, Harrison S, Gulabivala K (2001) Comparison of clinical outcome of periapical surgery in endodontic and oral surgery units at Eastman Dental Hospital – a retrospective study. *Oral Surg, Oral Med, Oral Pathol, Oral Radiol Endod* **91**, 700–9.

Rapp EL, Brown CE, Newton CW (1991) An analysis of success and failure of apicectomies. *J Endod* **17**, 508–12.

Regan JD, Gutmenn JL, Witherspoon DE (2002) Comparison of Diaket and MTA when used as root-end filling materials to support regeneration of the periradicular tissues. *Int Endod J* **35**, 840–8.

Reit C, Hirsch J (1986) Surgical endodontic retreatment. *Int Endod J* **19**, 107–12.

Rubenstein RA, Kim S (1999) Short-term observation of the results of endodontic surgery with the use of a surgical operation microscope and Super-EBA as root-end filling material. *J Endod* **25**, 43–8.

Rubenstein RA, Kim S (2002) Long-term follow-up of cases considered healed one year after apical microsurgery. *J Endod* **28**, 378–83.

Rud J, Andreasen JO, Möller Jensen JE (1972) A follow-up study of 1000 cases treated by endodontic surgery. *Int J Oral Surg* **1**, 215–28.

Rud J, Munksgaard EC, Andreasen JO, Rud V (1991) Retrograde root filling with composite and dentine-bonding agent, 2. *Endod Dent Traumatol* **7**, 126–31.

Tanzilli JP, Raphael D, Moodnik RM (1980) A comparison of the marginal adaptation of retrograde techniques: a scanning electron microscopic study. *Oral Surg, Oral Med, Oral Pathol* **50**, 74–80.

Zetterqvist L, Hall G, Holmlund A (1991) Apicectomy: a comparative clinical study of amalgam and glass ionomer cement as apical sealants. *Oral Surg, Oral Med, Oral Pathol* **71**, 489–91

Chapter 13

Management of acute problems

I Cross and R T Walker

One of the most rewarding aspects of endodontic treatment is caring for the patient in pain. This can normally be achieved in a short period of time without jeopardizing the overall treatment plan.

It is probably true to say that over 85% of patients attending the dentist in pain are suffering from pulpal or periradicular disease. The operator's aim, in providing emergency care, is to remove the pain and control the inflammation or infection that is present.

Endodontic emergencies that occur are essentially preoperative, operative and postoperative.

PREOPERATIVE EMERGENCIES

One of the major reasons for failed endodontic procedures is treatment of the wrong tooth. On many occasions patients arriving at the practice have been in pain for a number of days and have difficulty locating the tooth causing the pain. Inevitably patients arrive seeking emergency treatment at a time inconvenient to the busy practitioner. However, it is essential that a diagnosis be reached. Apart from the patient often not being able to locate the specific tooth causing the problem there are a number of pathological entities that will mimic

pain of odontogenic origin and in these cases endodontic procedures are obviously not indicated. A common cause for misdiagnosis is spasm of the lateral pterygoid muscle as seen in temporomandibular joint dysfunction syndrome. The use of an occlusal acrylic splint for diagnosis and treatment is often indicated (**13.1, 13.2**).

Pain of pulpal origin

The innervation of the dental pulp involves impulse transmission along myelinated A-δ-fibres and unmyelinated C-fibres. These fibres conduct pain of differing quality depending on the degree of pathological stimulus. Pulpal injury appears to cause a biphasic vascular response. There is an initial vasoconstriction followed by vasodilatation. The vasodilatation causes an oedema and a localized increase in tissue fluid. The resulting increase in tissue pressure in turn leads to a reduced regional blood flow and an increase in tissue carbon dioxide and acidity. The refined pulpal microcirculation (**13.3**), which contains arteriovenous shunts, attempts to divert blood away from the injured area to reduce this higher pressure. If the injury is severe enough to overcome this compensatory effect, then local

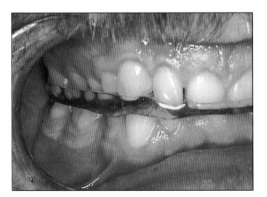

13.1 Splint therapy for TMJ dysfunction

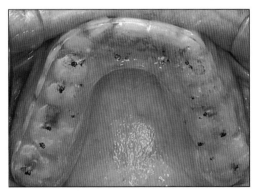

13.2 Palatal view of occlusal splint

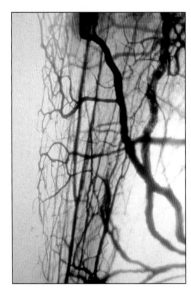

13.3
Pulpal
vasculature

ischaemia and tissue destruction can occur. This alteration in vascular flow is related to the altered sensitivity that is seen in cases of pulpitis.

Clinical reversible pulpitis is characterized by pain of short duration produced by extremes of temperature and sweet food. An increased vascular flow may contribute to a decrease in pain threshold of the larger A-δ-fibres leading to an increased responsiveness to hot and cold. The teeth do not tend to be sensitive to palpation or percussion. The pain is usually of dentinal origin in situations where there is exposed sensitive dentine, early dental caries, and leaking restorations. Radiographically there should be no widening of the periodontal ligament space unless the pulpitis is induced by occlusal trauma, creating inflammation within the periodontal ligament and pulp. Treatment involves removing the source of dentinal irritation. In the case of sensitive dentine, patent dentinal tubules may be treated using dentine-bonding agents to affect a seal. Fluoride varnish may also be applied to the affected area or desensitizing toothpaste may be prescribed. Dental caries and faulty restorations should be removed and replaced with a sedative dressing (**13.4**).

Persistent symptoms indicate clinical irreversible pulpitis. The pain tends to increase in duration and intensity and heat can become more reactive than cold, which may actually have a relieving influence. As further tissue injury occurs ischaemia can suppress the activity of the A-δ-fibres more than the C-fibres. There is a change in quality and intensity of the pain as the C-fibres become more involved and it is a sign that the pulpal tissues are irreversibly damaged. The pain is often spontaneous and lasts from several minutes to hours. The tooth may be difficult to locate until the periodontal ligament becomes inflamed, when it becomes tender to bite on. Early radiographic changes may be evident (**13.5**). Symptoms of irreversible pulpitis occasionally occur in teeth with primary periodontal lesions. Pain relief is achieved by root treatment but the long-term prognosis for the tooth depends on its periodontal status.

The ideal emergency treatment for irreversible pulpitis is to remove the diseased pulp completely and to clean and prepare the pulp canal system. Irrigating the pulp chamber with a 2.5–5.0% solution of sodium hypochlorite ensures disinfection before canal instrumentation. If time does not allow this, removal of pulp tissue from the pulp chamber and coronal part of the root canals is often effective. The use of corticosteroid preparations in vital root canals has been advocated in situations where complete instrumentation is inconvenient or impossible because profound anaesthesia cannot be secured.

Antibiotics have commonly been prescribed for irreversible pulpitis. An antimicrobial medication will have no effect on the inflamed pulp and is contraindicated. Advice regarding analgesics should be given.

A medical history needs to be taken to rule out possible drug hypersensitivity. However, generally pain can be controlled with self prescribed peripherally acting analgesics. Aspirin is widely used. However, it's efficacy is dose related, 1000–1200 mg four times per day providing greater analgesia than 500–600 mg four times per day. Dental pain is generally of short duration with analgesics only being taken for 24–48 hours and it is unlikely, therefore, that unwanted effects would occur. Non-steroidal anti-inflammatory drugs (NSAIDs), such as ibuprofen, can also be used. Ibuprofen has been shown to be one of the most effective analgesics at reducing pain; 400 mg four times per day appears to be the optimal dose. While paracetamol is often used by patients with sensitivity to aspirin and the other NSAIDs, it does not have the same anti-inflammatory properties.

Peripherally acting analgesics are often provided in combination with a centrally acting analgesic such as codeine. Evidence suggests that combined analgesics are more effective than the individual constituents alone.

Where there is a severe pain then the use of a NSAID and paracetamol in tandem can be considered. An initial dose of the NSAID can be given with paracetamol being taken 2–3 hours later. The NSAID can again be given two hours following this. The obvious risks are patients not understanding the drug regimen or using a proprietary analgesic with both an NSAID and paracetamol, and therefore possibly overdosing on the paracetamol.

Analgesics have been shown to more beneficial if they are taken before severe pain occurs. Patients should be advised that the analgesics should be taken if they feel pain developing and possibly to continue with a regular dose after the pain has subsided for a period of time.

The use of long-acting anaesthetics can be considered to give the patient pain relief while the analgesics start to act. Marcaine (0.5% bupivacaine with 1 : 200 000 epinephrine) when used as a regional block can give soft-tissue anaesthesia of 6–8 hours. Marcaine is not available in all countries in dental anaesthetic cartridges and in some areas is not licensed for dental use. Dental practitioners should satisfy themselves as to the local rules before administering it. Other preparations of bupivacaine are available such as Carbostesin (**13.6**).

If symptoms continue following pulpal extirpation, the presence of infected or inflamed pulpal tissue should be investigated, the root canal system examined again for the presence of an undiagnosed canal and the occlusal contacts of the tooth should be checked.

Teeth with undiagnosed fractures may cause symptoms of reversible and irreversible pulpitis. The degree of pain may vary considerably, depending on the extent of the fracture, from momentary pain on encountering heat and cold to spontaneous pain or pain on biting. Care should be taken that the correct tooth is diagnosed. It is possible for pain from a lower molar tooth to be referred to the premolar area. If reversible pulpitis is diagnosed, restorations should be removed from the suspected tooth, the dentinal fracture sought and the pulp protected from further insult by providing a restoration that reduces microleakage to a minimum and prevents the fracture propagating. Modern dentine bonding materials are useful in small cavities as an interim restoration before constructing a restoration giving occlusal protection (**13.7**). It is impossible to predict long-term events in this situation and patients must be warned that extraction following treatment is a possibility.

Where a fracture involves the pulp and symptoms suggest an irreversible pulpitis, all restorations should be removed from the tooth and the extent of the fracture examined. If the fractured portion of

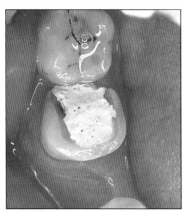

13.4 Dressed molar tooth

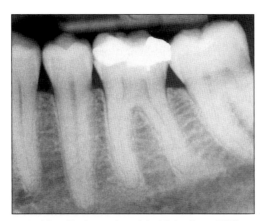

13.5 Mandibular molar with thickening of PDL space and sclerosing osteitis

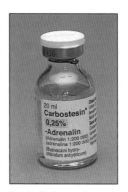

13.6 Carbostesin

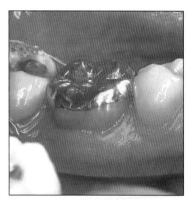

13.7 Gold partial coverage restoration giving occlusal protection

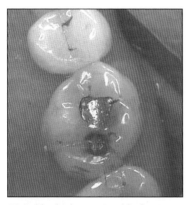

13.8 Vertical unrestorable fracture in maxillary molar

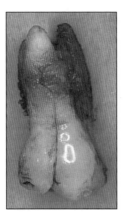

13.9 Maxillary molar following extraction

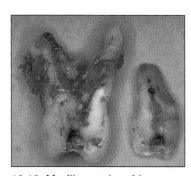

13.10 Maxillary molar with separated fractured segment

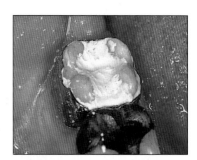

13.11 Molar tooth supported by an orthodontic band

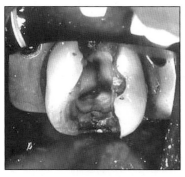

13.12 Fracture through floor of the pulp chamber of molar

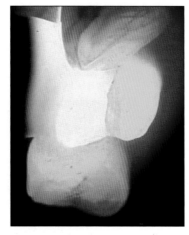

13.13 Use of fibre-optic light to illustrate the extent of an incomplete fracture (courtesy of Dr C C Youngson, Liverpool Dental Institute)

the tooth is mobile it should be removed, examined, and the possibility of restoring the remaining tooth substance established (**13.8**). Examination of the extracted fragment allows accurate assessment of the restorability of the tooth. Where the fracture runs into the apical periodontal attachment apparatus, as in this case, then extraction is the only option (**13.9, 13.10**). If the tooth is restorable root treatment may commence. Should the fracture line run through the floor of the pulp chamber then it is unlikely that the tooth will respond to treatment in the long term.

In cases where the tooth is fractured but the fracture is still incomplete the crown should be supported with a metal band (**13.11**) and root treatment commenced. The long-term prognosis of posterior teeth with oblique fractures above the alveolar crest and involving only the roof of the pulp chamber is higher than vertical fractures involving the floor of the chamber (**13.12**). A fibre-optic light is useful in locating and examining the extent of these fractures (**13.13**).

Emergencies of periradicular origin

Inflammation and infection of the periodontal tissues may cause pain. It is important to establish whether the pain and swelling involving the supporting tissues is of periodontal or pulpal origin. The cause is usually established by carrying out vitality tests (**13.14, 13.15**).

When dealing with a periodontal abscess emergency treatment will involve instituting drainage, prescribing antibiotics when required and debriding the pocket. Endodontic treatment should not be required.

Acute apical periodontitis is an acute inflammation of the periodontal ligament, generally related to pulpal inflammation but occasionally resulting directly from trauma. When endodontic treatment is initiated in a non-vital tooth with acute apical periodontitis the canal system should be cleaned thoroughly to remove all periodontal irritation and care must be exercised to prevent further insult to the periodontal tissues by over-instrumentation. Occlusal adjustment to remove contacts is also helpful.

An acute apical abscess (**13.16**) may develop from apical periodontitis. The tooth involved becomes exquisitely painful to touch. The tooth may be extruded from the socket and mobile. To relieve pain the priority is to establish drainage by opening the pulp chamber of the tooth (**13.17**). The tooth, if tender, should be stabilized while the access cavity is being cut. Any fluctuant swelling should be incised to establish drainage. The pulp chamber should be irrigated with sodium hypochlorite to remove superficial organic debris before commencing canal preparation. Following thorough cleaning of the canal system the tooth is sealed to prevent reinfection. Only when there is profuse, uncontrollable drainage should a tooth be left open to drain for a maximum period of 24 hours.

Where there is a spreading submandibular infection leading to swelling, serious consideration needs to be given to extraoral drainage achieved under general anaesthesia (**13.18**).

Antibiotics are indicated when patients have toxic systemic effects and a raised temperature. Increasingly, short-term antibiotics are being used. For patients who are not allergic to penicillin a two-dose regime of 3G amoxycillin can be used. Alternatively, for most patients, where drainage has been instigated, 2 or 3 days of oral antibiotics, given in a high dose, will suffice for acute dento-alveolar infections; amoxycillin 250 mg every eight hours. Metronidazole is active against anaerobic organisms, which are commonly found in acute dental infections. It is often given in combination with amoxycillin with good effect. However, it has also been shown to have good efficacy in isolation, possibly because the true nature of dental infections is not properly appreciated. Metronidazole (400 mg 2–3 times daily) is often preferred to penicillins due to

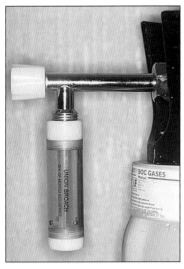

13.14 CO_2 cylinder for dry-ice vitality testing

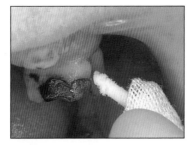

13.15 Dry-ice stick for vitality testing

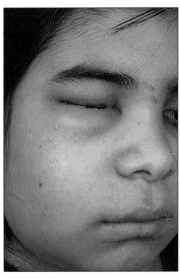

13.16 Acute apical abscess with facial swelling

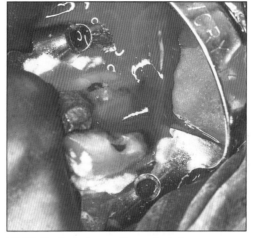

13.17 Tooth drainage of an apical abscess

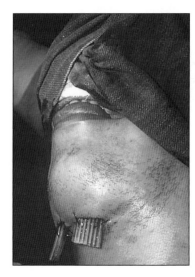

13.18 Extraoral drainage of a tooth abscess

causing fewer hypersensitivity reactions and the lack of bacterial resistance to it. It is advisable to review all patients within 24 hours.

Emergencies resulting from trauma

Trauma to young patients (**13.19**) and immature teeth are a common cause of dental emergencies. These injuries can leave patients requiring dental treatment for many years especially if the extent of the injury is not properly diagnosed and the correct treatment instigated. Traumatic incidents may result in luxation/avulsion injuries and fractures of the crowns and roots of teeth. The endodontic problems arising from these incidents can be managed successfully only after the following questions are answered:

1. *What is the nature of the injury?* It is important to assess the extent of both bony and soft-tissue injuries. The examination of lacerations and fractures should take precedence over the dental examination. The need for soft-tissue radiographs, antitetanus cover and referral to specialist colleagues should be established.

2. *Are the injured teeth preservable and restorable?* The extent of dental damage should be assessed and the efforts required to retain the teeth should be considered, in the light of the patient's overall treatment needs, in order to reach a balanced decision regarding the future of the teeth.

3. *Has the vascular/nutritive supply of the pulp been impaired?* What is the degree of this impairment? The assessment of vascular damage becomes particularly important if there is evidence of concussion and intrusive, extrusive, and lateral luxation of teeth.

4. *To what extent have the pulps of the teeth been contaminated with microorganisms? What is the potential for future contamination?* The endodontic penetration, and potential for further penetration, of bacteria and their toxins will have a profound influence on the immediate and long-term prognosis of fractured teeth.

5. *How mature is each tooth and is the root completely formed?* Immature teeth with large pulp spaces are structurally more difficult to restore and need long-term endodontic treatment although they are more likely to remain/re-establish vitality.

Treatment of fractured teeth

Crown fractures

Crown fractures may involve only the enamel or both the enamel and the dentine (**13.20**). The damaged tooth should be radiographed and vitality tested before protecting the exposed dentine with a liner and a bonded composite. It may be possible to use the fractured portion of the tooth as the restoration (**13.21**).

If injury to a mature tooth results in pulpal exposure root canal treatment is usually indicated. Partial removal of the pulp may be possible depending on the degree of bacterial contamination and necrosis. When the tooth involved is not fully formed and it is desirable to preserve the vital pulp, the treatment options are pulp capping or pulpotomy, as described in Chapter 1.

Pulp capping

Pulp capping is usually carried out only on very small and recent exposures. However, in healthy pulps, the size of the exposure has been shown to be of little consequence. The chronological/biological age of the tooth is of more importance. The chances of preserving a vital pulp are increased when there is a good blood supply. The tooth should be isolated and the exposure washed with saline. Haemostasis has to be secured. After the bleeding has stopped, traditionally, the area should be covered with calcium hydroxide and the tooth restored. The tooth should be reviewed clinically and radiographically for signs of disease.

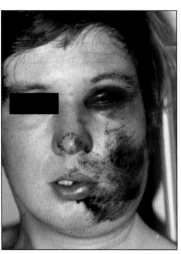

13.19 Young patient with head injuries

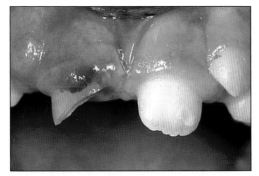

13.20 Maxillary incisor with complicated crown fracture (courtesy of Department of Child Dental Health, Leeds Dental Institute)

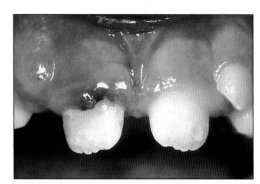

13.21 Subsequent restoration of maxillary incisor using fractured section (courtesy of Department of Child Dental Health, Leeds Dental Institute)

Pulpotomy

Pulpotomy procedures are performed in immature teeth with large exposures. The tooth is isolated with a rubber dam after administering local analgesia. A small portion of the coronal pulp is removed using a high-speed diamond bur under a cooling spray. The pulp stump is washed with saline and, after bleeding ceases, it is covered with calcium hydroxide and a zinc oxide preparation and the tooth is restored. As with pulp capping, other materials including mineral trioxide aggregate (MTA) are finding increasing favour. The key to success is prevention of microleakage and reinfection of the pulp. The tooth should be reviewed initially at 6 to 12 weeks and then at six-monthly intervals and annually until the root formation is considered complete. The tooth should be observed to establish the presence of a hard tissue barrier without abnormal calcification. If there is radiographic evidence of internal resorption root treatment should be commenced.

Crown–root fractures

The treatment of crown–root fractures depends largely on their position and the degree of mobility of the coronal portion. Fractures involving the gingival crevice and attachment may necessitate root treatment to stem the bacterial contamination that is likely to occur along the fracture line. Before root canal treatment is commenced it is wise to consider whether the fractured portion of the tooth is to be removed and how the tooth will be finally restored. The need for surgery to expose the margins of the fracture, orthodontic extrusion of the root to facilitate restorative procedures, and space maintenance to avoid later restorative problems should be borne in mind.

Root fractures

Traditionally root fractures below the level of the alveolar crest have been splinted for long periods, up to 12 weeks, to secure union of the fragments. This length of time for splinting may only be necessary in situations where there has been displacement and considerable mobility of the coronal fragment. Where no splinting is required, the tooth should then be reviewed clinically and radiographically at 3, 6 and 12 months. Vitality testing may be unreliable for a period of 2 to 6 months.

If the tooth remains firm and is vital no further treatment is necessary. Many undiagnosed fractures remain symptomless and cause no problems (**13.22**).

If vitality is lost, generally (in about 25% of cases) the coronal segment becomes necrotic (**13.23**). Root treatment is then performed to the fracture line. Calcium hydroxide is used as a long-term medicament to encourage calcification (**13.24**) and formation of a hard-tissue barrier against which the obturating material can be condensed (**13.25**). Alternatively MTA can be placed apically to act as a hard tissue barrier or, indeed, to act as the whole root-filling material. Root treatment of both fragments should be attempted rarely. When the whole pulp becomes necrotic, surgical removal of the apical portion may be a more manageable option.

Treatment of unfractured teeth

If there is evidence to suggest that the pulp of a luxated tooth has become necrotic, root treatment should be performed. Completely avulsed teeth that have been replanted should undergo root canal treatment 7 to 10 days following replantation. The possibility of replacement resorption (**13.26**) can neither be predicted nor treated.

Many types of splint are available for stabilizing replanted and fractured teeth. Vacuum-formed polyvinyl splints are inconvenient, require laboratory facilities (which delays their fitting) and tend to look rather bulky. Similarly, the use of foil and zinc phosphate cement is messy, rarely achieves what is aimed at and should be avoided (**13.27**). The use of etched enamel retained composite, and polymethacrylate reinforced with wire or nylon has also been advocated. Twistflex wire attached to the avulsed teeth and one tooth on either side with composite appears to be the current splint of choice (**13.28**). Reimplanted teeth are generally splinted for 7 to 10 days.

OPERATIVE EMERGENCIES

While the operator may consider an operative emergency as being unable to locate a canal or separated instrument within the root canal, other more serious complications can occur.

Medical emergencies

Hopefully a good medical history will have identified those patients who may be at risk from a medical emergency. There are very few, if any, medical conditions that preclude the possibility of endodontic treatment, especially as the alternative is often a tooth extraction with the entire attendant trauma. However, special arrangements may have to be in place to guard against possible problems. Diabetics may wish to be seen at a certain time of day so that their routines are not disturbed with the possibility of a hypoglycaemic attack occurring. Consultation with other specialists is often of benefit where the use of corticosteroids may be involved for those patients who have adrenal insufficiency. The prepositioning of intravenous access would allow a quicker and possibly less-panicked response in the case of an emergency.

While the treatment for vaso-vagal syncopy is to lay the patient flat, during pregnancy laying the patient flat can induce syncopy. Treatment is to remove the pressure of the foetus on the vena cavae by raising the patient forward.

Cardiovascular conditions in the mildest form would present as angina attack for which the patient should be able to self-medicate, although having a glyceryl trinitrate inhaler in the practice is advised. Patients exhibiting signs of a myocardial infarction should be given oxygen and the emergency services should be called.

One of the commonest medical emergencies in the practice is anaphylaxis. A patient can have an anaphylactic reaction to many materials. There has been a reported increase in reactions to latex. The use of rubber dams in endodontics makes this occurrence particularly important. A medical history showing food intolerance to bananas

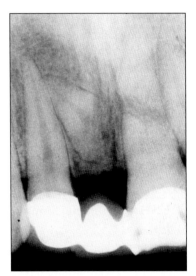

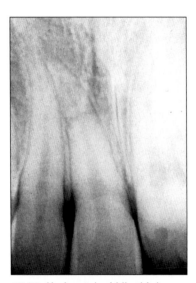

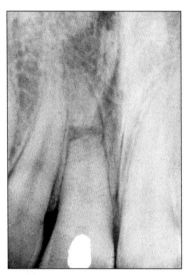

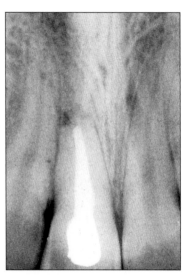

13.22 Symptomless, undiagnosed root fracture

13.23 Horizontal middle third fracture of maxillary incisor

13.24 Calcium hydroxide dressing to fracture line

13.25 Obturation of fractured incisor to fracture line

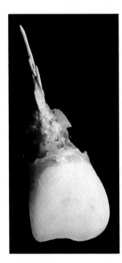

13.26 Replacement resorption affecting maxillary incisor (courtesy of Department of Child Dental Health, Leeds Dental Institute)

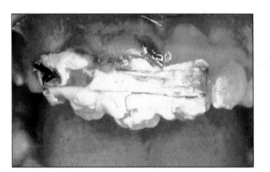

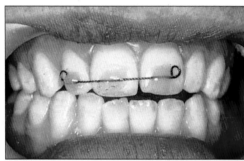

13.27 Foil and zinc phosphate cement splint – to be avoided (courtesy of Department of Child Dental Health, Leeds Dental Institute)

13.28 Twist-flex wire splint (courtesy of Department of Child Dental Health, Leeds Dental Institute)

Local analgesia

Local analgesia should be given at each appointment. There is a pre-conception that analgesia is not required in 'dead' teeth or teeth that are ready for obturation. However, necrotic pulps can contain nerve fibres still capable of transmitting pain while sealer extruded through the apex or lateral canals can cause pain.

Difficulties can often be encountered in trying to secure analgesia in irreversibly inflamed pulps or where there is acute infection. Failure of analgesia may be operator dependant (poor technique, choice of technique and/or solution) or patient dependant (anatomical, pathological or psychological).

The most commonly used analgesic solution for most endodontic procedures is lignocaine with adrenaline (epinephrine) (**13.29**). Providing the analgesic solution is given slowly with an aspirating technique then the adrenaline (epinephrine) is not a problem with most patients. Giving the analgesic slowly is not only less painful for the patient but there is evidence that the application of a slower injection speed is likely to produce deeper analgesia.

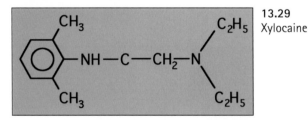

13.29 Xylocaine

and avocados may show a cross-reaction to latex. Patients can develop a reaction to latex with a number of exposures. Where patients show possible early signs, such as tingling of the lips, then latex-free rubber dams and gloves should be considered. Where there are the signs of an anaphylactic reaction adrenaline (epinephrine) (0.5–1 ml 1:1000 intramuscularly) and oxygen should be administered. The emergency services should be called even if the patient appears to recover following administration of the adrenaline (epinephrine).

The success rate for inferior alveolar block injections is over 90%. A practitioner who regularly fails with this method should reassess his/her technique.

If an inferior alveolar block fails and a repeat attempt also fails then an alternative technique should be considered. The Gow–Gates and the Akinosi techniques both attempt to anaesthetize the inferior alveolar nerve at a higher level. Both these methods are best reserved for cases where the conventional block fails as they can produce more complications than the standard approach – the higher the needle the closer it is to the maxillary artery and the pterygoid plexus.

Gow–Gates technique

This is a true mandibular block injection that provides analgesia of all the sensory divisions of the mandibular nerve including buccal, inferior alveolar, lingual and mylohyoid. The method relies upon the deposition of analgesic solution adjacent to the head of the mandibular condyle (**13.30**). The patient has the mouth wide open and a line is imagined from the corner of the mouth to the inter-tragic notch; this is the plane of approach. The needle is introduced from the direction of the contralateral mandibular canine tooth and directed over the ipsilateral second molar (**13.31**). The point of mucosal penetration is higher than for a conventional inferior dental block. The needle is advanced until bony contact is made with the head of the condyle, withdrawn slightly, aspiration is carried out, and a full cartridge of analgesic is delivered.

Akinosi technique

This is a simpler technique than the Gow–Gates method and is sometimes known as the closed-mouth technique. The patient has the mouth closed and a 35 mm needle is used. The syringe is advanced parallel to the maxillary occlusal plane at the level of the maxillary muco-gingival junction. The needle is advanced until the hub is level with the distal surface of the maxillary second molar (**13.32**). At this point a cartridge of analgesic solution is deposited. This technique does not rely on touching bone and this can be a disadvantage. However, the Akinosi technique allows provision of analgesia in a situation where all other methods of giving an inferior dental block would fail. Both motor and sensory analgesia are achieved allowing the patient to open the mouth.

Although it is generally considered that the sign of a successful block is a numb lip all that this indicates is that the nerves to the soft tissues of the lip have been blocked. It does not necessarily mean that there is pulpal analgesia. The presence of infection and inflammation can reduce the efficacy of analgesic solutions. In solution the local analgesic exists in two ionic forms, an uncharged anion (RN) and a positively charged cation (RNH$^+$). Both ionic forms of the solution are required for analgesia.

$$RNH^+ \leftrightarrows RN + H^+$$

Inflammation lowers the tissue pH and correspondingly the amount of the base form of the analgesic available to penetrate the nerve membrane. Consequently there is less of the ionized form within the nerve to achieve analgesia. In addition nerves arising in inflamed tissue have altered resting potentials and decreased excitability thresholds. These changes are not restricted to the inflamed pulp but affect the entire neural membrane.

Supplemental analgesia is often required when treating the 'hot' tooth. Accessory anatomy should not be discounted. Infiltrations, while not a replacement for inferior dental blocks, may be required to block input from the cervical plexus, together with the mylohyoid and lingual nerves. Cross innervation from the contralateral inferior alveolar nerve should also be considered. In the upper arch the posterior superior alveolar block to the upper molars can be considered while anterior superior alveolar nerve block can deposit analgesic at the opening of the infraorbital foramen – decussation of the fibres of the anterior superior dental nerve can provide innervation to the premolar teeth. When treating vital molar teeth serious consideration should be given to palatal infiltrations to block innervation from the greater palatine or nasopalatine nerve.

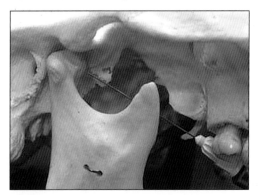

13.30 Position of deposition of local anaesthetic solution for Gow–Gates technique for inferior dental block

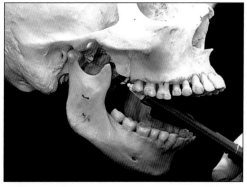

13.31 Gow–Gates technique for inferior dental block

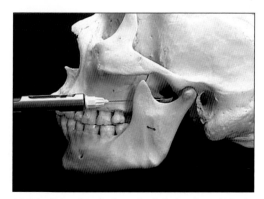

13.32 Akinosi technique for inferior dental block

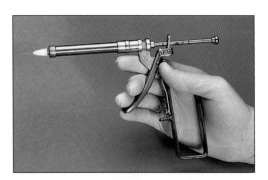

13.33 Articaine

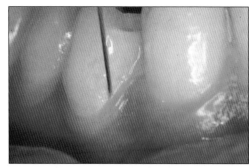

13.34 Peripress for intraligamental injections

13.35 Needle insertion for intraligamental injection

Articaine with adrenaline (epinephrine) (**13.33**) has gained favour as a local analgesic solution to use where lignocaine appears to have failed. Articaine differs from lignocaine as it has a thiophene ring as its lipophilic component rather than a substituted aromatic ring. Studies show that it is no more effective as an analgesic agent than lignocaine. However, it does have an increased propensity to diffuse widely, which may allow it 'unknowingly' to block accessory innervations. In addition, the change in structure may also account for its apparent increased success rate in some patients.

Further analgesia can be administered using intraligamental, intrapulpal or intraosseous techniques. Unfortunately, it is also associated with a higher frequency of persistent paraesthesia.

Intraligamental injections

Intraligamental injections are used to deposit analgesic directly into the periodontal ligament space and a number of specialized syringes (**13.34**) and small needles have been developed to facilitate this. The needle is inserted into the mesial gingival sulcus and in contact with the tooth (**13.35**). The needle is supported by fingers and positioned with maximal penetration between the root and crestal alveolar bone. Pressure is slowly applied to the syringe handle for 20–30 seconds. Backpressure has to be developed for this technique to work and blanching of the soft tissues would be sign of success. If analgesic solution flows readily out of the sulcus then analgesia will not be achieved. Pressure is necessary to force the solution into the marrow spaces to contact and block the dental nerves. The technique should be repeated on the distal surface of the involved tooth.

Intrapulpal injections

The major drawback of the intrapulpal injection is the need for the needle to be inserted into a very sensitive and inflamed pulp. The injection can, therefore, be painful. Additionally, the pulp has to be exposed to give the injection and analgesic problems may have occurred prior to this being achieved. The injection has to be given under strong backpressure. In the absence of backpressure, it is

difficult to achieve analgesia. It would appear that the analgesic agent is not solely responsible for intrapulpal analgesia. One technique to create the backpressure is 'stoppering' the cavity with gutta-percha to allow the backpressure to be created. Alternatively a small hole can be made into the pulp chamber with a half-round bur through which the needle can be introduced. If the pulp chamber has been opened then the needle can be advanced into the canal until it is wedged in place and the backpressure created. The needle may need supporting to prevent it buckling. If the backpressure cannot be created then a smaller gauge needle may be required. Buckling can be overcome by using the shorter and finer intraligamental needles.

Intraosseous technique

The intraosseous technique allows analgesic solution to be deposited directly into the cancellous bone around the apices of the tooth. It has a rapid onset and has shown extremely favourable results when used as a supplemental analgesic for the 'hot' mandibular molar. The mucosa overlying the injection site, either just mesial or distal of the tooth to be treated, is anaesthetized with a small infiltration. Special kits have been developed that facilitate drilling a small hole through the mucosa and cortical plate to allow injection of the anaesthetic solution into the cancellous bone. X-Tips (Prestige Dental, Bradford, UK) consist of a drill to perforate the cortical plate combined with a guide sleeve. When the drill is withdrawn the guide sleeve is left *in situ*. The analgesic solution can be injected through the guide sleeve, which is designed to accept an ultra-short 27-gauge needle (**13.36**). The guide sleeve can be left in place during the procedure so that the anaesthetic can be 'topped-up' if required (**13.37**). A small number of patients develop soreness at the injection site and a transitory increased heart rate can occur depending on the analgesic solution used.

The Wand (Milestone Scientific, USA) is a computer-controlled local analgesic delivery system that can facilitate all local anaesthetic techniques as well as introducing other possibilities (**13.38**). Essentially The Wand allows delivery of analgesic solution at a constant flow rate at low pressure. This has the advantage that a slow delivery of solution gives a less-painful injection. Although The Wand

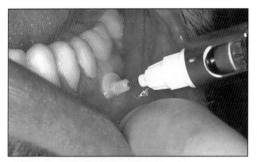

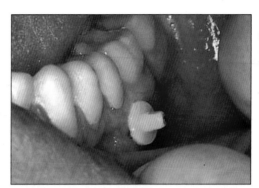

13.36 Intraosseous injection using X-Tips

13.37 Intraosseous guide sleeve left *in situ* until the end of the procedure

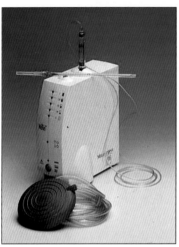

13.38 The Wand, computer-controlled local anaesthetic delivery system

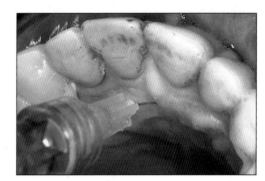

13.39 Blanching of the soft tissues while giving a palatal injection using The Wand

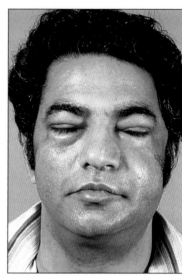

13.40 Soft tissue swelling following a sodium hypochlorite accident

can be used for all the conventional approaches to analgesia it is also possible to give larger volumes of analgesic palatally or via the periodontal ligament. Essentially, the periodontal ligament injection is given in the same conventional manner. As the analgesic solution is given slowly at low pressure, a larger quantity of solution can diffuse through the bone. Again, as the injection is given slowly larger volumes of analgesic can be delivered relatively painlessly into the palate. This allows a palatal approach when anaesthetizing the middle superior and anterior superior alveolar nerves, with the advantage of blocking a number of teeth with one injection when required. Blanching of the soft tissues is again a good indicator that analgesia has been achieved (**13.39**).

Sodium hypochlorite

Sodium hypochlorite remains the intracanal irrigant of choice for root canal work despite the possible accidents that can occur. Accidental injection of sodium hypochlorite into the periapical tissues can cause severe pain, swelling, and profuse bleeding (**13.40**).

It must be stressed that great care should be taken when using sodium hypochlorite. The bore of any needle used should be large enough to allow the free flow of the disinfectant without the application of undue pressure. A 'side-venting' needle should be used. It is always wise to check that it is securely fastened to the syringe and it is worth considering the placement of a rubber stop on the needle short of the working length. The needle should not bind in the canal and it should be possible to keep the needle moving within the canal. The irrigant should be expressed slowly and irrigation should be stopped if any resistance to the plunger is felt.

Where a hypochlorite accident does occur the patient should be calmed and reassured. The canal benefits from being washed with sterile water. Further analgesic may be administered to relieve pain. The tooth should be monitored over the next half an hour; there may be a bloody exudate. Drainage should be encouraged. The prescription of an antibiotic should be considered where root canal infection was present. Corticosteroids assist in limiting the swelling. The use of cold compresses for six hours will help to reduce pain and swelling. Following this, warm compresses will help to encourage healthy healing. The patient should be warned of swelling and consequent bruising.

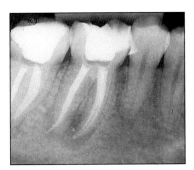

13.41 Root canal over-filling in mandibular molar

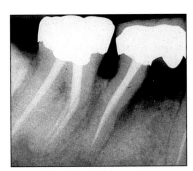

13.42 Radiographic appearance of root with vertical bone loss (courtesy of Mr A F Speirs, Leeds Dental Institute)

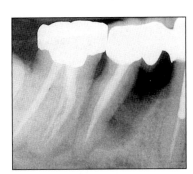

13.43 Further bone loss – suspected vertical fracture precipitated by the obturation procedure (courtesy of Mr A F Speirs, Leeds Dental Institute)

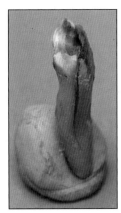

13.44 Extracted root with fracture (courtesy of Mr A F Speirs, Leeds Dental Institute)

INTERAPPOINTMENT AND POSTOPERATIVE EMERGENCIES

Patients may experience pain after canal preparation and cleaning or following obturation of the root canals.

Acute apical periodontitis occurs quite often following canal preparation. The common causes of this are over-instrumentation, leaving the tooth in traumatic occlusion, over-medication and incomplete cleaning. Teeth with pre-existing chronic lesions without sinus formation or symptoms can be particularly troublesome. It is as if the bacterial flora within the tooth reacts to the opening up of the tooth and an exacerbation of the chronic condition ensues, producing an acute apical abscess.

Treatment depends essentially on the preoperative diagnosis and the symptoms the patient is having. A previously vital case with complete cleaning and shaping generally does not require reopening. Where the case was vital and cleaning not completed then the canals should be cleaned with copious irrigation with sodium hypochlorite, dressed with calcium hydroxide and sealed. In previously necrotic cases where there is no swelling the canal should be reopened. Any exudates should be allowed to drain after which the canals should be gently instrumented and irrigated with sodium hypochlorite. A calcium hydroxide dressing is placed and the access sealed. In necrotic cases where there is swelling, incision and drainage should be considered. However, it is most important that the canals have been cleaned. If there is any doubt as to the initial cleaning then the canals should be reopened, instrumented and irrigated with sodium hypochlorite and a calcium hydroxide dressing placed. The access should be sealed; there are few indications for leaving cases on open drainage.

In all cases, the patient needs to be reassured and an appropriate analgesic prescribed. Antibiotics, again, should only be prescribed where required, in cases of rapidly spreading and diffuse swelling with pyrexia.

Interappointment discomfort is also encountered with leaking restorations, which allow recontamination of the canal system. The area of leakage must be found and the problem dealt with. Where a pre-existing crown has been retained and access gained through it to complete an endodontic procedure, its marginal integrity should be critically assessed.

The probable causes of pain occurring following obturation of the root canal system are traumatic occlusion, extrusion of irritant materials (**13.41**), inadequate cleaning of the root canal system and root fracture precipitated by the filling procedure (**13.42–13.44**).

Information about possible discomfort in the first few days following root canal work and advice regarding analgesics will reduce the patient's anxiety regarding postoperative pain. Where patients do require follow-up treatment, this may involve reassurance, advice on the use of analgesics (and possibly antibiotics), removal of the root filling and repreparation of the root canals, and surgical endodontics to remove overfilled material or resection of the tooth or root. There are a few cases where the symptoms do not respond to further therapy and extraction may be indicated.

Chapter **14**

Tooth resorption

P R Wesselink

Tooth resorption is a physiological or pathological process causing loss of either cementum or cementum and dentine.

The mineralized tissues of permanent teeth are not normally resorbed. They are protected in the pulp cavity by predentine and the odontoblasts and on the root surface by the precementum and the osteoblasts. If these protective structures are damaged or removed multinucleated cells, osteoclasts, will colonize the mineralized surfaces and root resorption will ensue. **Figure 14.1** shows multinucleated cells lying in a lacuna.

Resorption is considered to be *external* if the original site of the resorption is the periodontal ligament and *internal* if it starts in the pulp.

The aetiology of tooth resorption is unknown, although much is known about the histological process, and much work is needed before all types of resorption can be treated effectively.

INTERNAL RESORPTION

Internal resorption results from a chronic pulpitis, although why some teeth are affected more dramatically than others is not known. Trauma and infection are important aetiological factors.

The typical appearance is a smooth widening of the root canal wall (**14.2**, **14.9**). On rare occasions (when the pulp chamber is affected) it may appear as a 'pink spot' as the enlarged pulp is visible through the thin wall of the crown. Any tooth may be affected but the incidence is highest in incisors. The destruction of dentine may take years or may be very rapid. The pulp usually remains vital and symptomless for a long period of time, although it may become necrotic.

Diagnosis

In most cases diagnosis is simple but occasionally it may be difficult to differentiate between internal and external resorption. The diagram and radiographs (**14.3–14.5**) show external resorption as an irregular radiolucent area overlying the root canal; the canal outline remains visible and intact. A case of external resorption is shown in **Figure 14.6**, but it is not easy to diagnose from the radiograph, as the canal outline is indistinct. In internal resorption the outline of the canals is interrupted and usually appears as a smooth bulge, whereas with external resorption the canal outline can still be seen. If an angled radiograph is made the outline of the resorption defect is transported in relation to the pulp cavity (**14.7**, **14.8**).

Treatment

Since vital pulp tissue supplies the cells responsible for resorption its prompt removal is necessary in all diagnosed cases. The resorption ceases as soon as the chronically inflamed pulp is removed.

Access cavity

An access cavity is cut in the usual manner but it is not necessary to enlarge the access as this could weaken the tooth.

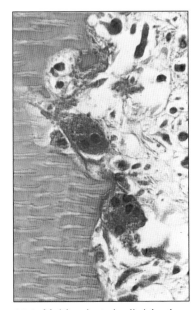

14.1 Multinucleated cells lying in a lacuna

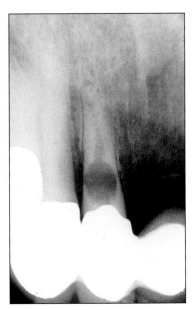

14.2 Internal resorption showing smooth widening of the root canal walls

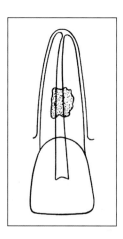

14.3 External resorption of an irregular radiolucent area overlying the root canal

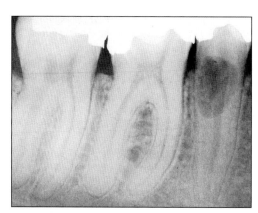

14.4 External resorption affecting a mandibular premolar

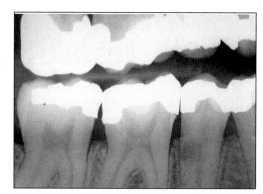

14.5 The same tooth as in **14.4**, one year earlier, showing that the resorptive process commenced outside the contour of the pulp canal

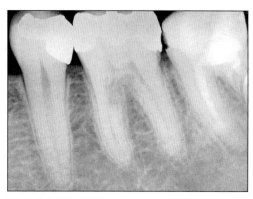

14.6 External resorption

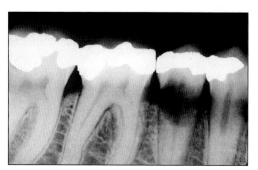

14.7 External root resorption that is centrally located over the root canal

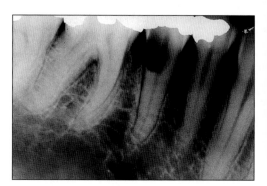

14.8 The same resorption as in **14.7**. The different-angle of this film has caused the radiolucency of the resorptive area to shift and appear closer to the periphery of the root

Debridement

Clinically, in teeth with internal resorption, pulp necrosis will be found in the pulp chamber and usually in the root canal to a level somewhere coronal to the resorption lacuna. The resorptive area and the root canal apical to this area will contain vital tissue. In some instances, the entire pulp may be necrotic. The resorptive process will then have stopped since vital cells are needed for the internal resorption to continue.

In root canals with vital tissue it may prove difficult to remove the tissue in the resorption lacuna, which are not easy to instrument. Debridement is carried out using copious amounts of 2–5% sodium hypochlorite, which may help dissolve organic material inaccessible to instrumentation. Ultrasonic agitation of the solution will improve the outcome.

Haemorrhage is a feature of internal resorptive tissue and may be difficult to control. Haemostasis is achieved only after the removal of all the pulp tissue. Continued bleeding after debridement may be an indication that there is communication between the root canal and the periodontal ligament, where the internal resorption has created a perforation.

Perforation

The canal should be checked for any perforation. An electronic measuring device will help to explore the walls of the canal using a file with a curve placed near the tip. The position of any perforation on the root wall should be noted. This assists in deciding whether the perforation is accessible for surgery.

After debridement, a root canal dressing of calcium hydroxide paste should be packed into the canal and the resorption lacuna (**14.9, 14.10**). Between appointments, this serves as a bactericide, necrotizes any remaining tissue in the lacuna and may help dissolve any remaining organic debris. The necrotic remnants are readily removed by irrigation with sodium hypochlorite at the next visit.

If there is no (or only a small) perforation the root may be obturated at the second visit, after the canal has been fully prepared. Care should be taken to obturate the resorption lacuna completely in order to seal any possible communication between the pulp cavity and the periodontium.

It is not uncommon to find vital granulation tissue and bleeding in the resorptive area at the second visit, indicating the presence of a root perforation. If a large inaccessible perforation is present

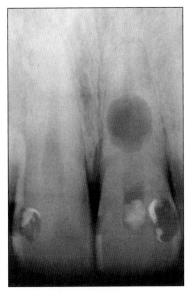

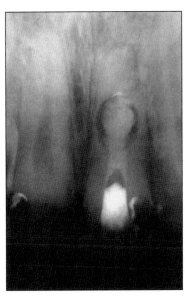

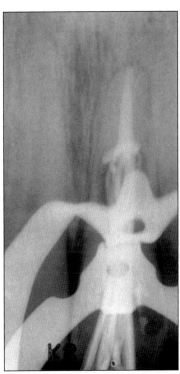

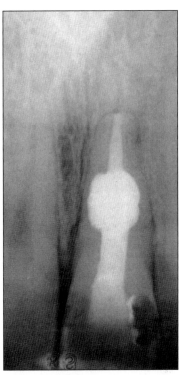

14.9 Internal resorption in a maxillary central incisor

14.10 Calcium hydroxide dressing

14.11 Apical part of the root canal obturated with laterally condensed gutta-percha and sealer

14.12 The resorption cavity and coronal part of the canal obturated with warm gutta-percha and sealer

long-term calcium hydroxide therapy should be instituted (see Chapter 9). It is unlikely that the perforation will heal completely. The inflamed area adjacent to the perforation will show signs of healing, with bone apposition and periodontal ligament formation along the defect. This healing facilitates control of haemorrhage and extrusion of filling material at the obturation session.

Root filling

A number of techniques may be used to fill the irregular root canal spaces. Warm lateral condensation may be used but a warm gutta-percha injection technique should ensure that the defect is well condensed (**14.11, 14.12**). Both methods are described in Chapter 10.

Surgery

A surgical approach is preferred if the perforation is large or the bleeding is uncontrollable. The root canal is cleaned, prepared and a flap reflected to expose the defect. The canal is then filled and the perforation sealed with a suitable restorative material.

EXTERNAL RESORPTION

The most common external resorption is the normal physiological process in primary teeth during eruption of the permanent dentition. Pathological resorption of the root surface following damage to the periodontal ligament and the cementum has many causes, including:

- impaction of teeth;
- luxation injuries;
- periapical inflammation due to a necrotic pulp;
- periodontal disease;
- excessive mechanical or occlusal forces;
- bleaching endodontically treated teeth;
- tumours and cysts;
- certain systemic diseases;
- radiation therapy.

This resorption may be transient or progressive.

Transient resorption

Transient resorption is seen after small luxation injuries, and orthodontic treatment. After a small luxation injury some periodontal ligament cells may become necrotic, and are removed by phagocytes. This phagocytic process may be accompanied by a degree of cementum and dentine resorption. As the periodontal ligament heals and resorption ceases the root becomes covered by cementum, without the replacement of the lost root tissue (**14.13, 14.14**). This type of resorption is also referred to as *surface resorption.*

In orthodontic treatment pressure may cause damage or even necrosis of periodontal ligament cells. Removal of this sterile necrotic tissue followed by resorption of bone and tooth may be considered as unwanted side-effects of pressure. As soon as the treatment stops, the resorption ceases (**14.15**). Occasionally this type of resorption can be very severe (**14.16**).

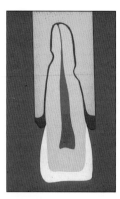

14.13 Surface resorption – diagram

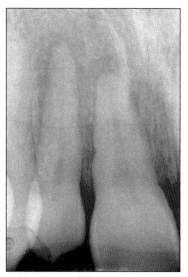

14.14 Surface resorption

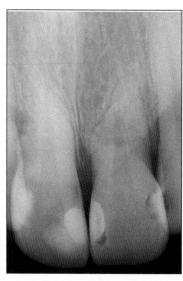

14.15 Apical surface resorption after orthodontic treatment

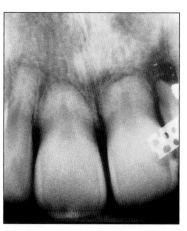

14.16 Extensive apical resorption after orthodontic treatment

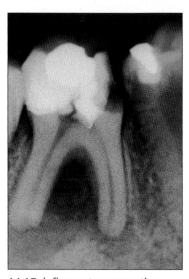

14.17 Inflammatory resorption associated with a necrotic pulp and apical periodontitis

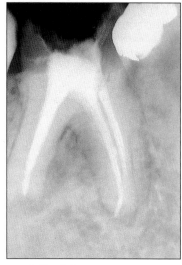

14.18 Tooth in **14.17** one year after root canal treatment. Bony repair has occurred and the resorption has not progressed

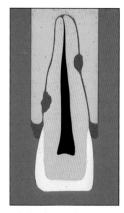

14.19 Lateral inflammatory root resorption following luxation injury – diagram

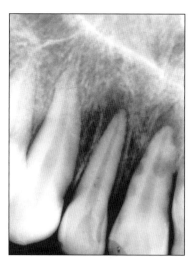

14.20 Lateral inflammatory root resorption following luxation injury

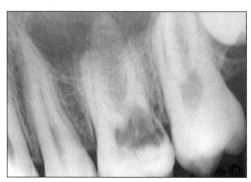

14.21 Cervical inflammatory tooth resorption

Progressive resorption

Progressive resorption may be classified as:

- inflammatory;
- cervical;
- replacement (ankylosis).

Inflammatory

This type of root resorption may be present either in the apical (**14.17,14.18**), lateral (**14.19, 14.20**) or cervical (**14.21**) area of the root.

Apical inflammatory resorption This is a phenomenon that accompanies apical periodontitis caused by the presence of infected necrotic pulp tissue. It usually only occurs at a microscopic level and is not visible on an intraoral radiograph.

Radiographic apical external inflammatory root resorption is characterized by a persistent and progressive radiolucency adjacent to the region of root resorption. Even when observed radiographically, root canal treatment has a good prognosis in cases of this inflammatory resorption (**14.18**). The only problem that may arise is difficulty in establishing an apical stop when the apical constriction is missing. This may be overcome by:

- long-term dressing with calcium hydroxide;
- use of the chloroform-dip technique to provide for a good fit in the apical 2–3 mm of the canal;
- The application of MTA prior to obturation to prevent the extrusion of filling material into the periradicular tissues.

Lateral inflammatory resorption This is initiated by trauma affecting the periodontal ligament, usually a luxation injury, and is maintained by the presence of an infected necrotic pulp.

Injury to the periodontal ligament results in phagocytosis of damaged periodontal ligament cells that may be accompanied by resorption of the root cementum covering the root dentine, and

even dentine resorption. If the pulp is necrotic and infected, micro-organisms or microbial products may pass through the dentinal tubules into the tissue surrounding the root since the protective layer of cementum, which would prevent this, is no longer intact (**14.22, 14.23**). Inflammatory products stimulate the resorptive process resulting in a rapidly progressing resorption. On the radiograph bowl-shaped radiolucent lesions on the lateral root structure are seen in association with the occasional loss of adjacent lamina dura (**14.20, 14.24**). Root canal treatment will remove the microbial component of this process. Thereafter the resorption process will cease and healing will occur or, in the case of extensive resorption, replacement resorption may follow (**14.25**).

Cervical

The cause of (invasive) cervical root resorption has not been clearly established but it may be due to inflammation within the periodontal ligament following injury to the epithelial cervical attachment apparatus and to the area of the root surface just apical to it.

The injuries can be differentiated into physical and chemical types. Physical injuries, which occur to non-endodontically and endodontically treated teeth, typically include all forms of tooth trauma, surgical procedures, orthodontic treatment, bruxism and periodontal root planing and scaling. Chemical injury can occur from agents used within the root system such as aggressive internal bleaching solutions, such as 30% hydrogen peroxide leaching through cervical dentinal tubules. Resorption is sited in the cervical area of the tooth and may present clinically in two different forms: a wide shallow crater (**14.26**) or a burrowing type (**14.27**). Single, rather than multiple teeth are affected and the process tends to be slow. Cervical resorption is usually asymptomatic and found on routine radiographic examination. The pulp is not involved until the condition is well advanced (**14.28**). 'Pink spot' is more likely to be due to the burrowing type of cervical resorption than to internal resorption. **Figure 14.29** shows a pink spot on the buccal aspect of a maxillary lateral incisor.

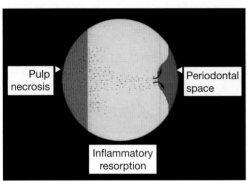

14.22 Diagram illustrating that microorganisms or microbial products pass through dentinal tubules into surrounding tissues after loss of cementum

Pulp necrosis

Periodontal space

Inflammatory resorption

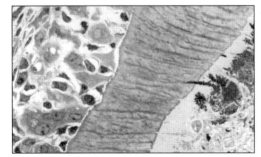

14.23 Light micrograph showing multinucleated cells together with neutrophilic granulocytes at resorbed external dentine surface with microorganisms extending into dentinal tubules on the pulpal side

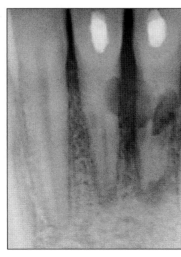

14.24 External root resorption after luxation and pulp necrosis

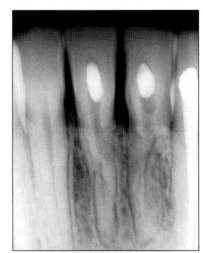

14.25 Three months after cleaning the root canals of the teeth in **14.24**. The inflammatory resorption is followed by replacement resorption

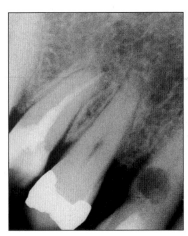

14.26 Cervical resorption with a shallow crater

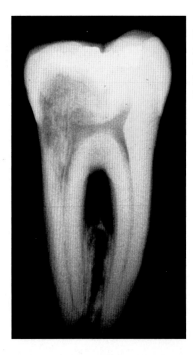

14.27 Burrowing external tooth resorption – radiograph

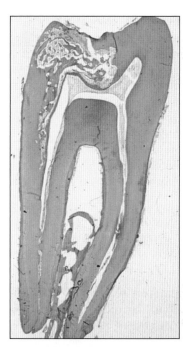

14.28 Burrowing external tooth resorption – histological section – note that the pulp cavity is not involved

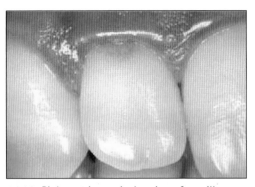

14.29 Pink spot in cervical region of maxillary lateral incisor

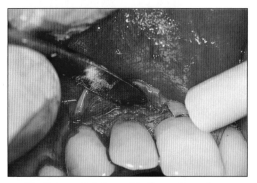

14.30 Extent of defect with flap reflected

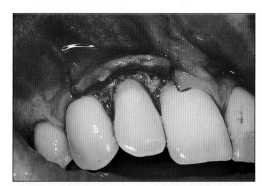

14.31 Defect repaired with glass ionomer cement

Treatment involves exposing the lesion, removing the resorptive tissue and inserting a restoration (**14.30, 14.31**). Severe cases may require orthodontic extrusion or extraction. It is often difficult to decide whether the defect is fully accessible to surgery before a flap is raised. A confident decision can be made only with experience and by taking radiographs using the parallel technique from different angles.

As a rule the pulp is not involved in the early stages. When a flap is raised and the extent of the defect can be seen the decision on whether or not to carry out root canal treatment can be made.

Replacement resorption (ankylosis)

Replacement resorption is caused by damage to the periodontal ligament cells covering the root surface, usually by luxation injuries. If large areas of the periodontal ligament are lost or damaged healing occurs from the alveolar side of the socket and leads to deposition of alveolar bone tissue on the root instead of periodontal ligament

cells, such as cementoblasts and fibroblasts. Once this union between alveolar bone and root surface has taken place, the cells involved in the remodelling of bone are not able to distinguish between root cementum, dentine and bone. **Figures 14.32–14.34** show an osteoclast present with its border in close proximity to all three tissues suggesting that osteoclasts can resorb distinct mineralized tissues at the same time. The tooth root is thus incorporated into the remodelling process of the alveolus and is gradually replaced by bone. The rate of progression of ankylosis is directly related to the initial damage to the root surface and the age of the patient.

The condition may be transient if the damage is limited but in more extensive cases it is progressive, finally resulting in complete loss of the root (**14.35, 14.36**). The progress of ankylosis is very rapid in young individuals. Clinically, the tooth is asymptomatic. The most significant clinical feature is a high-pitched or metallic response to percussion compared to that of the adjacent teeth. Other clinical signs that may be present include infraocclusion, incomplete

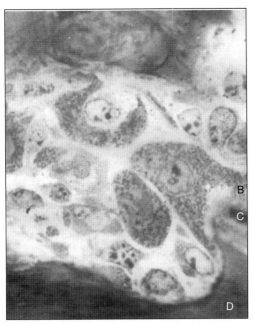

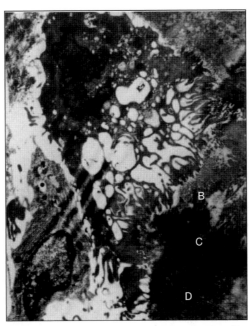

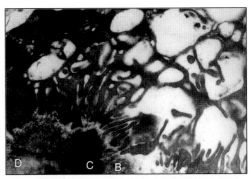

14.34 Electron micrograph showing the ruffled border of the osteoclast like cell in **14.32** along dentine (D), cementum (C), and alveolar bone (B) (× 19000)

14.32 Light micrograph of an osteoclast-like cell in close apposition to dentine (D), cementum (C) and alveolar bone (B) (× 100)

14.33 Electron micrograph of the osteooclast like cell in **14.32** with its ruffled border along dentine (D), cementum (C), and alveolar bone (B) (× 5000)

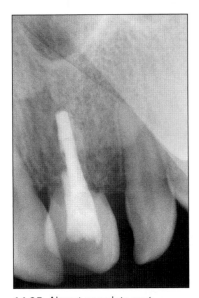

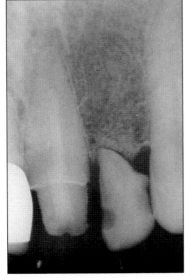

14.35 Almost complete root resorption with gutta-percha remaining in bone tissue after ankylosis

14.36 Complete loss of root structure 13 years after traumatic luxation

pulp is necrotic an overlying inflammatory resorption may be present. Removal of the infected pulp may aid bony repair (**14.38, 14.39**). This appearance, however, does not guarantee long-term resolution (**14.40**)

Replacement resorption is preventable but not treatable. Extraction should be considered to prevent interference with alveolar growth. In avulsion cases the tooth should be replanted as soon as possible or transported in milk to a healthcare worker. The pulp should be removed within 10 days after the trauma if the apex is mature, and root treatment carried out. The pulp of an immature root apex should be monitored with radiographs and pulp testing.

IDIOPATHIC RESORPTION

A striking type of root resorption is that of the distal root of the first mandibular molar seen in **Figures 14.41 and 14.42**. In the history there seems no explanation for this root resorption, which did not appear to progress during a twelve-year period. Since it is associated with a vital pulp no root canal treatment is indicated (**14.43**); contrary to the type of inflammatory root resorption seen in **Figure 14.17**, where a necrotic pulp and periodontitis were present. Some cases of external resorption involving multiple teeth but with no systemic disease do not fit into any of the above categories. The case illustrated (**14.44, 14.45**) is a 50-year-old Caucasian woman who presented with no symptoms, no systemic disease and a normal blood picture. The patient had never had any orthodontic treatment. The only teeth affected were the mandibular molars.

alveolar process development, and lack of a normal mesial drift. A history of trauma particularly avulsion with a prolonged extraoral time and dry storage during this period, may confirm the diagnosis.

Radiographically, there is a disappearance of the periodontal ligament space with associated progressive resorption (**14.37**). If the

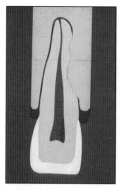

14.37 Ankylosis with a direct union between bone and tooth structure

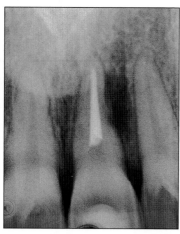

14.38 Inflammatory root resorption after luxation injury and root canal treatment

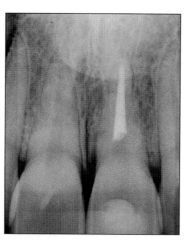

14.39 Apparent bony repair of tooth in **14.38** with some ankylosis two years after root canal treatment

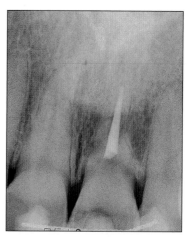

14.40 Extensive resorption and ankylosis of tooth in **14.38** twenty-one years after treatment. There have been no clinical symptoms

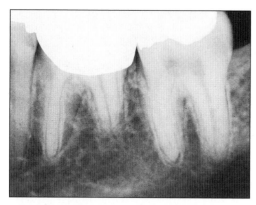

14.41 Root resorption of distal root of first mandibular molar

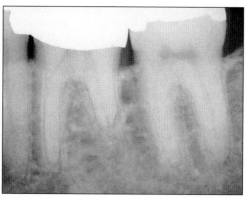

14.42 Tooth of **14.41** twelve years later. Notice that resorption has not progressed

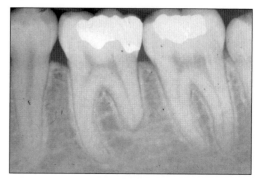

14.43 Root resorption of distal root of first mandibular molar with a vital pulp

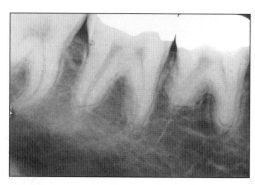

14.44 Idiopathic root resorption affecting the mandibular molars – right side

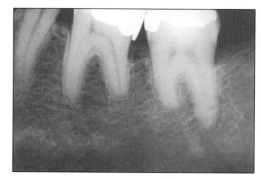

14.45 Idiopathic root resorption affecting the mandibular molars – left side

Further reading

Heithersay GS 1999 Treatment of invasive cervical resorption: an analysis of results using topical application of trichloracetic acid, curettage, and restoration. *Quintessence Int* **30**, 96–110.

Ne RF, Witherspoon DE, Gutmann JL 1999 Tooth resorption. *Quintessence Int* **30**, 9–25.

Trope M 2002 Root resorption due to dental trauma. *Endod Topics* **1**, 79–100.

Tronstad L 1988 Root resorption-etiology, terminology and clinical manifestations. *Endod Dent Traumatol* **4**, 241–52.

Chapter 15

Root canal retreatment

C J R Stock and Y-L Ng

CAUSES OF FAILURE

Failure of root canal treatment is generally attributed to either residual or resistant intraradicular microorganisms surviving the chemomechanical cleaning procedures or new microorganisms invading the canals via coronal microleakage, vertical fracture of the tooth, perforation or accessory canals which communicate with the oral cavity. In rare instances, persistent lesions may be sustained by an established extraradicular infection in cases associated with a long-standing sinus, foreign body reaction to extruded root dressing/filling material or apical true cyst.

TYPES OF BACTERIA INVOLVED IN FAILURE CASES

There is increasing evidence that the microbial flora of root-filled teeth differs significantly from that reported in untreated teeth. In the former cases, the number of strains and species of microorganisms is lower and facultative anaerobes predominate. The Gram-positive facultative bacterium, *Enterococcus faecalis* has been frequently recovered from such cases and this has significant implications for the choice of antibacterial medication during retreatment. The combined use of sodium hypochlorite and iodine irrigant has been recommended for such cases.

The outcome of root canal retreatment is less favourable than the initial treatment with the success rates ranging from 56 to 88%. The low success rate might be attributed to the different type of microorganisms associated with failed cases or lack of access to the infection.

INDICATIONS FOR RETREATMENT

When failure is demonstrated by:

- presence of clinical signs (swelling, sinus, tenderness to percussion) and/or symptoms (pain of endodontic origin);
- enlargement of existing periradicular radiolucent lesion associated with the tooth;
- development of new periradicular radiolucent lesion associated with the tooth;
- persistence of periradicular radiolucent lesion associated with the tooth which had root canal treatment four years ago or more.

When a new restoration is required for the root filled tooth, of which:

- the root filling is adequate, but has been contaminated with saliva for longer than 30 days (**15.1**);
- the root filling is inadequate (**15.2**).

DECISION-MAKING PROCESS FOR RETREATMENT

When failure of the previous treatment is confirmed and retreatment is indicated, the general and local factors (**Box 15.1**) affecting the prognosis and feasibility of non-surgical retreatment should be assessed carefully. The patient should be informed about the prognosis of the tooth and the available treatment alternatives and participate in the choice of treatment. The operator should make a decision about the point at which the case should be better managed surgically, the tooth extracted or the patient referred to a specialist,

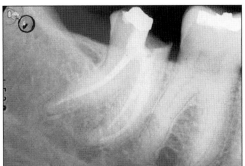

15.1 Adequate root filling, but lost coronal restoration

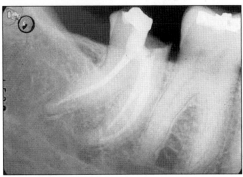

15.2 Inadequate root filling

Box 15.1 Factors affecting prognosis and feasibility of non-surgical retreatment

Patient's general factors:
- awareness and expectation;
- time and financial commitment;
- medical condition;
- access (two fingers opening) (15.4).

Local factors:
- type and condition of coronal restoration;
- type and condition of post;
- type of root filling material;
- presence of blockage due to packed dentine debris or sclerosed canals;
- presence of ledges;
- presence and location of fractured instruments;
- presence and location of perforations.

according to the degree of complexity of the operative procedures (on a scale of 0–10)(**15.3**), the set-up in the dental practice, his/her experience and capability as well as the patient's inclination.

PLANNING TREATMENT

When carrying out retreatment, the most common error is destruction of part of the remaining dentine with consequent further weakening of the tooth. It is important to use some form of magnification – if you can see it, you can probably do it, for example removing a trough of dentine around a post or fractured instrument requires good magnification (**15.5, 15.6**), good lighting, and a steady hand. Longer appointments are required for retreatment cases, in particular for removal of foreign material from root canals. Ultrasonic units and tips (**15.7–15.10**) are very useful equipment for cutting a trough around embedded metallic material. There is equipment specifically designed for removal of coronal cast restorations (**15.11**), posts (**15.12–15.14**) and fractured instruments (**15.15–15.19**).

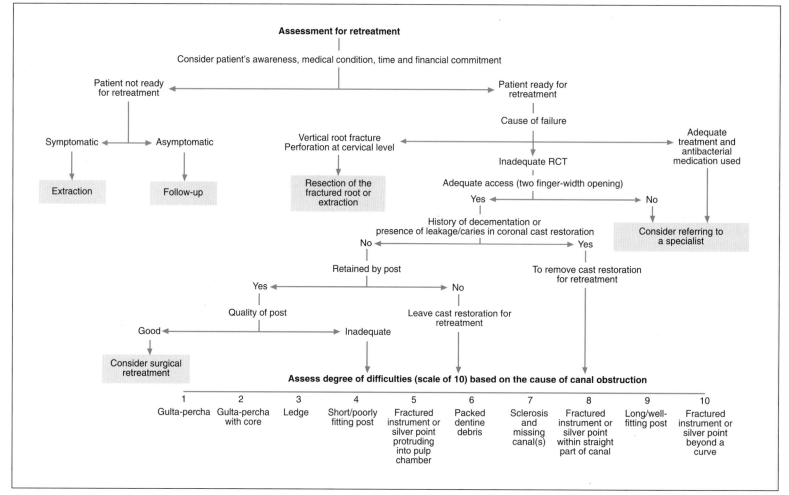

15.3 Decision-making tree for retreatment

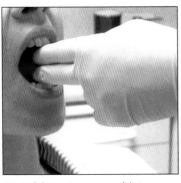

15.4 Adequate access with two-finger opening

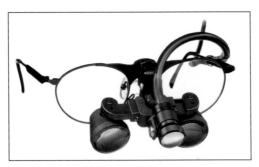

15.5 Loupes with light attachment

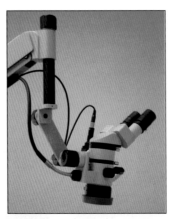

15.6 Microscope

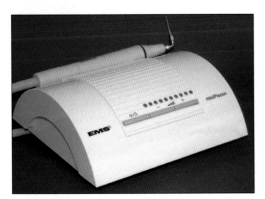

15.7 Ultrasonic unit

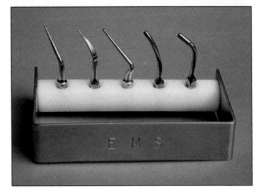

15.8 Ultrasonic tips

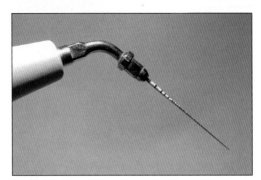

15.9 Ultrasonic file holder with size 15 K-file

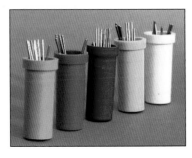

15.10 A range of ultrasonic files from size 15 to 35

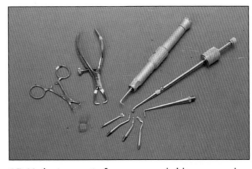

15.11 Instruments for crown or bridge removal

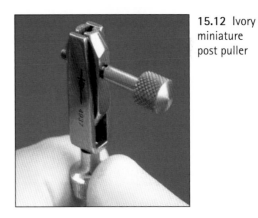

15.12 Ivory miniature post puller

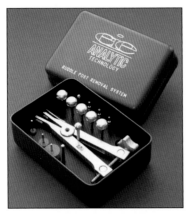

15.13 Ruddle post-removal kit

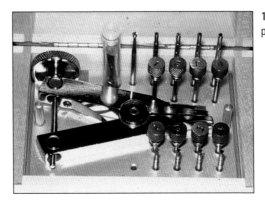

15.14 Thomas post-removal kit

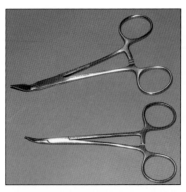

15.15 Steiglitz and endodontic fine-beaked forceps

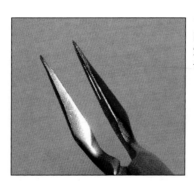

15.16 Beaks of Steiglitz forceps

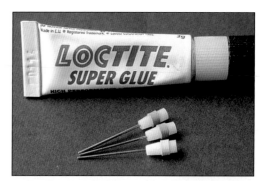

15.17 Cancellier tubes and cyanoacrylate glue

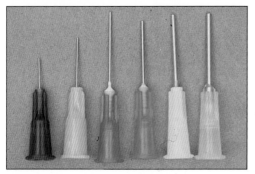

15.18 Ultradent tubes as an alternative to Cancellier tubes

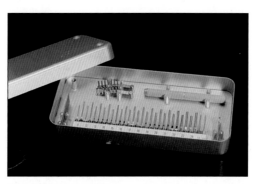

15.19 Masserann kit

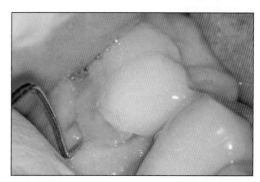

15.20 Leaking crown beneath buccal margin

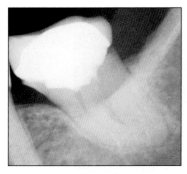

15.21 Leaking beneath distal margin of crown
15.22 Access

RETREATMENT PROCEDURES

Removal of coronal restorations

All coronal restorations should be removed prior to treatment if they are either leaking or if caries is present (**15.20, 15.21**). This also applies to full coverage crowns. If the restoration is sound it is better to leave it in place during treatment and access the pulp chamber through the restoration. It is easier to place a rubber dam and to keep the operating field dry by cutting through an existing restoration (**15.22, 15.23**).

It is difficult, or impossible, to remove a crown that is seated on a near parallel preparation and is well fitting, without damaging it beyond repair. It is always well worth trying to ease off a crown by inserting a large excavator under the margin and lightly twisting as it may be loose.

Removal of bridges

Any bridge that has become decemented must be removed. In most cases when an abutment tooth requires retreating it will mean that a new bridge has to be constructed. If a new bridge is planned then it is immaterial if the bridge is damaged during its removal, providing it can be used as a temporary crown. The easiest method of removing a bridge is to make a vertical cut through the crown on the buccal aspect and then break the cement lute with an instrument such as a Mitchell's trimmer by inserting it into the cut and twisting the blade. There are, however, many devices (**15.11**) which can be used to remove bridges most of them causing both the operator and patient some aggravation.

Removal of posts

There are many different gadgets on the market specifically made for the removal of posts. See **Figures 15.8, 15.12–15.14**.

Currently, first attempts at post crown removal are usually performed by the use of ultrasound. The crown is first removed by cutting a vertical slot to allow leverage and expansion of the margins. Excess cement is then taken away. A solid curved tip is inserted in the ultrasonic handpiece and rubbed gently around the incisal edge of the core (**15.24**). The power is varied while the ultrasonic tip is in contact with the core to achieve the maximum effect. When the right power setting is reached, cement particles may be observed vibrating at the base of the core. If this does not loosen the post after

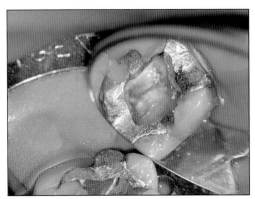

15.22 Access through restoration with no caries

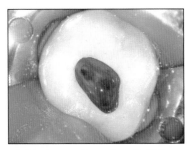

15.23 Access through well-fitting crown

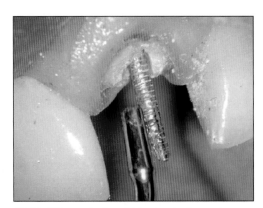

15.24 Ultrasonic tip rubbing against a post

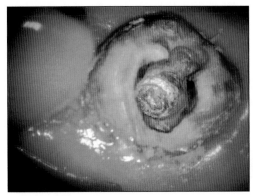

15.25 Post fractured at canal orifice

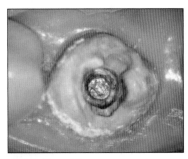

15.26 Troughing cut around post with ultrasonic file

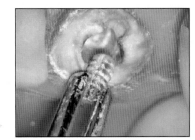

15.27 Loosened post removed with fine-beaked forceps

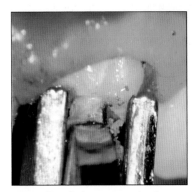

15.28 Post being removed using miniature post puller

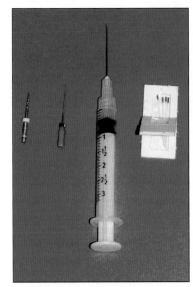

15.29 Nickel–titanium orifice openers, Hedstrom files and chloroform are useful for gutta-percha removal

a few minutes, a fine tip can be used to cut a narrow trough around the post to reduce the retention (**15.25, 15.26**). The first step is repeated with the blunt tip. This procedure will remove the majority of posts (**15.27**). In the case of an excessively long, non-threaded post, one of the post-pulling devices may have to be used (**15.28**).

Removing gutta-percha

Many retreatment cases fail because of poor root canal preparation techniques. It should always be remembered that the thorough disinfection, cleaning and shaping of the root canal(s) remain primary goals.

The first stage of gutta-percha (GP) removal involves gaining access to the pulp chamber and clearing it. This may be accomplished with a high-speed bur and excavators. A GP root-filling that has been in place for many years tends to become brittle and hard, making it more difficult to remove. Nickel–titanium orifice openers, Hedstrom files and chloroform are useful for removing gutta-percha (**15.29**). There are three stages to the procedure:

1. A simple way to remove the bulk of the GP is to use a nickel–titanium rotary instrument for example an Orifice Shaper (Maillefer®) or Orifice opener (Kerr) run at double the normal speed (600–700 rpm) to provide frictional heat. The appropriate sized file is chosen to fit the canal (**15.30–15.32**).

2. Most of the remaining bulk of the GP can be removed with Hedstrom files (**15.33**). An appropriate-sized file that is unlikely to bind on the canal wall is placed in the canal and rotated by hand to engage the GP. The depth of penetration can be judged from the preoperative radiograph.

3. The final stage is to wick out the remaining tags of GP. The canal is flooded with chloroform from a disposable dispenser (**15.34**). The chloroform should not overflow the pulp chamber otherwise the rubber dam will be dissolved. The chloroform is then stirred using a small hand file to ensure the solution mixes with the canal contents (**15.35**). The largest paper points that fit into the canal are then selected. Wicking is achieved by inserting several points one after the other into the canal (**15.36**). When the canal is dry it can be seen if any GP remains. If there is, the wicking procedure is repeated. The canal is then thoroughly washed with irrigant.

Removing gutta-percha with central core (Thermafil®)

The initial stage is to remove the plastic core, using a nickel–titanium rotary instrument preferably an Orifice Shaper. The file is run at 600–700 rpm. The size selected is small enough to allow the tip to engage the GP between the core and the canal wall. Once the core is removed the remaining GP may be removed by using the wicking technique.

Negotiating a ledge

When the previous root-filling is short of the working length of the root there may be either a ledge or debris packed tight into the canal. It is often possible to predict a ledge if the preoperative radiograph is examined (**15.37**). If the apical extent of the root-filling is not in the centre of the root but on the outer side of the curve this strongly suggests that there is a ledge. This may be negotiated once the coronal portion of the canal has been cleaned by inserting a size-10 handfile which has a small curve placed at the tip (**15.38**).

Packed dentine debris

When the root-filling is short, dentine debris may have been packed into the apical portion of the root canal (**15.39**). There is no easy method of displacing the debris except by the patient use of a small file in a light picking motion. Copious amounts of irrigant agitated by a small file in an ultrasonic handpiece may help to loosen the debris (**15.40–15.42**). The danger is that when the debris is packed very tightly it may be as hard as the surrounding dentine and attempts to remove it might result in a false canal being cut and, therefore, create a possible perforation.

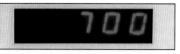

15.32 Set handpiece speed at 700 rpm for gutta-percha removal

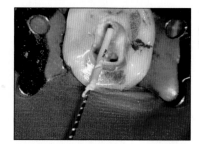

15.33 Apical portion of gutta-percha removed with Hedstrom file

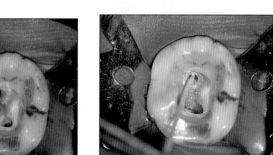

15.30 Gutta-percha in distal canal

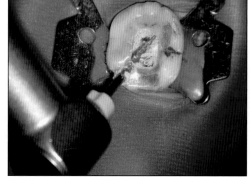

15.31 Orifice opener removing gutta-percha with handpiece – speed at 700 rpm

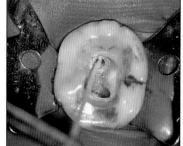

15.34 Chloroform placed in canal entrance using a syringe

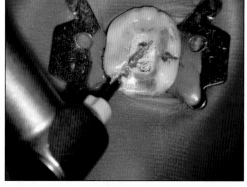

15.35 File placed in canal to mix chloroform and gutta-percha then wicked with paper points

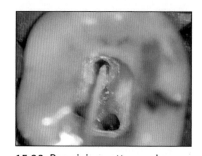

15.36 Remaining gutta-percha dissolved in chloroform and wicked with paper points

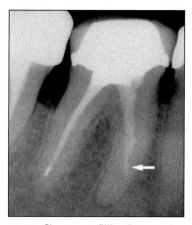

15.37 Short root-filling in curved canal suggesting ledge present (arrowed)

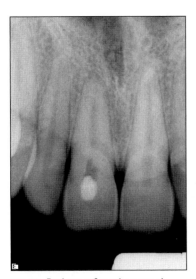

15.38 Ledge bypassed placing a curve at the tip of small file. Rubber stoppers with marking to indicate orientation of the curve

Sclerosed canals

Very fine canals may be found in the teeth of elderly patients, teeth that have been subjected to trauma, or in those teeth, which have had large restorations or have been associated with marginal periodontitis for many years. Where secondary dentine has been laid down due to irritation in the crown of the tooth the canal may be fine in the coronal portion and widen out towards the apex. Negotiation of these canals is carried out initially using a size-8 or 10 handfile with a lubricant containing EDTA. A watch-winding, backwards and forwards, movement is used. When the file begins to meet resistance a larger file is taken and the procedure repeated, the steps are size 10, 15, 20 and then back to size 10. The size 10 will find its way further into the canal as it is no longer constricted in the coronal few millimetres. See **Figures 15.43–15.46**.

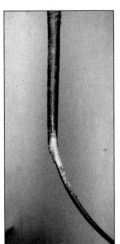

15.39 Plastic block ledged and packed with debris

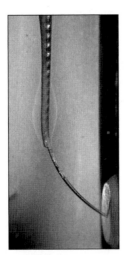

15.40 Size 15 ultrasonic file used in wet canal to dislodge debris

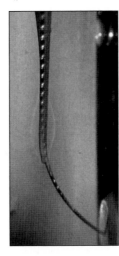

15.41 Size 10 K-file with curve at the tip bypasses the ledge

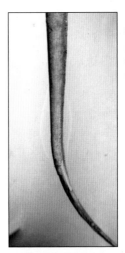

15.42 Canal preparation completed using hand instruments

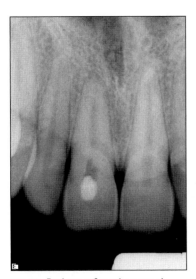

15.43 Patient referred as canal could not be located

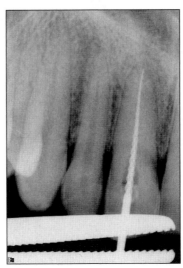

15.44 Increasing resolution of radiograph showing canal is patent

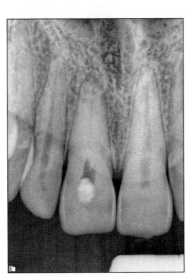

15.45 Canal located and negotiated as described in text

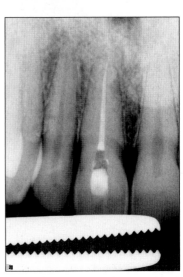

15.46 Canal preparation completed and obturated

Removal of metal instruments and silver points

It should be emphasized that a fractured instrument itself does not cause failure. It does not endanger the health of the patient nor produce any symptoms providing it lies within the canal system. If, however, it is preventing the negotiation of the canal, which may be infected, then it should, if possible, be removed. A preoperative radiograph will show where the metallic object is situated. The simple classification below will help the operator decide how best to proceed. Examples are presented in **Figures 15.47–15.49**.

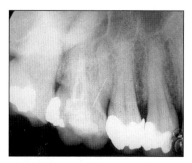

15.47 Fractured instrument in coronal portion – often possible to remove

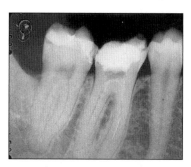

15.48 Fractured instrument in middle portion – may be able to remove

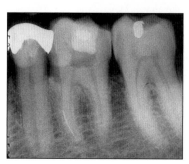

15.49 Fractured instrument in apical portion – difficult to remove

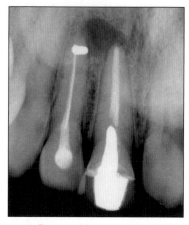

15.50 Fractured instrument embedded in retrograde amalgam in the 12

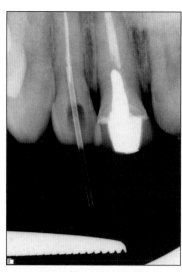

15.51 Cancellier tube fitted over instrument

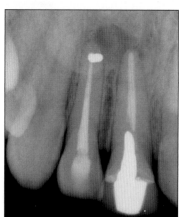

15.52 Cancellier tube in position tapping out with artery forceps

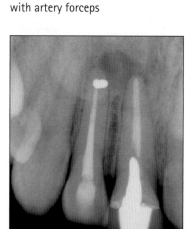

15.55 Canal prepared and obturated

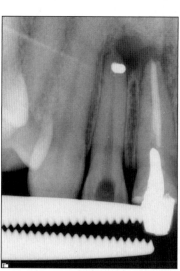

15.53 Fractured instrument successfully removed

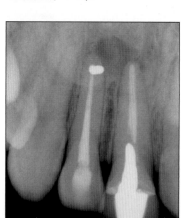

15.54 Hedstrom file securely glued in Cancellier tube

Class 1 *lies in the canal but protrudes into the pulp chamber.* These are simple to remove using a Steiglitz or a small pair of locking forceps

Class 2 *lies within the straight part of the canal.* An attempt is made to bypass the obstruction with a small hand file and lubricant. If the canal can be negotiated to the working length and prepared it may not be necessary to remove the metallic object but obturate the canal so that the object is embedded within the filling material.

If the object cannot be bypassed a narrow trough is cut around the embedded object with an ultrasonic tip. When the coronal 2.0 mm is exposed it can be removed using an extractor (**15.50–15.55**).

Great care has to be taken when ultrasound is used to remove a silver point or nickel–titanium instrument. Silver is soft and the ultrasonic tip rather than cutting a trough around the point will cut into it; in the case of nickel–titanium the ultrasonic tip will shatter small pieces from the fractured instrument making it more difficult to remove. Avoiding the silver point or nickel–titanium instrument requires excellent vision and good magnification as well as a steady hand.

Class 3 *lies beyond a curve in the canal.* The majority of these metallic objects cannot be removed. An attempt is made to bypass using a fine handfile with a lubricant. A small curve is placed at the tip of the instrument to help locate a passage past the object. Canals are not round and, therefore, there should be a gap between the metal and the wall of the canal. Once the instrument can be bypassed, larger instruments are used until the canal is prepared to the desired shape (**15.56–15.58**).

Perforations

Perforations may occur due to internal/external resorption or operator error. The success of a repair will depend on the site and size of the perforation, and the risk of contamination. A perforation enclosed within bone is more likely to be successful (**15.59**) than one that is in contact with the oral cavity. The perforation should be repaired as soon as possible to prevent contamination, providing it can be accessed through the coronal cavity. There have been many different materials recommended for repair of perforations. Zinc oxide/engenol-based cements such as IRM® and EBA® have frequently been used for their antibacterial properties. Glass ionomer cement (GIC) is preferred if communication with the oral cavity is present. **Figures 15.59–15.64** show perforation repair using GIC. In some cases, an iatrogenic perforation located at the apical third of the canal can be treated as a separate canal and obturated with guttapercha. Mineral trioxide aggregate (MTA) is the current material of choice (**15.65–15.68**). It has good biocompatibility, although it has a tendency to be dissolved away in the presence of saliva.

Surgical repair of a perforation is indicated when access through the canal is impossible.

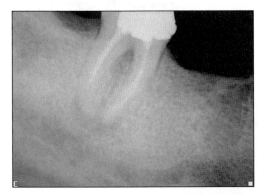

15.56 Fractured instrument lies beyond a curve in the canal

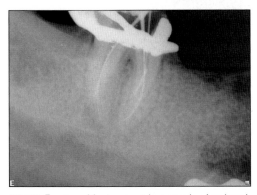

15.57 Fractured instrument bypassed using hand instruments and then dislodged with ultrasonic 15 K-file

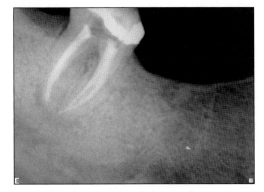

15.58 Canal prepared and obturated

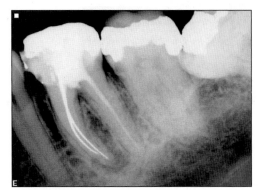

15.59 Silver point in mesial canal – perforation in pulp chamber

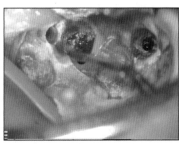

15.60 Perforation visible. Endodontic probe placing glass ionomer cement (GIC) at the perimeter of the perforation

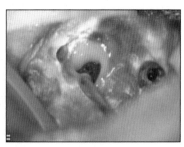

15.61 Building GIC bridge without touching periodontal tissue

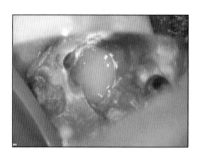

15.62 GIC bridge completed

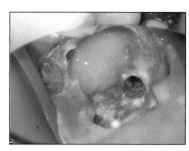

15.63 Additional GIC placed to prevent material being pushed into periodontal tissue

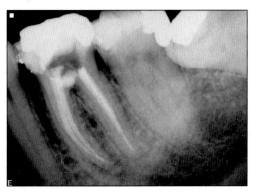

15.64 Postoperative radiograph

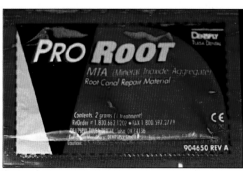

15.65 Sachet of mineral trioxide aggregate (MTA)

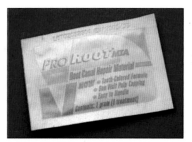

15.66 White MTA – recently introduced and with better handling properties

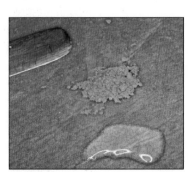

15.67 MTA and sterile water mixed

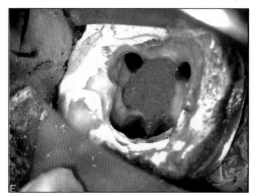

15.68 MTA placed on floor of pulp chamber to seal perforation

Chapter 16

Restoration of the root-treated tooth

K Gulabivala

Much has been written about restoration of the root-filled tooth, in part because root-treated teeth are often severely damaged and require novel and ingenious methods of restoration. Very wide ranges of dowel or retention systems are available to aid restoration but significant research to support all the claims of manufacturers is lacking. That root-treated teeth are more susceptible to fracture is a widely held clinical impression and they, therefore, may require different considerations when restoring them compared to vital teeth. The high fracture rate of endodontically treated teeth (**16.1a & b, 16.2a & b**), especially those restored with mesio-occlusal-distal (MOD) amalgams, has been documented. The three main reasons advanced to explain this high fracture rate are:

1. *Altered physical properties of tooth tissue* The idea that root-treated teeth are brittle has long been propagated as an explanation for the apparently higher fracture rate of such teeth but no convincing evidence has been found to support the theory.
2. *Weakening due to loss of tooth tissue* Many studies have evaluated the effect of pattern of tooth-tissue loss as a cause of tooth weakening. The loss of marginal ridge integrity is probably one

of the most important factors. The width of occlusal isthmus and depth of cavities compound the situation. Loss of roof of the pulp chamber has been considered to be an important contributory factor in the weakening effect and there is some evidence to support this contention. Its importance probably lies in its contribution to the increased depth of the cavity, making the cusps more susceptible to flexure (**16.3, 16.4**). Loading of such cusps may lead to unfavourable stress concentration at the cervical region making the cusps prone to fracture (**16.5, 16.6**).

3. *Loss of proprioception* Loss of the dental pulp may deprive the tooth of some of its mechano-receptive properties. Teeth without pulps have a higher 'load perception' threshold and may take up to twice the load of a tooth with vital pulp before registering discomfort. Although no definite proprioceptors have been found in the dental pulp, there is evidence for A-β-nerve fibres, which are reputed to serve a proprioceptive function. Despite lack of clear evidence, this concept is plausible and, together with tooth weakening, offers an attractive explanation for the high rate of mechanical failure of root-treated teeth (**16.7**).

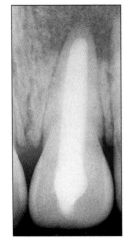 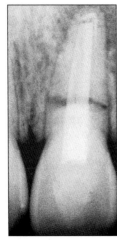

16.1a Root-filled maxillary central incisor

16.1b Middle third fracture of the same tooth

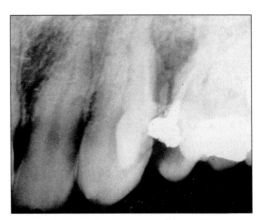

16.2a Radiograph of root-treated maxillary premolar

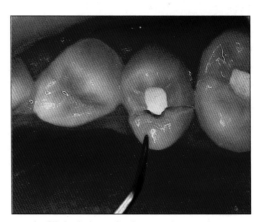

16.2b Clinical view of a fractured premolar

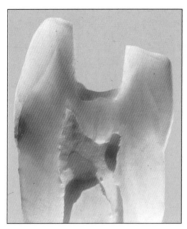

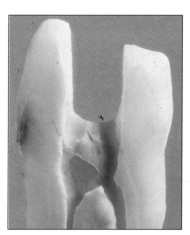

16.3   16.4

16.3–16.4 Deeper proximal boxes and lack of roof of pulp chamber render cusps more prone to flexure

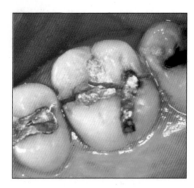

16.7 Mesio distal fracture of maxillary molar

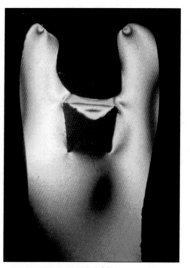

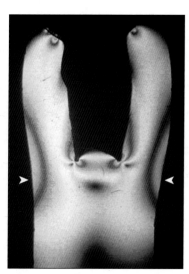

16.5   16.6

16.5–16.6 Photo elastic model showing concentration of stress increases at the base of the cusps (arrowed) when the roof of the pulp chamber is removed

PRINCIPLES OF RESTORATION OF ROOT-TREATED TEETH

The same principles, which govern the restoration of all teeth, also apply to root-treated teeth. However, in view of the discussion above, it is important to pay special attention to two factors:

● preservation of remaining tooth tissue;
● reduction of stress and its favourable distribution within the remaining tooth tissue.

The most conservative restoration design compatible with acceptable aesthetics and function should, therefore, be selected. Occlusal loads can only be assessed subjectively from the history: breaking restorations or teeth; occlusal tooth-tissue loss due to attrition; mobility and drifting; and the size and activity of the muscles of mastication are indicators of high loads. A young individual with a thickset jaw, well-developed muscles of mastication and marked faceting on occlusal contact areas is likely to exert greater occlusal loads. Restoration design is dictated not only by the pattern of residual tooth tissue but also by the properties of the restorative materials used. Consideration of these and the occlusal demands of the individual case together with meticulous execution of the clinical procedures should lead to a successful restoration.

RESTORABILITY OF THE TOOTH

The restorability of the tooth should always be determined before endodontic treatment as part of a general restorative treatment plan. Space available should be sufficient to place an aesthetic, functional restoration with cleansable contours, which will optimize the health of the periodontal tissues and adjacent teeth. Often the tooth requiring endodontic treatment is severely broken down and movement of neighbouring teeth may result in occlusal (**16.8**) and proximal (**16.9, 16.10**) loss of space, which may occasionally be corrected by orthodontic movement but this is not always a practical solution. Even when the tooth is not to be restored but used as an overdenture abutment, an assessment of the space for a denture is important (**16.11, 16.12**). A denture with thin metal framework may fracture (**16.13**).

An adequate amount of remaining tooth tissue is necessary in addition to space. Although it is difficult to describe strict limits, a cast restoration encompassing at least 2 mm of sound dentine around the circumference would make the longevity of the restoration more predictable (**16.14**).

In the absence of sufficient coronal tooth tissue it may be possible to gain retention from the root. Under such circumstances it is critical to evaluate the length, width, shape and curvature of the root, to assess the potential use of a dowel. In the absence of sufficient coronal dentine, under exceptional circumstances, it may be possible to extrude the tooth orthodontically. In some procedures, the supporting alveolar and periodontal tissues are extruded with it, which must then be recontoured surgically prior to restoration (**16.15–16.18**). Rapid extrusion may allow the tooth to be extruded without the periodontal supporting tissues, circumventing the need for surgery.

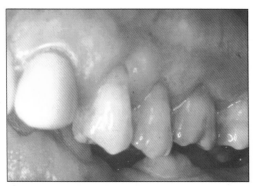

16.8 Occlusal loss of space

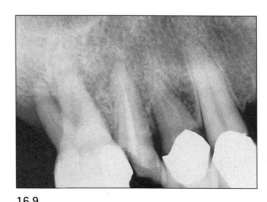

16.9

16.9–16.10 Proximal loss of space

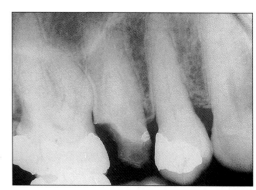

16.10

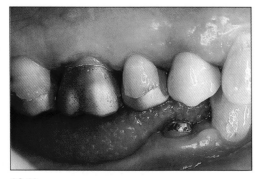

16.11

16.11–16.12 Occlusal space considerations for overdenture situation

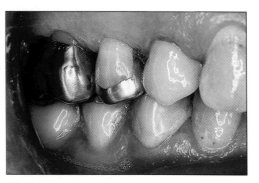

16.12

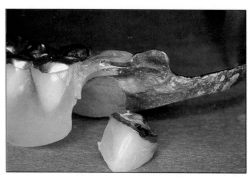

16.13 Fracture of denture due to thinness of framework

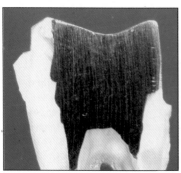

16.14 The margins should be finished on sound tooth tissue

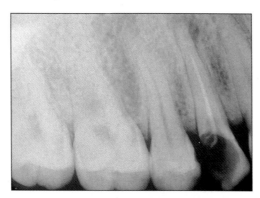

16.15

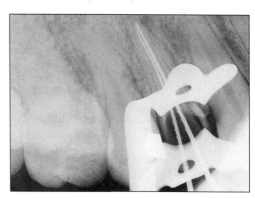

16.16

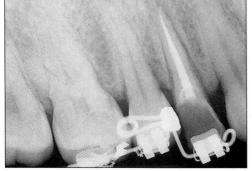

16.17

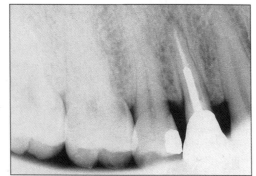

16.18

16.15–16.18 Orthodontic extrusion and periodontal surgery are necessary to make tooth tissue supragingival for restoration

WHEN TO RESTORE AFTER ENDODONTIC TREATMENT

The decision to place expensive restorations on teeth immediately following completion of root canal treatment may sometimes be difficult because of the uncertainty of success of root canal treatment. It may take several years for a periapical lesion to heal but it is not practical to wait this long before a permanent restoration is placed: indeed an early permanent coronal seal is an important final stage in the completion of endodontic treatment so as to prevent recontamination of the root-canal system and ensure success. Fortunately, the success rate of root canal treatment is relatively high (85%), so it is not necessary to review the tooth for longer than an arbitrary period of a couple of weeks before providing the permanent restoration. During this time, there should be no sinus, no tenderness to palpation of the soft tissues over the apices or to percussion of the tooth. Any tooth with an uncertain postoperative endodontic status may require a longer review period prior to restoration. Teeth with multiple factors that compromise success should be reviewed for longer before provision of the permanent restoration, e.g. symptomatic teeth with large periapical lesions and extruded root-filling material.

Anterior teeth

Unfortunately, severely broken down anterior teeth require immediate restoration of aesthetics and provision of predictable function. Three compromises may be considered to achieve this:

1. *A temporary post crown* may be suitable if the post has adequate length and is well-fitting. Otherwise, its decementation not only causes inconvenience but also allows coronal leakage, further compromising the prognosis.

2. *A permanent post and core* may be cemented permanently if there is a risk of losing the temporary post-crown (**16.19**), followed by placement of a temporary crown (**16.20**). This reduces the chances of coronal leakage and should periapical surgery be required (**16.21**), allows modification of the margin for a permanent crown once the gingival margin has stabilized (**16.22**).

3. *A temporary overdenture* instead of post-crowns allows the temporary seal to remain intact (**16.23, 16.24**). If the roots ultimately need extraction, the overdenture also serves as an immediate replacement. The disadvantages include additional cost, time and acceptability to the patient.

Posterior teeth

In posterior teeth, the amalgam core can serve as the temporary occlusal surface. The cores should have adequate proximal and occlusal contacts (**16.25, 16.26**).

TEETH WITH ADEQUATE TOOTH STRUCTURE FOR RETENTION WITHOUT AUXILIARY AIDS

Restoration of the root-treated tooth should achieve satisfactory aesthetics, form and function while preserving and protecting the maximum amount of tooth tissue. In any given situation a number of design options are available. The choice depends on the structural integrity of tooth, aesthetic and protective requirements. In order to place these in perspective a number of clinical cases have been used to illustrate the application of these principles. The examples will again be considered separately for posterior and anterior teeth, as the requirements are different.

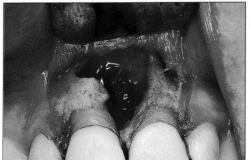

16.21

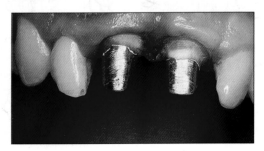

16.22

16.21–16.22 If surgery is required, the preparation margins may be modified after healing to avoid exposure of the crown/tooth junction

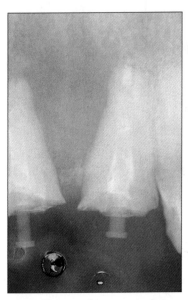

16.19 The use of temporary post crowns may be complicated by recontamination of the root canal system

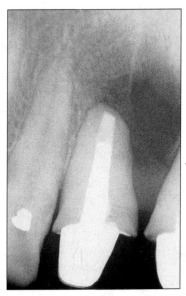

16.20 Permanently cemented post, core and temporary crown

Posterior teeth

Relatively intact teeth

Endodontic treatment is sometimes necessary on a tooth that has not previously been restored or that does not have caries. The pulp may become compromised by periodontal disease (**16.27**), trauma (**16.28**) or accidental severance of the blood supply during surgery (**16.29**). Following root canal treatment, restoration of the access cavity may be carried out with a plastic restorative material such as amalgam or posterior composite, provided there is no evidence of cracks in the tooth or signs of heavy occlusal loading (**16.30, 16.31**).

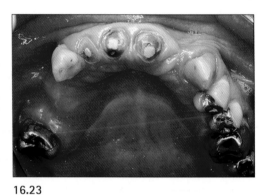

16.23

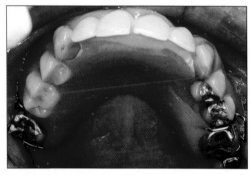

16.24

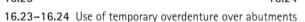

16.23–16.24 Use of temporary overdenture over abutments

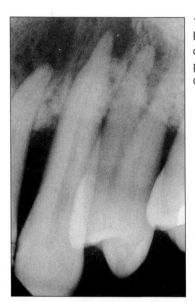

16.27 Pulp death caused by periodontal disease

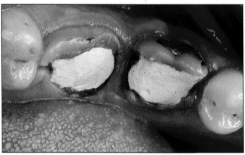

16.25

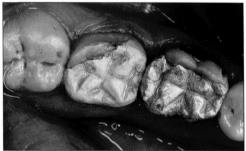

16.26

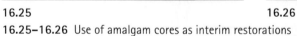

16.25–16.26 Use of amalgam cores as interim restorations

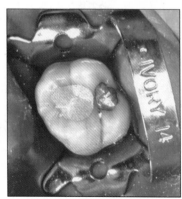

16.28 Trauma to the first molar caused by a cricket ball resulting in root fracture

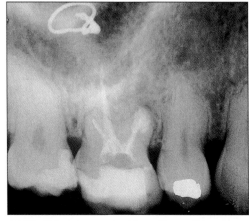

16.29 Pulp compromised by orthognathic surgery

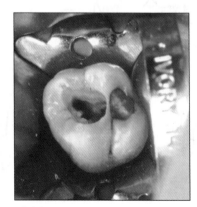

16.30

16.31

16.30–16.31 Simple restoration of access cavity

The presence of cracks across marginal ridges or cusps (**16.32, 16.33**), together with signs of heavy occlusal loading, indicates the need for cuspal protection – in the short term with a cemented orthodontic band (**16.34**) and in the long term preferably using a cast partial veneer gold restoration (**16.35, 16.36**). The design of such a restoration may be challenging. The problem is to provide adequate retention and resistance form and to maintain the margins in the proximal areas away from contact areas to enable their direct examination and access for cleaning. The nature of proximal contact dictates whether it is possible to maintain the margin above the contact or below it: the latter effectively means cutting a minimal proximal box (**16.37, 16.38**).

Provided that a sufficient wrap-around effect is achieved and the preparation is minimally tapered, a satisfactory degree of retention and resistance form may be obtained. Where it is considered to be insufficient, cast pins may be employed to increase retention (**16.39, 16.40**).

Recent suggestions include the use of adhesive techniques, retaining the composite materials by acid-etching enamel and dentine-bonding agents to increase the strength of the tooth. Although

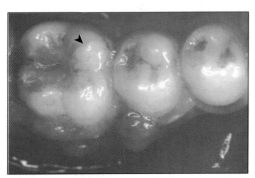

16.32 Fracture line – mesio lingual cusp

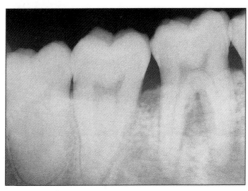

16.33 Radiograph of molar in 16.32

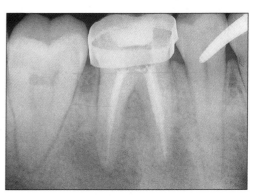

16.34 Cemented orthodontic band

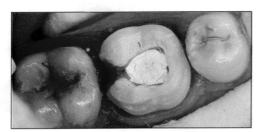

16.35 Modified onlay preparation

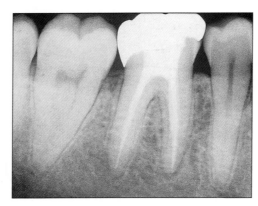

16.36 Radiograph of tooth with root canal treatment completed and a restoration with occlusal coverage

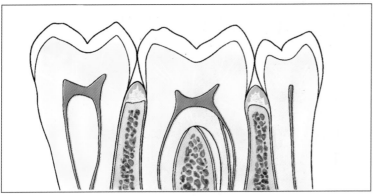

16.37

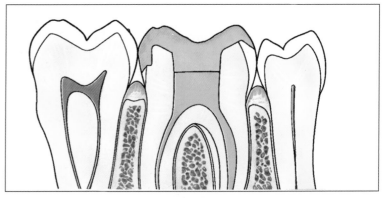

16.38

16.37–16.38 Effect of proximal contacts on preparation design – mesial margin above and distal margin below contact point

supported by laboratory studies, the durability of such bonding remains to be clinically proven. The technique has been recommended as a temporary means of reinforcing a tooth after endodontic treatment. Caution should be exercised in restoring large cavities with this technique because of the potential for cusp deformation and fracture caused by curing shrinkage of the composite material (**16.41, 16.42**). Where cuspal coverage is required, it may be possible to bond a base-metal alloy occlusal restoration to the prepared occlusal surface. The use of a precious metal alloy is made possible by plating or heat treatment (**16.43a & b**). In the case shown, occlusal surfaces eroded by acid and attrition were restored by bonding heat-treated gold castings to the occlusal surfaces. Minimal tooth preparation consisted of a bevelled margin of 1 mm depth around the circumference. This is a conservative and preferred method for restoring relatively intact root-filled teeth.

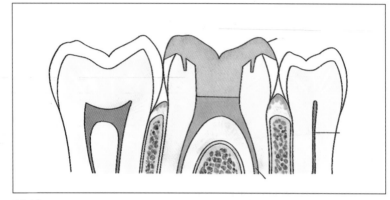

16.39

16.40

16.39–16.40 The use of cast pins to aid retention of cast onlay

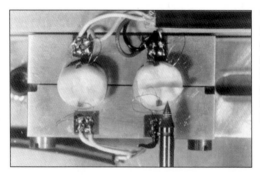

16.41 Experimental measurement of cusp deformation caused by curing composite material in a mesio-occlusal distal cavity, using an adhesive technique (courtesy of Prof. N Meredith)

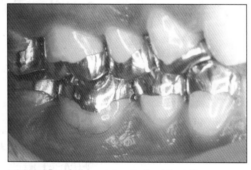

16.43a Bonded heat-treated gold castings – buccal view

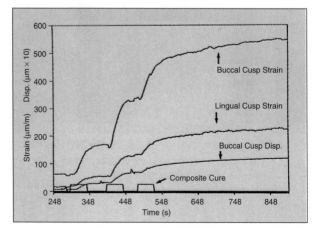

16.42 Strain in buccal and lingual cusps with time after curing and displacement of the cusps (courtesy of Prof. N Meredith)

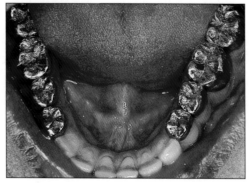

16.43b Bonded heat-treated gold castings – occlusal view

Teeth with proximo-occlusal cavity

The case of a root-treated tooth with an existing proximal box needs different consideration (**16.44**). The restoration in this case will depend on the width and depth of the box and the occlusal loading. In a tooth with a moderately wide, shallow proximal box and no signs of severe occlusal loading, a plastic restorative material may suffice (**16.45**). A tooth with a similar-sized cavity but signs of heavy occlusal loading, or which provides lateral excursive guidance that cannot be eliminated, may benefit more from a cast partial veneer metal restoration (**16.46, 16.47**). A plastic restoration would be inadequate in a tooth with a wide, deep box with signs of heavy occlusal loading but a cast metal cuspal coverage restoration would help to reduce such stresses and protect the tooth from fracture (**16.48**, a photo-elastic-model representation of the situation shown in **Figure 16.6**, under identical conditions but with a cuspal coverage restoration). The model remains relatively stress-free even when the load is doubled. **Figures 16.49–16.52** illustrate restoration of a case with a plastic restorative material core followed by cuspal coverage restoration. The premolar has been restored initially using composite on the buccal wall of the undermined cusp to prevent discolouration by amalgam and the rest was filled with amalgam (**16.50**). The tooth was then prepared for a partial coverage cast onlay (**16.50–16.52**).

Teeth with MOD (mesio-occluso-distal) cavities

The presence of two proximal boxes almost makes it mandatory that cuspal protection is used, unless there is no opposing tooth or if the tooth occludes against a tissue-born denture. Treatment options include plastic restorative materials or cast restorations.

Amalgam may be used to provide cuspal protection by reducing cusp height and building the entire occlusal surface. Although this is a relatively cheap method of restoring a compromised tooth it is a method that takes considerable practice to develop correct occlusal contacts and more occlusal reduction is required to provide adequate strength for the amalgam. The method is suitable for those teeth already lacking considerable tooth tissue (**16.53–16.55, 16.56a & b, 16.57a & b**).

Composite resin materials suffer from the disadvantages discussed above, particularly when the cavity is large (**16.58**). The problem of

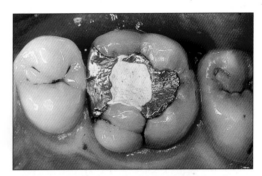

16.44 Root-filled tooth with moderately sized mesio-occlusal amalgam restoration

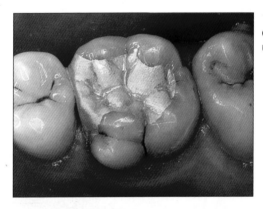

16.45 Restoration of tooth in **16.44** using new amalgam

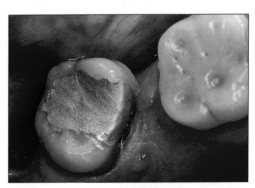

16.46

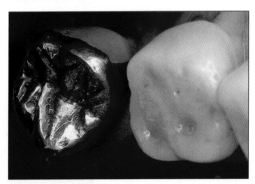

16.47

16.46–16.47 Restoration of a tooth with moderately sized mesio-occlusal amalgam with cast onlay restoration

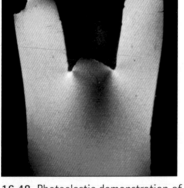

16.48 Photoelastic demonstration of absence of cervical stress concentration due to capped cusp cast onlay restoration (courtesy of Dr P O'Neilly)

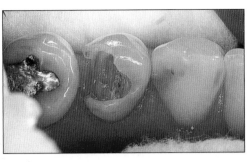

16.49

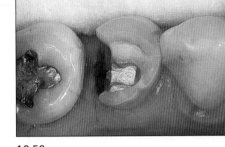

16.50

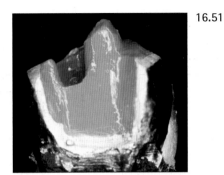

16.51

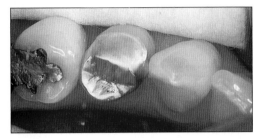

16.52

16.49–16.52 Restoration of root-filled mandibular premolar with capped cusp cast onlay restoration

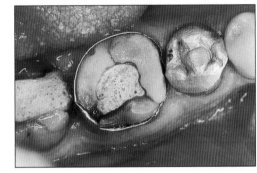

16.53

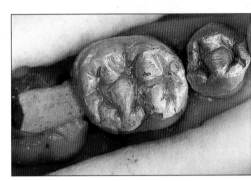

16.54

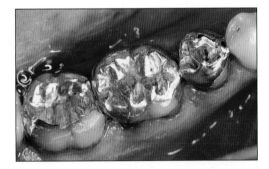

16.55

16.53–16.55 Restoration of a severely damaged premolars and molars using capped cusp amalgam restorations

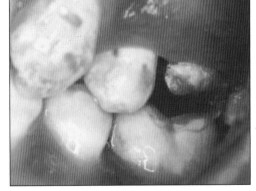

16.56a

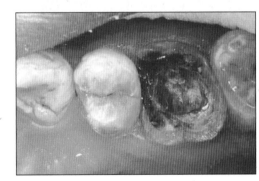

16.56b

16.56a & b Clinical views of broken down maxillary molar

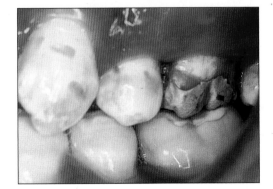

16.57a

16.57a & b Maxillary molar restored with amalgam

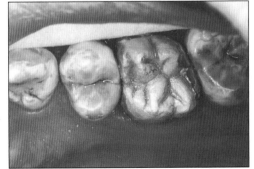

16.57b

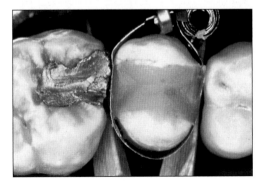

16.58 Composite used to restore mesio-occlusal distal cavity in a root-filled premolar

curing shrinkage and its unfavourable stressing of residual tooth tissue may be partly overcome by using indirect composite or porcelain inlays/onlays (**16.59a–c**). The problem with these is that the cement bond between the restoration and luting agent may fail allowing microleakage.

The most conservative option is to consider (where appropriate) the use of partial veneer onlays (**16.60a–c**) which help to minimize

sacrifice of tooth tissue and provide adequate cuspal protection with proper design. On a mandibular tooth, the need for a functional cusp bevel and occlusal shoulder on the buccal aspect means greater metal coverage of the buccal surface (**16.61**). On a maxillary tooth, the extent of metal coverage of the buccal cusp may be minimized (**16.62, 16.63**). Aesthetics may be improved by sandblasting the surface to reduce shine. The design may be modified

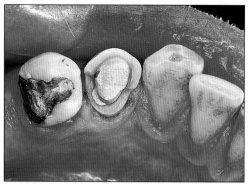

16.59a

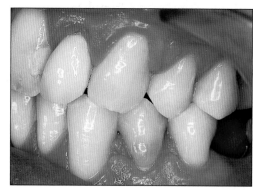

16.59b

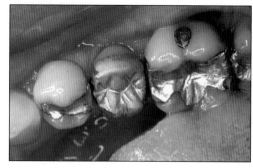

16.59c Restoration in place

16.59a & b Preparation of mandibular premolar for porcelain onlay

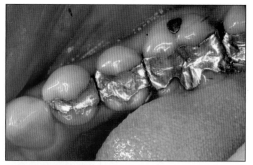

16.60a Mandibular second premolar with an MOD amalgam requiring occlusal protection

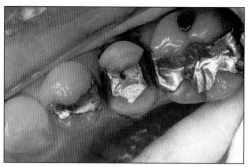

16.60b Preparation for partial veneer onlay

16.60c Gold onlay in place

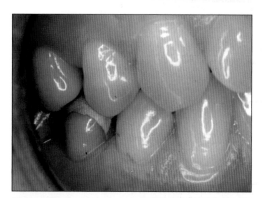

16.61 Restoration covering the functional cusp of the premolar

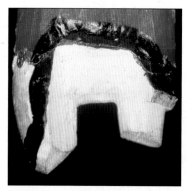

16.62 Silver die of preparation for restoration of a maxillary premolar with a capped cusp cast onlay

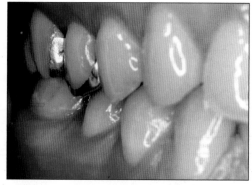

16.63 Buccal view of the cemented cast restorations

to suit the situation if additional tooth tissue is missing (**16.64, 16.65**). However, if the preparation is executed inadequately the restoration will be retained poorly, resistance form will be reduced and the aesthetics compromised.

The aesthetics of an extensive gold restoration may not be acceptable to some patients who may prefer a full coverage ceramometal restoration. However, before considering such a restoration the amount of tooth tissue likely to be lost in providing space for the dual thickness of metal and porcelain should be considered. The minimum thickness required is 1.3 mm. This may weaken the tooth further but may be an acceptable risk in order to secure the aesthetic requirements. As long as extracoronal tooth-tissue loss is minimal the preparation of an access cavity in addition to sacrifice of dentine for a ceramometal restoration may leave enough tooth tissue for retention and resistance form (**16.66**). The preparation of the upper premolar shown in **Figure 16.67** for a ceramometal crown resulted in a pulp exposure but root canal treatment through a coronal access cavity left enough tooth tissue (**16.68**) for retention and resistance form without resorting to a post/core.

Anterior teeth

Relatively intact teeth

Unrestored anterior teeth may require endodontic treatment because of pulp necrosis caused by traumatic injury (**16.69**), severance of blood supply during surgery (**16.70**) or tooth transplantation (**16.71**). Restoration of such teeth would normally be confined to the access cavity (**16.72**) and may be achieved satisfactorily with composite restorative material. In such cases 'reinforcement' of the tooth by placement of a post or dowel remains controversial (**16.73**). The rationale for post placement is based on the belief that the root-treated tooth is inherently weak and that the post would provide a degree of reinforcement by distributing some of the stresses to the root. The scientific support for this is equivocal. It appears that whether a tooth is made more resistant to fracture by placement of a dowel is dependent on the type of loading. It is widely accepted that where a post is not required to aid retention then it should not be placed. If one is placed then it should be at the expense of the minimal amount of tooth tissue. The need for a post

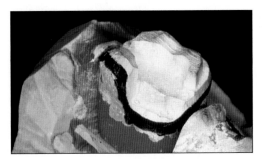

16.64 Die for modified cast onlay preparation

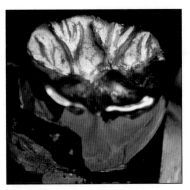

16.65 Cast onlay preparation on the die

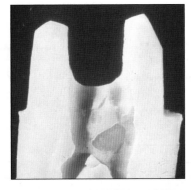

16.66 Following access for root canal treatment and preparation for a ceramometal restoration, remaining tooth tissue must be adequate for retention and resistance form

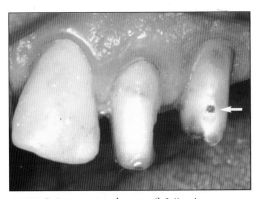

16.67 Pulp exposure (arrowed) following preparation for a ceramometal crown

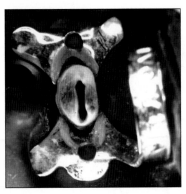

16.68 Adequate tooth tissue remains after access for root canal treatment

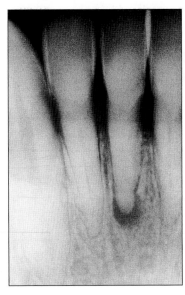

16.69 Pulp necrosis following trauma

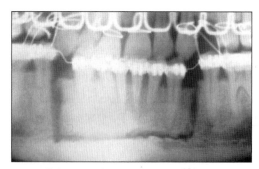

16.70 Pulp necrosis caused by orthognathic surgery

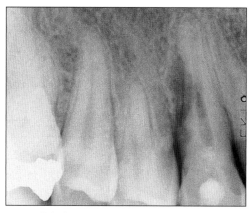

16.71 Pulp in 3| damaged by transplantation

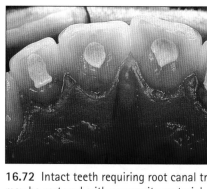

16.72 Intact teeth requiring root canal treatment may be restored with composite material

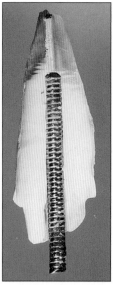

16.73 'Reinforcement' of intact root-filled teeth prepared for crowns is unnecessary

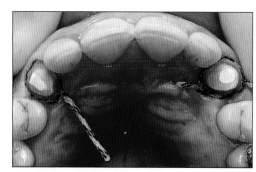

16.74 Adequate dentine cores remaining after crown preparation of root-filled canines render posts or cores unnecessary

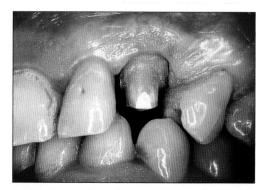

16.75 Buccal view of prepared left canine

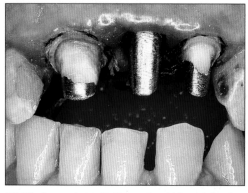

16.76 As much tooth tissue should be retained as possible, supplemented with a metal core as necessary

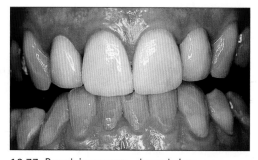

16.77 Porcelain veneers – buccal view

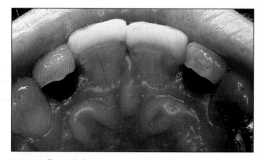

16.78 Porcelain veneers – palatal view

is a subjective clinical assessment based on the amount and distribution of remaining dentine after preparation of the tooth for the selected restoration. In **Figures 16.74 and 16.75**, sufficient dentine cores remained after crown preparation to render post/cores unnecessary; whereas in **16.76**, loss of tooth tissue in the three teeth was variable. The gold posts and cores supplemented residual dentine cores. The idea of 'reinforcement' has recently been resurrected with the possibility of using adhesive luting cements to bond posts made of materials similar in physical properties to dentine (according to claims, carbon-fibre posts). There is, as yet, no long-term clinical evidence to support this concept.

Previously unrestored, root-treated teeth sometimes require more extensive restoration than simple access filling, for example if the crown requires realignment or if its discolouration cannot be dealt

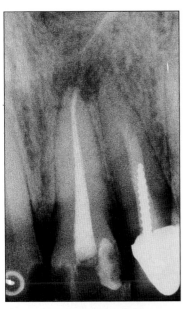

16.79
Mesial, distal and access cavities leave a band of tooth tissue missing

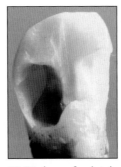

16.80 Loss of palatal tooth tissue when mesial, distal and access cavities exist

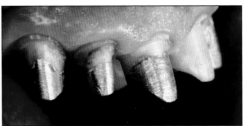

16.81–16.82
Use of post cores to supplement retention

16.81

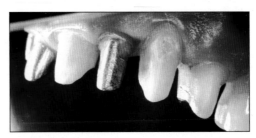

16.82

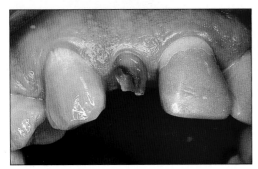

16.83 Following preparation for a crown, spicules of tooth tissue that do not contribute to the strength of the tooth should be sacrificed

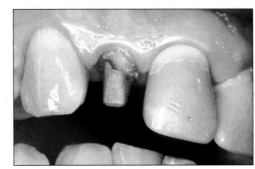

16.84 This also makes post/core construction easier

with by bleaching alone. The most conservative restoration likely to satisfy aesthetic and functional requirements should be selected, so as not to weaken the tooth further. Such restorations may include composite or porcelain veneers (**16.77, 16.78**), with or without tooth preparation according to the prevailing preoperative condition. The least conservative preparation is for a ceramometal crown but, even using this design, the tooth should be prepared to review the need for supplementation of retention by a dowel.

Teeth with proximal cavities

A common clinical situation is one in which an anterior tooth has mesial and distal cavities or restorations (**16.79**). The addition of an access cavity leaves such a tooth with a band of missing tooth tissue across the middle of its crown (**16.80**). Provided that the labial enamel plate is intact, relatively strong and unblemished by discolouration or surface deformities such as pitting, the tooth may be satisfactorily restored with composite restorative materials. A crown may give a better aesthetic result, particularly if adjacent teeth also need to be crowned, but will not necessarily confer greater strength or durability on the tooth. The presence of additional

cavities/restorations or tooth-tissue loss would strengthen the case for full coverage cast restorations.

TEETH WITH INADEQUATE TISSUE FOR RETENTION WITHOUT AUXILIARY AIDS

Anterior teeth

A full coverage cast restoration may be desirable if extensive tooth surface has been lost due to erosion, abrasion or attrition. Poor aesthetics due to large restorations and severe discolouration may also make a full crown more desirable. In such circumstances, the 'rooftop' preparations once recommended are now considered too destructive. It is considered better to prepare the tooth for the required restoration according to the requisite space demands and make good the tooth tissue deficit for retention and resistance form with a metal core retained by a dowel (**16.81, 16.82**). Spicules of tooth tissue that would not contribute to the strength of the tooth and may jeopardize uncomplicated construction of a core may be sacrificed at this stage (**16.83, 16.84**). In this way a more conservative restoration may be constructed.

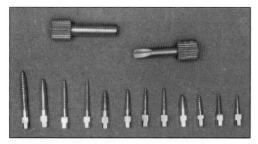

16.85 Dentatus

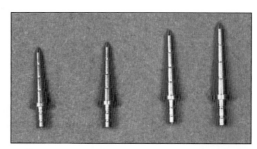

16.86 FKG pivots

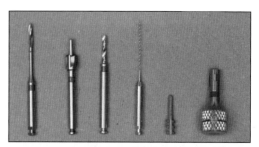

16.87 Maillefer radix Anker – Long (titanium alloy)

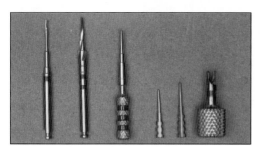

16.88 Maillefer Cytco (titanium alloy)

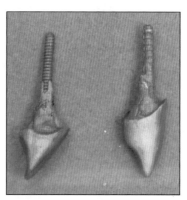

16.89 Custom-made post and cores

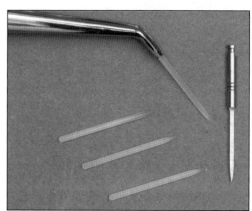

16.90 Dentatus Classic Post System

Characteristics of dowels

Dowels may be selected from a range of prefabricated designs (**16.85–16.88**), may be custom made (**16.89**) or may be customized from prefabricated designs (**16.90**). Dowels are selected on their properties of retention, stress distribution, ease of application and cost. The characteristics determining retention and stress distribution include shape, length, diameter, surface configuration and the presence of a diaphragm.

Shape

Dowels may be parallel-sided or tapering (**16.91**). The parallel-sided dowels provide better retention per unit length than the tapered dowels. An increase in taper reduces retention. The stress-distributing characteristics of the two designs differ during installation and functional loading. Tapered dowels generate the least stress during cementation (**16.92**), parallel-sided dowels generate greater stress by virtue of the hydraulic pressure developed (**16.93**). However, the parallel-sided posts perform better in function (**16.94**) because tapered posts generate a wedging force (**16.95**). This may be alleviated if the shoulder rest is firm but this would concentrate stress at the shoulder.

Although parallel-sided dowels are considered more desirable, the natural tapering shape of roots and prepared root canals mitigate against a dowel parallel along its entire length. Inevitably the dowel will be tapered in the coronal portion and parallel-sided apically (**16.96**) but this carries a danger of apical root perforation (**16.97**). One solution to this problem has been to taper the apical portion (**16.90**). Despite the relatively poorer retention and stress distribution characteristics of the tapered post it has been used successfully in many cases, which often makes it a more conservative choice. Parallel-sided posts require preparation of the canal to a matching shape, which can render their use less conservative. A compromise is to select the narrowest parallel-sided post compatible with adequate retention and strength of post and root (**16.98**).

Length

Length is as important a determinant of post retention as it is for crown preparations. Longer posts provide better retention and stress distribution for all types of posts in function. Unfortunately, an increase in length also leads to greater stresses during installation, particularly of the parallel-sided dowels. This can be eased to an extent by ensuring that the post is vented (**16.99**).

Determinants of dowel length

1. *Root filling length* The need for a minimum length of root filling may limit the achievement of optimal post length in cases where the root is of insufficient length to satisfy both requirements. There is no common agreement about the

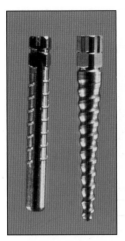

16.91 Parallel-sided or tapering dowels

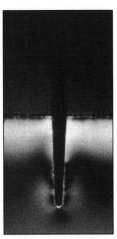

16.92 Tapered dowels generate least stress during cementation (courtesy of Mr P O'Neilly)

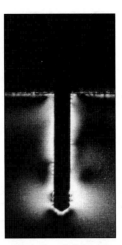

16.93 Parallel dowels generate greater stress during cementation (courtesy of Mr P O'Neilly)

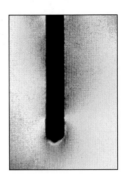

16.94 Parallel dowels provide better stress distribution in function (courtesy of Mr P O'Neilly)

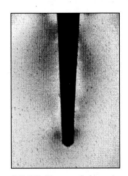

16.95 Tapered dowels generate a wedging force during function (courtesy of Mr P O'Neilly)

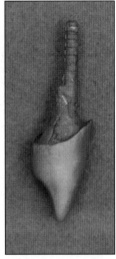

16.96 Dowel tapered coronally but parallel apically

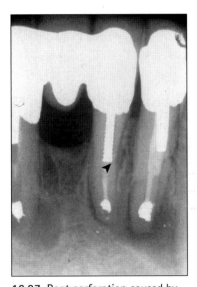

16.97 Root perforation caused by the parallel post in a mandibular incisor (arrowed)

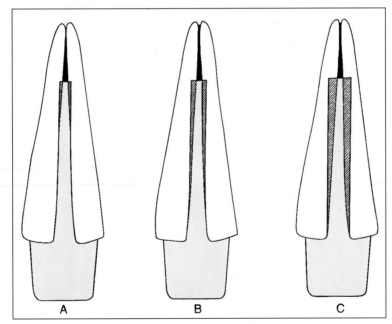

16.98 Selection of appropriate diameter of parallel-sided post: B = optimum for retention and root strength

16.99 Vented post

minimum length of root filling that should remain in the apical portion of the root: lengths from 3 to 7 mm have been suggested. There is little firm clinical evidence to provide guidance, but what there is indicates that apical filling material of less than 3 mm is more likely to be associated with periapical disease. The remaining root filling should be at least 3 mm long and preferably as long as the minimum length of post consistent with retention will allow it to be.

2. *Root morphology* This also influences dowel length. The degree and position of root curvature (**16.100, 16.101**) and the cross-sectional size and shape of the root will limit the length and diameter of the post (**16.102, 16.103**).

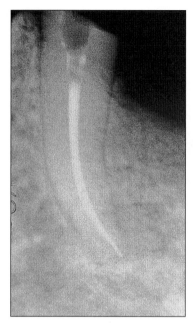

16.100 Curved mandibular premolar prior to restoration

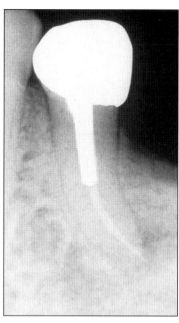

16.101 Postrestoration radiograph indicating the influence of the degree of curvature of the root on the length of the post

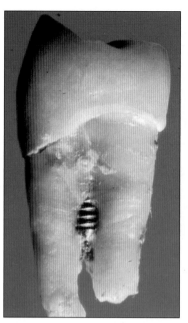

16.102 Lack of appreciation of the cross-sectional profile of the root leads to perforation

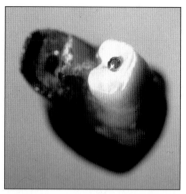

16.103 Extracted tooth showing the relationship between the post and the cross-sectional shape of the root

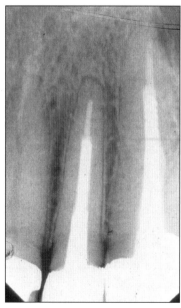

16.104 Long posts

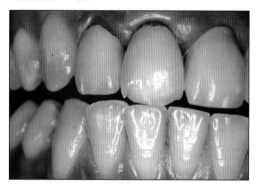

16.105 Decementation of unfavourably loaded long posts – note fractured porcelain on upper right central incisor

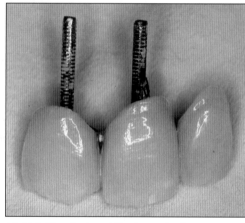

16.106 The displaced fixed prosthesis

3. *Clinical yardsticks* These have been advocated for determining post length, including 'various fractions of root length, 1/3, 1/2 and 2/3' (**16.104**), 'of similar length to the crown', 'in teeth with loss of periodontal support the post should extend apical to the alveolar bone'. Of these guidelines the last two are widely accepted. The required length of post for retention has to be weighed against occlusal loading. If the loading is unfavourable, restorations, retained even by long posts, may become uncemented (**16.105, 16.106**) but if occlusal loading is minimal, extremely short posts may suffice (**16.107**). It is sometimes argued that many roots are not long enough to accommodate optimum lengths of both post and root filling and that the length of one or the other needs to be compromised. The choice is a matter of clinical judgement.

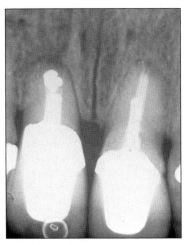

16.107 Survival of favourably loaded short posts

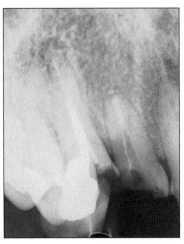

16.108 Deformation of post (courtesy of Mr P King)

16.109 Fracture of post (courtesy of Mr P King)

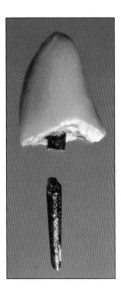

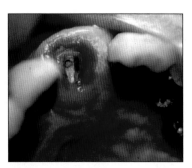

16.110 Fractured post in central incisor

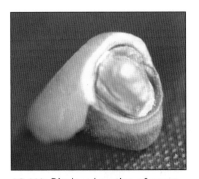

16.111 Displaced portion of crown and fractured post

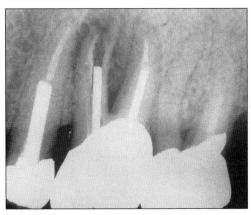

16.112 Wide posts may cause root fracture because of the amount of dentine sacrificed

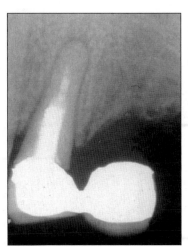

16.113 Unfavourable restoration designs increase the risk of root fracture

Diameter

Posts must be of a minimum diameter to be strong enough to resist deformation (**16.108**) but the design of the restoration also contributes to the fatiguing of the post and even a wide post will fracture if poorly designed (**16.109–16.111**). The diameter of a cast post should be greater than that of a wrought post made of the same alloy if it is to be as strong. In narrow roots, posts made of wrought metal should therefore be considered. Wider posts provide only slightly better retention and their use also means thinner and weaker residual root dentine which may be prone to fracture (**16.112**). If the restoration is badly designed, the chances of root fracture increase (**16.113**). The minimum post diameter compatible with adequate strength and retention should be considered.

Surface configuration

The surface of posts may be smooth, roughened, serrated or threaded and in addition may be modified for venting. Surface characteristics influence seating and retention. Rough or uneven surfaces increase retentive capacity. Threaded posts have the best retentive properties. Prefabricated posts with a variety of thread designs are available. They may be threaded along their entire length or only on a restricted portion. Threaded posts generate the greatest stresses, as demonstrated by the concentration of stresses around the threaded portion of the post shown in **Figure 16.114**. The stresses increase when the post is loaded (**16.115**). The manner of placement of the post also influences the stress generated. The stress associated with the threads upon conventional placement is shown in **Figure 16.116**.

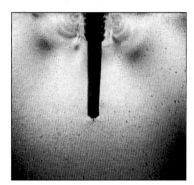

16.114 Higher stresses are associated with threads (courtesy of Mr P O'Neilly)

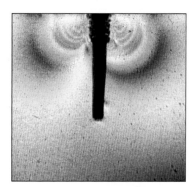

16.115 Further increase in stresses upon loading (courtesy of Mr P O'Neilly)

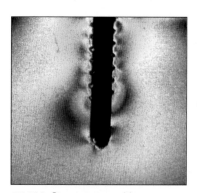

16.116 Stresses caused by placement of a threaded parallel post (courtesy of Mr P O'Neilly)

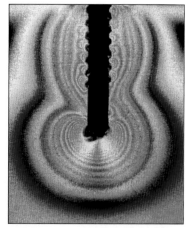

16.117 Increase in stresses if the post is tightened by a quarter turn (courtesy of Mr P O'Neilly)

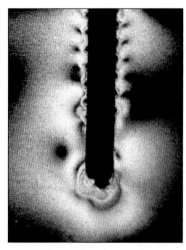

16.118 Loosening the post by tapping and cementing in place also reduces stresses (courtesy of Mr P O'Neilly)

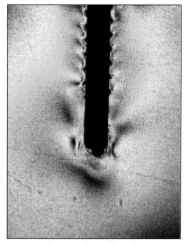

16.119 Upon loading the stresses are considerably reduced (courtesy of Mr P O'Neilly)

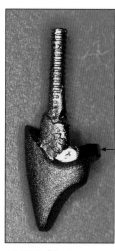

16.120 Diaphragm built into post/core (arrowed)

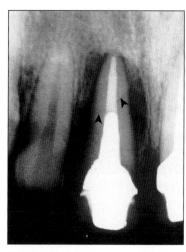

16.121 Root fracture associated with the tip of the post (arrowed)

If the post is tightened by an extra quarter turn, the stress increases tremendously (**16.117**). Upon loading, the stresses increase further, but are proportionately much lower than those due to over-tightening. Removing the post and tapping the threads before replacement decreases the stresses considerably. Loosening the fit of the post by removing and replacing it and then cementing it in place also reduces the stress (**16.118, 16.119**). Serrations on the posts are also associated with increased stresses but not to the same extent as threads. Loading once again increases stresses. The improved retention due to serrations and threads should, therefore, be weighed against the disadvantages of increased stress concentration. The surface of the post may also be modified with cutaway portions or channels, which act as escape routes for luting cement during installation and allow better seating and improved retention.

Diaphragm

A diaphragm or an apron, usually placed on the palatal aspect, may help to brace the tooth and distribute stresses more favourably (**16.120**). It is also useful for making good lost tooth tissue. When there is inadequate coronal tooth tissue, a correctly designed and placed diaphragm prevents concentration of stresses around the apical portion of a post which can lead to horizontal or oblique fractures of the root (**16.121**).

Posterior teeth

Teeth requiring root canal treatment are often broken down to the extent that retention for a restoration is compromised (**16.122**). Restoration then requires installation of a core to replace the lost dentine before a full or partial coverage cast restoration can be placed on the tooth (**16.123**).

Retention for the core may be achieved in a number of ways, including the use of grooves and slots, dentine pins and dowels. Slots and grooves cut into residual dentine require favourable distribution of the remaining dentine. The depth and size of these retentive devices depend on the physical properties of the core material. Most of the currently available plastic materials require reasonable bulk to provide strength, which limits their clinical application.

The use of dentine pins in root-treated teeth is controversial. The presence of a pulp chamber and root canals should provide adequate retention. Rarely, a pin may be useful to help retain an interim amalgam restoration while root-canal treatment is being performed (**16.124**). Placement of dentine pins is associated with complications such as perforation (**16.125**) and induction of stresses in the dentine possibly leading to cracks (**16.126**) and fractures. Induced stresses are greatest with threaded (**16.127**) and friction-grip pins and least with cemented pins but the latter require greater length for equivalent retention. Stresses due to pins may be reduced by:

- pinhole preparation with a sharp drill using a speed reducing handpiece and minimum number of passes so as not to cut the hole eccentrically;
- using pins with minimal mismatch between size of pinhole and pin;

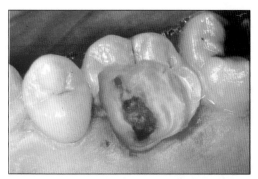

16.122 Tooth requiring a core to retain a cast restoration

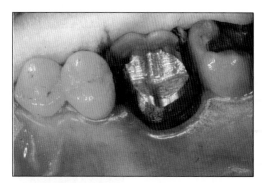

16.123 Amalgam core in place

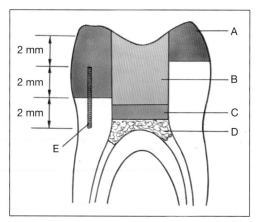

16.124 Use of dentine pins to retain an interim restoration: A = amalgam; B = access restoration; C = gutta percha; D = cotton wool; E = pin

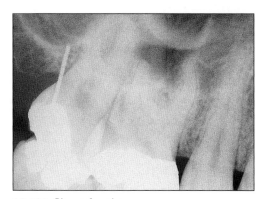

16.125 Pin perforation

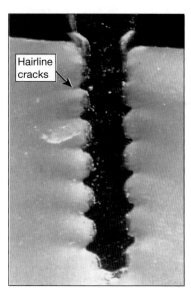

Hairline cracks

16.126 Stress-induced dentinal fractures

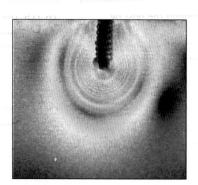

16.127 Threaded pins generated the greatest stress (courtesy of Mr P O'Neilly)

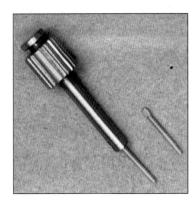

16.128 Hand wrench for the insertion of pins

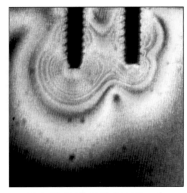

16.129 Pins placed close together cause stresses to accumulate (courtesy of Mr P O'Neilly)

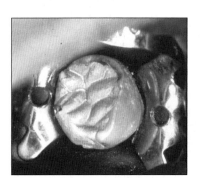

16.130 Nayyar amalgam core

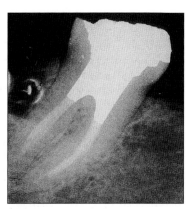

16.131 Radiograph of the Nayyar amalgam core

- inserting the pin using a handwrench (**16.128**) and unwinding it by at least a quarter turn so as not to engage the bottom of the pinhole;
- using a threaded pin at least 4 mm long with 2 mm in dentine, 2 mm in restorative material and with 2 mm of restorative material above the tip of the pin (**16.124**);
- using pins with sharper threads minimizes stresses during installation (but these potentially increase stresses in function);
- using pins made of alloys softer than dentine, such as titanium which may induce less stress;
- using only one pin per cusp because pins placed close together result in interaction of stresses and an increased potential for fracture (**16.129**).

The pulp space may be used for retention in a number of ways. The most conservative is the Nayyar amalgam dowel core (**16.130, 16.131**). This involves placing amalgam in the pulp chamber. It was originally believed that the amalgam should extend into the root canals to a depth of about 3 mm to retain the amalgam but it is better to seal the coronal aspect of the root canals with zinc oxide/eugenol and use only the pulp chamber. The coronal amalgam may be designed to act as the final capped-cusp restoration (**16.132, 16.133**) or the core may be cut down for placement of a cast restoration (**16.134–16.136**). The shortness of the dowel reduces the disturbance of the root filling. Adequate remaining tooth tissue is essential and should be judged in terms of:

- depth of pulp chamber (**16.131, 16.137**);
- distance from floor of pulp chamber to furcation (**16.137**), floor to amelo–cemental junction (**16.137**), floor to alveolar crest (**16.131**) and the projected margin of the crown (**16.134–16.136**);
- thickness of dentine at the level of the crown margin (**16.14**).

Nayyar cores are more rarely placed in premolars. When the remaining coronal dentine is not enough to support such a core, retention may be gained by placing a dowel into one of the canals, usually the one with the largest and straightest root (the palatal

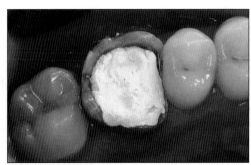

16.132 Root-treated maxillary molar

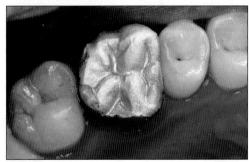

16.133 Molar restored with Nayyar-based amalgam restoration

canal in an upper molar and the distal canal in a lower molar) (**16.138–16.140**). The dowel and the residual coronal dentine can then provide the retention for the core. Multiple roots make it possible to place multiple posts, which do not have to be as long as in single-rooted teeth.

CORE MATERIALS

Amalgam

Amalgam remains the material of choice for cores because of its strength, versatility, availability and dimensional stability. Its one drawback was the slowness of set, making it difficult to prepare the

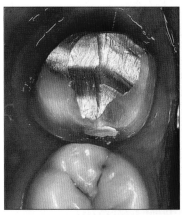

16.134 Mandibular molar with Nayyar core

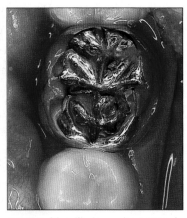

16.135 Mandibular molar restored with cast restoration

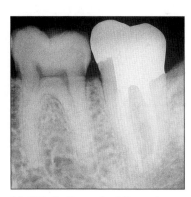

16.136 Radiograph of the molar showing the extent of the core and cast restoration

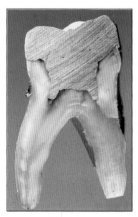

16.137 Sectioned molar with Nayyar core in place

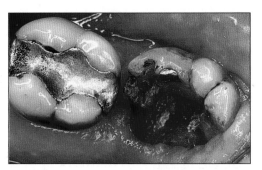

16.138

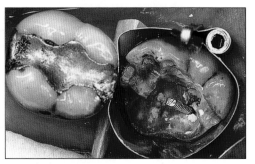

16.139

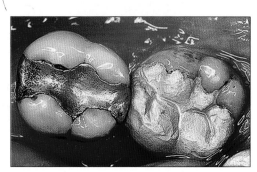

16.140

16.138–16.140 Stainless steel post/amalgam core in mandibular molar

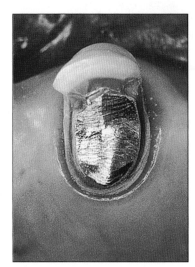

16.141 Partial veneer preparation in a maxillary premolar

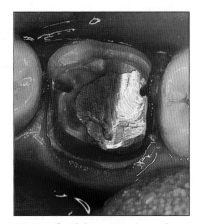

16.142 Partial veneer preparation in a mandibular molar

Composite

Composite cores became popular because they set rapidly and were strong. However, they have now largely fallen out of favour because they tend to absorb moisture and are dimensionally unstable, because eugenol temporary cements tend to soften the core and because moisture in the core affects the physical properties of acid-based permanent luting cements, such as zinc phosphate, glass ionomer or polycarboxylate.

Cermets

Cermets or metal reinforced glass ionomers have also been recommended as core materials, but their strength does not compare with that of amalgam or composites. They are suitable only for use as a space-filler to reduce the amount of metal in the cast restoration. They should not be used as a structural core that provides the principal retention and resistance form.

Once placed, the cores may serve as interim restorations before being prepared for cast restorations. If aesthetic requirements allow, a conservative partial veneer restoration such as a three-quarter crown is preferable (**16.141, 16.142**). The margins of the casting should always be placed on sound tooth tissue.

core for a cast restoration at the same visit. However, new faster-setting alloys have largely overcome this disadvantage. Reports of systemic problems caused by amalgam seem to be unfounded.

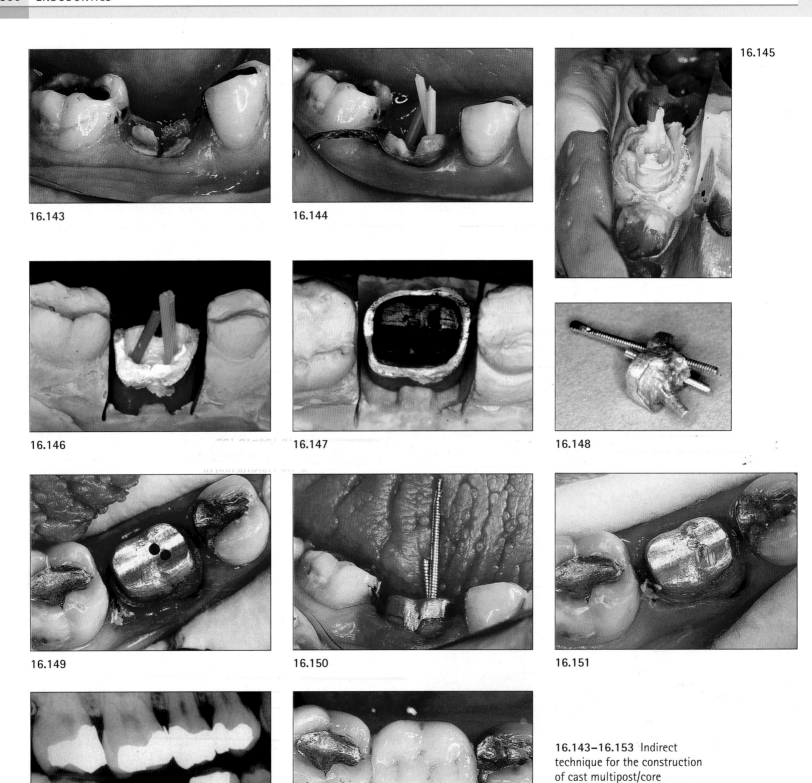

16.143

16.144

16.145

16.146

16.147

16.148

16.149

16.150

16.151

16.152

16.153

16.143–16.153 Indirect technique for the construction of cast multipost/core

Cast cores

Cast multiple posts or cores may be used in multirooted teeth with little remaining coronal tooth tissue by constructing only one of the posts integral with the core and cementing the remaining post(s) into their respective canals through the core. This method can be applied using either indirect or direct techniques.

In the indirect technique an impression of the tooth (**16.143**) and post canals (**16.144**) is taken using preformed plastic patterns and rubber-base impression material (**16.145**). A model is constructed with a die (**16.146**), on which the post and core is waxed with withdrawable posts in two canals (**16.147, 16.148**). The cast post and core is tried in the mouth for fit (**16.149**) and the removable posts are inserted through their respective channels (**16.150**). The post and core system is cemented with zinc phosphate (**16.151, 16.152**). The final crown is constructed with margins on sound tooth tissue (**16.153**).

Where some coronal tooth tissue remains it may interfere with the path of insertion of the core. The canal providing the path of least resistance may be selected for the principle post to help preserve tooth tissue and place a partial veneer cast restoration. If a substantial amount of tooth tissue needs to be sacrificed to provide a path of insertion for the core, it may be better to cement preformed posts into the canals and build up a core with plastic restorative materials.

The direct technique may also be used to construct a multiple post and core system using preformed plastic patterns and acrylic resin (**16.154, 16.155**). The method is more difficult to perform than the indirect technique but is more suitable in some circumstances.

ROOT TREATED AS ABUTMENTS

It is generally accepted that the stresses on an abutment tooth are different from, and likely to be more severe than, those on a single unit (**16.156**). There may be a higher tendency for root-treated (**16.157a & b**) abutment teeth and their restorations to fail mechanically than vital abutments. For this reason many operators avoid using root-treated teeth as abutments. However, it is also documented that such teeth can survive despite acting as abutments (**16.158, 16.159**). The truth probably lies somewhere inbetween. The potential for failure is a function not only of endodontic status but also of the amount of remaining dentine, restoration design and occlusal loading. The bridge shown in **Figures 16.158 and 16.159** would not be expected to survive, yet it has been in place for at least

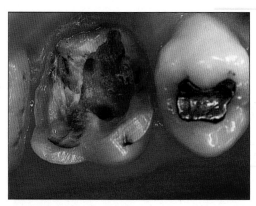

16.154

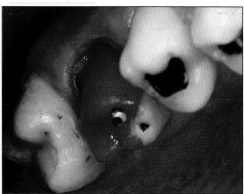

16.155

16.154–16.155
Direct technique for the construction of multipost core

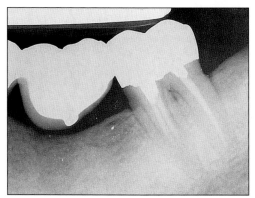

16.156 Stresses are likely to be more severe on an abutment tooth

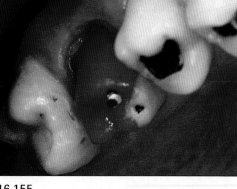

16.157a Failed anterior cantilever bridge carried by a non-vital abutment

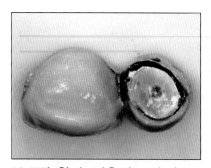

16.157b Displaced fixed prosthesis

ten years. Different bridge and denture designs impose different stresses on the teeth and it is important to select a design likely to reduce such stresses. Fixed–fixed bridge designs distribute stresses equally between abutments, whereas, the minor retainer in a fixed–movable design takes the lower load. The terminal abutment for a free-end saddle design is likely to take greater loads than an abutment for a bounded saddle. Crown to root ratios, bracing, type of retention and rest seat design all influence lateral loading of abutment teeth. The number of remaining teeth and potential for bracing from other teeth and soft tissues may also dictate overall loading. The denture design selected should attempt to minimize stresses on root-treated teeth.

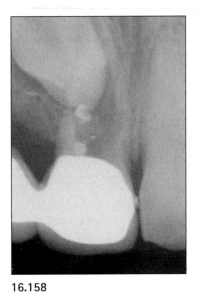

16.158

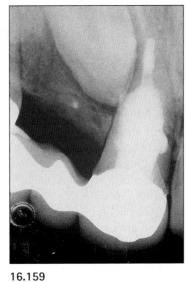

16.159

16.158–16.159 Survival of severely weakened tooth as a bridge abutment

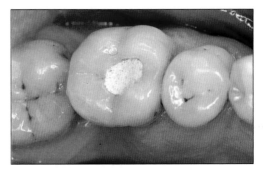

16.160 Molar requiring root resection

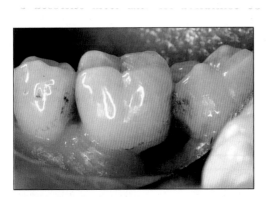

16.161 Tooth post resection

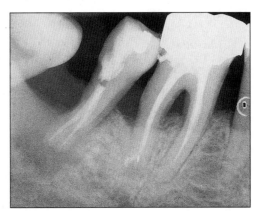

16.162

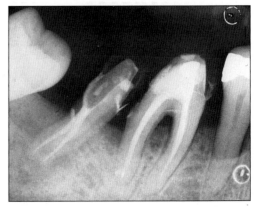

16.163

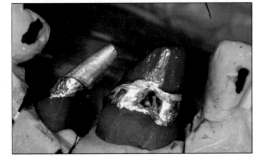

16.164

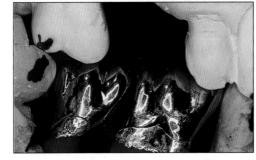

16.165

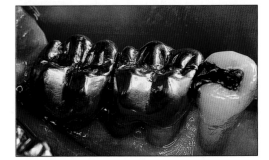

16.166

16.162–16.166 Restoration of hemisected mandibular second molar and first molar

OCCLUSAL LOADING

Occlusal loading is difficult to control. It is dependent not only on the occlusal contacts but also on eating and chewing habits, parafunctional activity and the state of the masticatory musculature. There is only limited scope for influencing the nature and magnitude of occlusal forces. Adequately designing the intercuspal, excursive and closure contact relationships of teeth can achieve this. Lateral forces are often regarded as being the most damaging and, therefore, designing excursive occlusal contacts to preferentially load adjacent vital and more robust teeth may be useful.

RESTORATION OF A TOOTH WITH A RESECTED ROOT

If the crown of a tooth scheduled for root resection is intact, the only restorations required are the amalgam seal in the canal of the root to be resected and the access restoration (**16.160**, **16.161**). If the tooth already has a restoration with stable interproximal and occlusal contacts, no further restoration should be required. In the absence of stable contacts a suitable restoration should be constructed (**16.162–16.166**).

RESTORATION OF A HEMISECTED TOOTH

Teeth may be hemisected for various reasons, such as tooth fracture or furcal involvement. The procedure may be followed by extraction of one of the roots and restoration of the remaining one as a premolar. Restoration is made difficult by the root morphology in the furcation (**16.167**). Rarely both roots may be restored as independent premolar units but the procedure is fraught with difficulties mainly related to controlling the margin placement in the furcation (**16.168**).

TREATMENT OF TOOTH DISCOLOURATION

Non-vital teeth may be discoloured by various factors including, caries, restorations, secondary calcification and contamination of dentinal tubules by blood or food products. Removal of the cause, usually removes the discolouration, except in the case of severe secondary calcification, which gives a dense, opaque yellow discolouration (**16.169**, **16.170**). Options for treatment include:

- vital bleaching;
- non-vital bleaching;
- labial/buccal veneers;
- crowns.

Vital bleaching

Vital bleaching may be considered for vital teeth sclerosed by secondary calcification but it is unlikely to be successful. Use of home-bleaching products is regarded by some as potentially harmful and is the subject of legal action as commercial products with greater than 0.1% hydrogen peroxide cannot be prescribed by a practitioner in the EU (Dental Defence Union 2002).

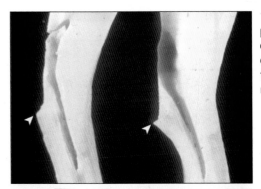

16.167 Margin placement and contouring difficulties caused by the shape of the tooth in the furcal region (arrowed)

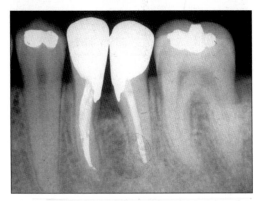

16.168 Difficulties of contouring restorations in the furcation

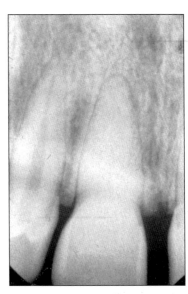

16.169 Obliteration of the pulp

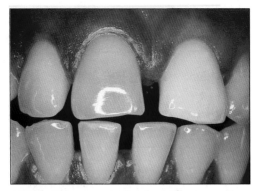

16.170 Dense opaque discolouration due to the obliteration of the pulp

Non-vital bleaching

The use of bleaching agents in the access cavity under rubber dam isolation is quite effective (**16.171–16.178**). Bleaching may be performed at the chair-side by placing hydrogen peroxide in the pulp chamber. Bleaching is usually performed after the pulp chamber has been prepared by removing all restorative and root-filling material to the cervical level (**16.172**) and covering it with a layer of zinc phosphate (**16.173**). The dentine is then etched for 30 seconds with phosphoric acid (**16.174**), washed away and the cavity dried. Hydrogen peroxide is flooded into the canal, taking care to ensure that there is no overflow (**16.175**). After 5–10 minutes, the access cavity is gently dried and a paste of sodium perborate mixed with water (**16.176**) is applied. The access cavity is properly sealed to prevent loss of dressing between appointments. There may be some improvement at this stage (**16.177**). One week later, further improvement is seen due to the 'walking bleach' technique (**16.178**).

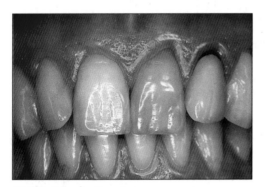

16.171 Preoperative view

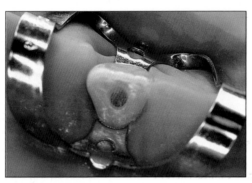

16.172 Removal of root-filling material

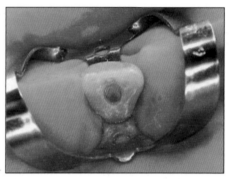

16.173 Zinc phosphate base

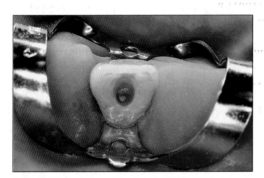

16.174 Thirty-second etching of dentine

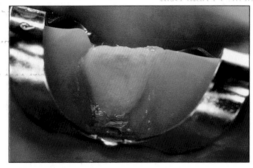

16.175 Hydrogen peroxide placed with cotton pledget

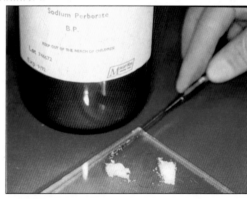

16.176 Mixing paste of sodium perborate

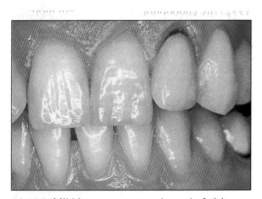

16.177 Mild improvement at the end of visit

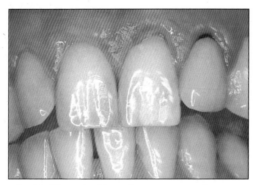

16.178 More significant improvement after one week

Composite or porcelain veneers

These can effectively mask discolouration provided that it is not severe and that an adequate thickness of masking material is used. A combination of bleaching and veneering may help if neither method alone is sufficient to eliminate discolouration.

Ceramometal or ceramic crowns

These are capable of providing excellent aesthetics but require an adequate thickness of porcelain, which means sacrificing more tissue in an already weakened tooth.

Further Reading

Bergman B, Lundqvist P, Sjogren U, Sundqvist G. (1989) Restorative and endodontic results after treatment with cast posts and cores. *J Prosth Dent* **61**(1), 10–15.

Burke FJT (1992) Tooth fracture in vivo and in vitro. *J Dent* **20**, 131–9.

Carter JM, Sorensen *et al.* (1983) Punch shear testing of extracted vital and endodontically treated teeth. *J Biomechanics* **16**, 841–8.

Cavel WT, Kelsey WP, Blankenall RJ (1985) An in vivo study of cuspal fracture. *J Prosth Dent* **53**(1), 38–41.

Dental Defence Union 2002 *Legal position with regard to teeth bleaching.* Advice leaflet GDP/014/1002.

Eakle WS, Maxwell EH, Braly BV (1986) Fractures of posterior teeth in adults. *J Am Dent Assoc* **112**, 215–18.

Gher ME, Dunlap RM, Anderson MH, Kuhl LV (1987) Clinical survey of fractured teeth. *J Am Dent Assoc* **114**, 174–7.

Guzy GE, Nicholls JI (1979) In vitro comparison of intact endodontically treated teeth with and without endopost reinforcement. *J Prosth Dent* **42**(1), 39–44.

Hansen EK (1988) in vivo cusp fracture of endodontically treated premolars restored with MOD amalgam or MOD resin fillings. *Dent Mat* **4**, 169–73.

Hansen EK, Asmussen E (1990) In vivo fractures of endodontically treated posterior teeth restored with enamel-bonded resin. *Endod Dent Traumatol* **6**, 218–25.

Hansen EK, Asmussen E (1993) Cusp fracture of endodontically treated posterior teeth restored with amalgam. Teeth restored in Denmark before 1975 versus after 1979. *Acta Odontol Scand* **51**, 73–7.

Hansen EK, Asmussen E, Christiansen NC (1990) In vivo fractures of endodontically treated posterior teeth restored with amalgam. *Endod Dent Traumatol* **6**, 49–55.

Hatzikyriakeos AM, Reisis GI, Tsingos N (1992) A 3-year postoperative clinical evaluation of posts and cores beneath existing crowns. *J Prosth Dent* **67**, 454–8.

Helfer AR, Melnick S, Schilder H (1972) Determination of the moisture content of vital and pulpless teeth. *Oral Surg* **34**(4), 661–70.

Heling I, Gorfil C, Slutzky H, Kpolovic K, Zalkind M, Slutzky-Goldber I (2002) Endodontic failure caused by inadequate restorative procedures, review and treatment recommendations. *J Prosth Dent* **87**, 674–8.

Hommez GM, Coppens CR, De Moor RJ (2002) Periapical health related to the quality of coronal restorations and root fillings. *Int Endod J* **35**, 680–9.

Howe CA, McKendry DJ (1990) Effect of endodontic access preparation on resistance to crown-root fracture. *J Am Dent Assoc* **121**, 712–15.

Huang TG, Schilder H, Nathanson D (1991) Effects of moisture content and endodontic treatment on some mechanical properties of human dentine. *J Endod* **189**(5), 209–15.

Kantor ME, Pines MS (1977) A comparative study of restorative techniques in pulpless teeth. *J Prosth Dent* **34**, 405.

Kvist T, Rydin E, Reit C (1989) The relative frequency of periapical lesions in teeth with root canal-retained posts. *J Endod* **15**(12), 578–80.

Lagouvardos P, Souvai P, Douvitasas G (1989) Coronal fractures in posterior teeth. *Op Dent* **14**, 28–32.

Lawson TD, Douglas WH, Geistfeld RE (1981) Effect of prepared cavities on the strength of teeth. *Op Dent* **6**, 2–5.

Lewinstein I, Grajower R (1981) Root dentine hardness of endodontically treated teeth. *J Endod* **7**, 421–2.

Nayyar A, Walton RE, Leonard LA (1980) An amalgam coronal-radicular dowel and core technique for endodontically treated posterior teeth. *J Prosth Dent* **43**(5), 511–15.

Panitvisai P, Messer HH (1995) Cuspal deflection in molars in relation to endodontic and restorative procedures. *J Endod* **21**, 57–61.

Papa J, Cain C, Messer HH (1994) Moisture content of vital vs endodontically treated teeth. *Endod Dent Traumatol* **10**, 91–3.

Randow K, Glantz PO (1986) On cantilever loading of vital and non-vital teeth – An experimental clinical study. *Acta Odontol Scand* **44**, 271–7.

Reeh ES, Messer HH, Douglas WH (1989) Reduction in tooth stiffness as a result of endodontic and restorative procedures. *J Endod* **15**(11), 512–16.

Sedgeley CM, Messer HH (1992) Are endodontically treated teeth more brittle? *J Endod* **18**(7), 332–5.

Sorensen JA, Martinoff JT (1984) Intracoronal reinforcement and coronal coverage. A study of endodontically treated teeth. *J Prosth Dent* **51**, 780–4.

Sorensen JA, Martinoff JT (1984) Clinically significant factors in dowl design. *J Prosth Dent* **52**, 28–35.

Trabert KC, Caputo AA, Abou-Rass M (1978) A comparison of endodontic and restorative treatment. *J Endod* **4**(11), 341–5.

Chapter 17

Endodontic treatment of primary teeth

C Mason

Retention of the primary dentition until the time of natural exfoliation is important for several reasons. There are clear psychological advantages of conserving rather than extracting teeth. In addition, primary teeth have important roles in mastication, appearance, speech development and space maintenance for the permanent successors.

Endodontic treatment of primary teeth differs from that of permanent teeth for two main reasons – tooth morphology and pulp pathology. Techniques and medicaments differ due to these factors and the processes of physiological root resorption and exfoliation.

MORPHOLOGY OF PRIMARY TEETH

The enamel and dentine are thinner and the pulp chamber, with its extended horns, larger in proportion than in permanent teeth (**17.1**).

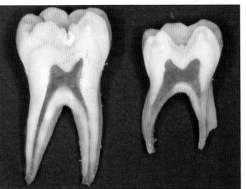

17.1 Comparison of adult and primary molars

more rapid inflammatory changes

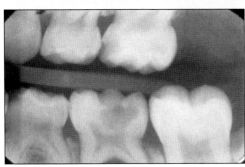

17.2 Caries and intraradicular bone loss in primary molars

Caries progresses relatively more rapidly to the pulp in the primary dentition.

Primary molars have irregularly shaped ribbon-like root canals with lateral branches. The floor of the pulp chamber is thin and there are numerous accessory canals in the interradicular area. The permeability of the dentine in this region often leads to interradicular rather than periapical bone loss associated with infected primary molars (**17.2**).

The roots of the primary teeth are in close relationship to the developing permanent successor and will undergo physiological resorption during the process of exfoliation (**17.3**). Materials used within the root canal system must, therefore, be resorbable. The close proximity means that trauma to, or infection of, primary teeth may affect the developing successor. Possible sequelae include enamel defects, arrested development or cyst formation.

PULP DISEASE IN PRIMARY TEETH

Inflammatory changes in response to carious attack occur more rapidly in the pulps of primary teeth compared to permanent teeth. These changes are soon irreversible and extend throughout the coronal pulp. Symptoms arising from pathological changes in primary teeth may not be severe until the later stages of necrosis and abscess formation (**17.4**).

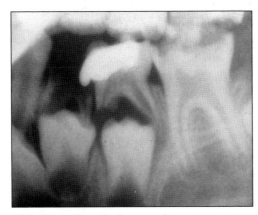

17.3 Resorption of primary molar

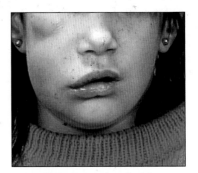

17.4 Abscess associated with primary molar

Diagnosis of pulp disease in young children is difficult since they are usually poor historians and respond unpredictably to subjective clinical tests. Certain techniques used in the management of pulp disease in permanent teeth cannot, therefore, be reliably used in the primary dentition. Methods of objectively measuring inflammatory changes in the pulps of primary teeth by prostaglandin assays are currently being researched.

TECHNIQUES OF PULP THERAPY

Indirect pulp capping

Carious lesions should usually be fully excavated before teeth are restored. A clinical dilemma is sometimes presented by deep caries in an asymptomatic tooth, without clinical or radiographic evidence of pulp disease. This situation may be in a child whose cooperation or attention span would not allow the treatment to progress to pulpotomy. Indirect pulp capping may be used in such instances. Its success relies on the basis that the advancing front of the carious lesion contains very few cariogenic bacteria. Provided that the overlying infected dentine is removed, a small amount of softened dentine may be left in the deepest part of the cavity and covered by a thin layer of setting calcium hydroxide. In its classical application, the tooth would have been dressed with zinc oxide/eugenol cement for several weeks and then further excavation of the dentine would have been performed. This has now been replaced by covering the calcium hydroxide with a layer of hard-setting cement, restoring the tooth definitively and reviewing clinically and radiographically for pulp disease. This avoids a second operative visit, which is an obvious advantage for children.

Direct pulp capping

This technique is generally contraindicated for the primary dentition. Pathological changes progress rapidly within the pulps of primary teeth and their healing ability is limited. Pulpal inflammation usually persists and progresses to pulpal necrosis or internal root resorption, particularly if calcium hydroxide has been placed on the exposed pulp (**17.5**). The only circumstance where the technique may be used is for a small traumatic exposure during cavity preparation in an area of otherwise sound dentine. Haemorrhage from the exposure should be minimal and easily controlled. Further haemorrhage indicates pulpal inflammation and pulpotomy is the treatment of choice. If the bleeding stops easily, calcium hydroxide is placed and the tooth restored.

Vital pulpotomy

This technique involves the removal of the inflamed coronal pulp tissue and the fixation of the vital radicular pulp tissue. Formocresol is still the medicament of choice for the fixation of pulp tissue in primary teeth, although alternatives will be discussed later in the chapter. The one-stage formocresol pulpotomy technique has a high success rate in correctly selected cases. Since there have been concerns regarding the safety of formocresol, the technique has been modified over the years and alternatives are constantly being researched.

The constituents of the original Buckley's formocresol were:

- tricresol   35%;
- formaldehyde   19%;
- glycerol   15%;
- water   31%.

It is now recommended that a 1/5 dilution be used, for example:

- Buckley's formocresol   1 part;
- glycerol   3 parts;
- water   1 part.

Indications for pulpotomy:

- restorable tooth;
- no history of spontaneous or persistent pain;
- absence of abscess or sinus;
- no interradicular bone loss;
- no internal resorption;
- medical – to avoid extraction, e.g. in area of haemangioma or child with bleeding disorder.

Contra-indications for pulpotomy:

- unrestorable tooth;
- spontaneous or persistent pain;
- abscess or sinus;
- interradicular bone loss;
- internal resorption;
- permanent tooth close to eruption;
- medical – immunocompromised or at risk of endocarditis.

Procedure:

1. Adequate local analgesia and isolation, preferably with a rubber dam, are essential. All peripheral caries should be removed prior to entering the pulp chamber. The pulp chamber is then entered via the exposure (**17.6, 17.7**).
2. The roof of the pulp chamber is removed, ensuring no overhangs are left which could cause difficulty in removal of pulp tissue. It is important at this stage that the bur is not taken any deeper into the cavity, since this would endanger the thin floor of the pulp chamber (**17.8, 17.9**).
3. The coronal pulp is removed using a large sharp excavator or round bur. The chamber is irrigated and dried with cotton wool pledgets to control haemorrhage and identify pulp stumps (**17.10, 17.11**).
4. A small pledget of cotton wool is dipped in the 1/5 dilution of formocresol and squeezed in gauze to remove excess. This is then applied to the radicular pulp for four minutes (**17.12, 17.13**).

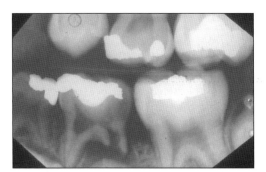

17.5 Internal root resorption

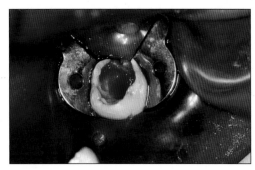

17.6 Caries removal

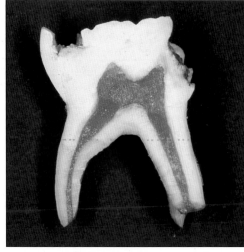

17.7 Sectioned primary molar

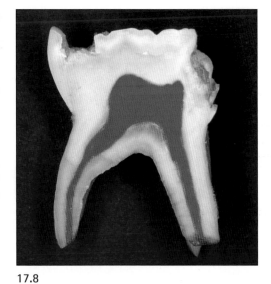

17.8

17.8–17.9 Access preparation

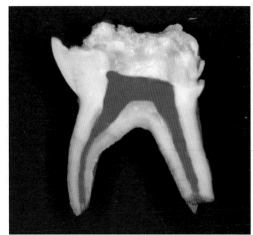

17.9 Removal of root of pulp chamber

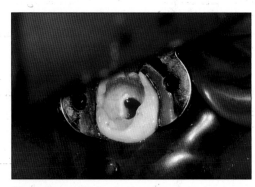

17.10 Removal of pulp chamber contents

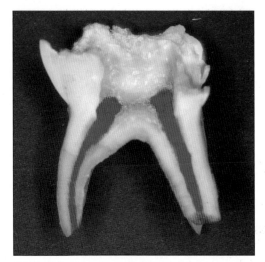

17.11 Pulp stumps remaining

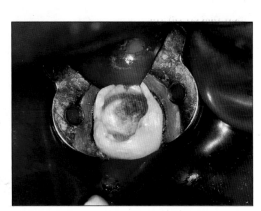

17.12 Application of formocresol

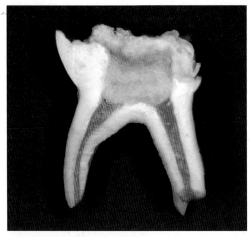

17.13 Formocresol in contact with pulp stumps for four minutes

5. On removal of the cotton wool, the radicular pulp stumps should appear dark brown and there should be no haemorrhage (**17.14, 17.15**). If there is a little oozing, the formocresol may be reapplied for a couple more minutes. Persistent haemorrhage indicates radicular inflammation and the need for either a two-visit technique (sealing in a pledget of cotton wool with formocresol for 1 week) or pulpectomy.

6. When haemorrhage has been arrested, the chamber is filled with zinc oxide/eugenol cement and the tooth definitively restored, ideally with a stainless-steel crown (**17.16, 17.17**).

When the pulp is infected with necrotic tissue or pus in the canals or there is swelling, sinus or radiographic evidence of bone loss, other techniques are required – 'non-vital pulpotomy' and pulpectomy. The medical indications and contraindications are the same as for vital pulpotomy techniques.

'Non-vital pulpotomy' (disinfection technique)

This method has largely been replaced by the pulpectomy technique. However, it will be briefly described since it may still be useful in situations of acute infection associated with non-vital primary teeth.

The cavity is prepared and the coronal pulp chamber and access to the root canals thoroughly cleaned. A cotton wool pledget moistened with formocresol, camphorated monochlorophenol or beechwood creosote is placed into the pulp chamber. This is sealed in with a dressing for 7–10 days and, in the absence of signs and symptoms of infection, the tooth is then restored as following pulpotomy.

Pulpectomy

The basis of this method is to remove as much necrotic and infected material from the root canal system as is possible. Since the root canal system is complex with many fine accessory canals, it is not possible to completely clean and fill the system. The roots will undergo physiological root resorption and for these reasons, the techniques employed differ from those used for the permanent dentition.

Procedure:

1. Adequate local analgesia must be ensured and the tooth isolated with a rubber dam. The caries is removed from the tooth and the exposure site identified. As in the pulpotomy technique, the roof of the pulp chamber is removed taking great care not to extend preparation to the floor (**17.18, 17.19**).

2. The openings to the root canals are identified and the canals filed to within 1–2 mm of the apices. The working lengths can be estimated from a preoperative radiograph. In a cooperative child, a diagnostic radiograph may be taken with files in situ, but this is optional since the lengths do not have to be exact. The canals are filed up to the maximum size 30 (**17.20**).

3. The canals are dried with paper points and a pledget of cotton wool moistened with formocresol is applied for four minutes to fix any remaining tissue. If there is an acute abscess, with or without cellulitis, or purulent discharge from the canals, the pledget may be sealed in for a week. This is then a two-visit pulpectomy, and the stages below would be on the second visit.

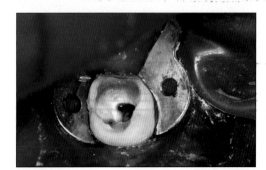

17.14 Removal of cotton wool

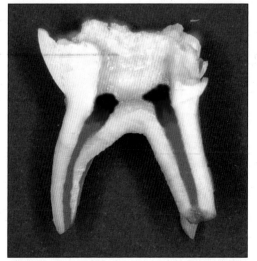

17.15 Pulp stumps appear dark brown

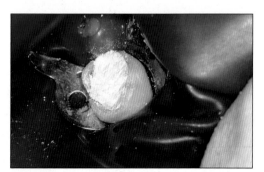

17.16 Zinc oxide restoration

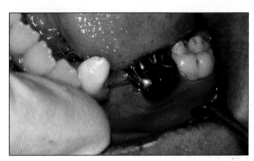

17.17 Stainless-steel crown

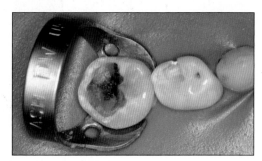

17.18 Removal of caries

4. A spiral filler (a size smaller than the last file used) is modified by cutting it to half its length (**17.21**). This makes it easier to handle in a small mouth and helps prevent extrusion of material through the apex. A slurry of pure zinc oxide/eugenol is then spun into the canals (**17.22**).
5. When the canals have been filled, the pulp chamber is filled with zinc oxide/eugenol cement and the tooth restored with a stainless steel crown (**17.23**).

Alternative medicaments for pulp therapy in primary teeth

For many years there have been concerns regarding the use of formocresol. Both formocresol and formaldehyde have been shown to be cytotoxic, mutagenic and carcinogenic in laboratory and animal experiments. Alternatives have been investigated and are briefly outlined below.

Glutaraldehyde

Glutaraldehyde is used as a fixative and disinfectant. It has been reported that the fixative properties are better than those of formaldehyde and it is less penetrative, thus less able to diffuse into periapical tissues. Clinical studies have shown high success rates (82–98%) using a 2% solution. Toxicity and mutagenicity studies have been conflicting and neither glutaraldehyde nor formaldehyde is consistently safer.

Calcium hydroxide

Calcium hydroxide is advocated for pulpotomy techniques in permanent teeth. However, when used in primary teeth, internal resorption occurs. Factors thought to play a role in the pathogenesis are the presence of a blood clot between the amputation site and the material and the inflammatory status of the pulp. It is the latter factor which is so difficult to assess in the primary dentition. There have been promising results in situations where these factors have been controlled, and, particularly in its pure powdered form, this material could be a useful alternative.

Ferric sulphate

Ferric sulphate has been shown to be effective in primary molar endodontic treatment. The success rate in some studies has not been as good as that of formocresol or glutaraldehyde. The advantage is that the solution only needs to be applied for a few seconds, compared to four minutes with alternative medicaments. This obviously would have advantages when dealing with young children. Other studies have shown a good success rate and this medicament warrants further long-term clinical trials.

Iodoform

In several studies, iodoform paste has been shown to be as effective as zinc oxide/eugenol as a resorbable filling material following

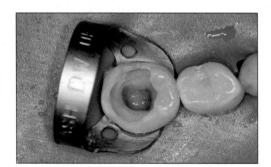

17.19 Removal of roof of the pulp chamber

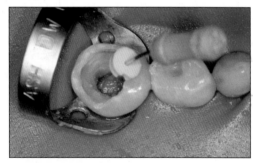

17.20 Canal filing

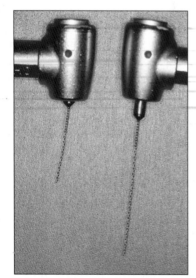

17.21 Spiral filler cut to length

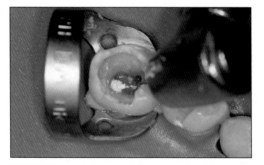

17.22 Slurry of zinc oxide/eugenol applied

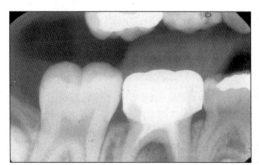

17.23 Radiograph of final restoration

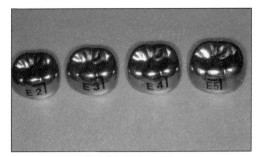

17.24 Stainless-steel crowns

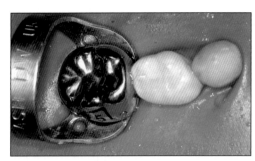

17.25 Stainless-steel crown being fitted

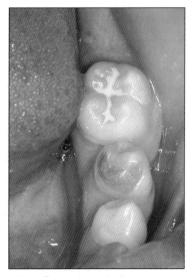

17.28 Turner hypoplasia

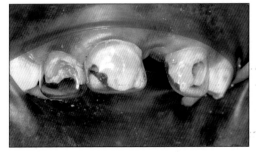

17.26 Resin crown formers in place

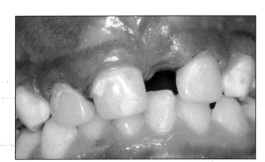

17.27 Resin crowns

pulpectomy of primary teeth. The adequate cleaning of the canals and underfilling rather than overfilling are the key factors for success whichever of the two materials is used.

Bone morphogenic proteins

With the techniques of molecular biology, progress has been made in the purification of factors with bone inductive properties. The generic term for this family of proteins is bone morphogenic proteins or BMPs. If BMPs induce dentine as well as bone a true biological pulp capping and pulpotomy agent will be available.

Other methods

Pulpotomy techniques have been developed using electrosurgery, argon laser and CO_2 laser. However, results have been conflicting when compared to the success of the formocresol pulpotomy. Further research is required into these newer methods.

Restoration of endodontically treated primary teeth

When primary teeth have been endodontically treated, they are weakened by the destruction of tooth tissue during preparation. It is important that the definitive restoration has the necessary strength to support the tooth structure. In addition, the success of the endodontic treatment will rely on an adequate seal. For these reasons, the most suitable restorations are stainless-steel crowns for posterior teeth and composite-resin strip crowns for anterior teeth

(**17.24–17.27**). The reader is referred to other texts for details of the techniques (e.g. Duggal *et al.* 1995).

Follow-up and complications

When a primary tooth has been endodontically treated, it must be regularly reviewed clinically and radiographically. The primary tooth may develop signs and symptoms of infection, acute or chronic. These may manifest as swelling, sinus formation, tenderness to percussion, or mobility. Radiographically, pathological root resorption must be distinguished from physiological root resorption. Areas of bone loss may appear on follow-up or fail to heal following pulpectomy. Cyst formation may occur or there may be arrested development of the permanent tooth. An infected primary tooth may give rise to a hypoplastic permanent tooth, sometimes known as a 'Turner tooth' (**17.28**).

In the majority of cases, when treatment fails, extraction is the preferred option, rather than subjecting the underlying successor to greater risk.

ACKNOWLEDGMENT

Mrs Noushin Attari for assistance with the pulpectomy series and the photographs of strip crowns.

Reference

Duggal MS, Curzon MEJ, Fayle SA, Pollard MA, Robertson AJ 1995 *Restorative Techniques in Paediatric Dentistry*. Martin Dunitz, London.

Chapter **18**

Reducing the risk of legal action in endodontics

C J R Stock

INTRODUCTION

A letter from a solicitor alleging that a patient has been treated negligently has a dramatic and lasting impact on any dental practitioner however experienced or well qualified. Unfortunately, these letters are arriving with ever-increasing frequency, in line with the increasing frequency of claims against health professionals. This chapter is designed to help the dental practitioner, particularly when carrying out endodontic treatment, to reduce the risk of receiving such letters.

Although the chapter has been written from the English law perspective it should be emphasized that some of the recommendations given may differ in other jurisdictions. While the law may differ slightly between countries there is no doubt that provided a dentist carries out endodontic treatment to the best of his ability, explains the treatment to the patient, keeps careful records, and maintains good communication at all times the chances of litigation will be greatly reduced.

According to the insurers and indemnity organizations during recent years, endodontic treatment is a common source of claims for compensation, and of allegations of professional misconduct to dental regulatory bodies.

The main type of complaints received by defence bodies include:

- poor communication;
- unsatisfactory treatment;
- failure to make an appropriate diagnosis;
- incorrect or unnecessary treatment;
- fee dispute;
- post-treatment complication.

NEGLIGENCE

A dentist assumes a duty of care under common law when a patient is accepted for treatment. If the dentist is negligent and infringes that duty of care, with the result that the patient suffers avoidable harm the patient is entitled to be compensated for the loss and damage sustained. To succeed in an action for negligence the patient must prove, on the balance of probabilities, that the dentist owed them a duty of care, breached that duty by some act or omission, and that, as a direct consequence of the breach of duty, some loss or damage followed.

To prove the practitioner acted negligently the patient must prove he/she departed from what is considered to be standard practice by a responsible dental body. If the dentist has acted in accordance with an accepted view on endodontics then it is unlikely that he/she will be found negligent. However, one of the problems in dentistry, and in particular in endodontics, is that there may be more than one responsible body and each may hold a different view. It is the responsibility of the dentist to keep up to date with advances in endodontics and to be aware that the view they are following is current.

RECORDS

A dentist must always obtain a medical history from a patient before commencing treatment and check the history for any changes at subsequent visits. Full contemporaneous records are also a prerequisite for responding constructively to a complaint, or successfully defending a disciplinary action or negligence claim. If, for example, a patient alleges that the treatment was unnecessary or inappropriate the patient records including X-rays will almost invariably prove essential to refute such an allegation by confirming the investigations leading to the decision to undertake endodontic treatment. Likewise, radiographs may be essential to refute allegations of unsatisfactory treatment.

The use of apex locators is now well established in endodontics, but pre- and post-treatment radiographs are still necessary to demonstrate both the tooth and supporting tissues and the quality of the final root canal treatment.

In the absence of such adequate clinical records to corroborate the dentist's account of events, the courts may be more likely to accept the patient's evidence than that of the dentist. This is because the court may well consider the patient's recollection of a single event or a limited number of consultations to be more reliable than that of the dentist, who may have cared for many hundreds or thousands of patients during the interval since the treatment in question.

Digital radiographs are acceptable dento-legally, but care should be taken to ensure that the software system prevents tampering with the images. Similarly, computer held records are acceptable dento-legally, provided the software incorporates suitable safeguards to protect the integrity of the data. Digital data should be backed up to prevent loss in the case of damage or theft of computer equipment.

Clinical records should include the following;

- patient's complaints and symptoms;
- relevant medical, dental, and social histories;
- clinical signs;
- special tests, such as percussion tests, vitality tests, radiographs, and radiographic findings;
- diagnosis and treatment plan;
- local analgesia type and amount given;
- working-length measurement(s);
- instrumentation and preparation;
- type of root-filling material used;
- number of radiographs taken;
- temporary restorations;
- any complications or mishaps.

CONSENT

Dentists must obtain valid consent from their patients prior to treatment. It is very common nowadays for a dissatisfied patient or their advisor to attack a dentist not only in the performance of the endodontic treatment itself, but also in having failed to obtain valid consent.

The need to obtain consent is an ethical/professional duty, as well as a legal duty. The General Dental Council's guidance to dentists *Maintaining Standards* states:

A dentist must explain to the patient the treatment proposed, the risks involved and alternative treatments and ensure that appropriate consent is obtained.

If a general anaesthetic or sedation is to be given, all procedures must be explained to the patient. The onus is on the dentist to ensure that all necessary information and explanations have been given either personally or by the anaesthetist/sedationist. In this situation written consent must be obtained.

The three principles of consent are:
- giving the patient adequate information;
- competency/capacity of the patient (i.e. his/her understanding of the information supplied);
- non-coercion of the patient into giving the consent (i.e. the consent must be given freely).

To satisfy the first principle the dentist must ensure that the patient has adequate information and fully understands the intended treatment:

- the purpose;
- the procedures involved;
- how the procedures will be carried out;
- the feasible options such as osseo-integrated implants, given their long-term success rates, where this is a viable and reasonable choice – equally, if extraction alone, or in combination with some other form of prosthesis, is a reasonable option the patient should be informed, so they can make a balanced judgement;
- the significant risks; and
- the prognosis.

The provision of adequate information in relation to the risks that must be highlighted to a patient has seen a shift in recent years in many jurisdictions throughout the world. The previously held (and still held in certain jurisdictions) 'professional standard' was that the patient should be forewarned of all substantial risks as deemed appropriate by responsible and relevant bodies of professionals. In many countries, including the USA and Australia, this has moved towards a 'patient standard' by which practitioners should forewarn of *all risks* that might influence the patient's choice not to consent to a specific procedure. Accordingly, if one is in doubt as to whether to warn about a potential complication or risk, it would be sensible to err on the side of caution and so inform the patient. Furthermore, the giving of such warnings should be noted in the records.

If the treatment proposed is complex, and arguably all endodontic treatment is complex, or if several treatment options are available, the discussions with the patient should be clearly documented in the records. Indeed the General Dental Council requires a written treatment plan and fee estimate for all expensive and/or extensive treatments. The advice is to issue a patient with the treatment plan in duplicate and ask the patient to sign and return one copy, confirming agreement to the treatment and fees. The signed copy of the plan should be retained in the records but always be aware that the signed plan will only be one piece of documentary evidence that may help to prove that consent was obtained. It should not be used as a substitute for a two-way dialogue with the patient and notes of such discussions in the records.

Note that written consent is required by the General Dental Council for any treatment under any form of sedation or general anaesthesia.

TREATMENT COMPLICATIONS

Fracturing an endodontic instrument during treatment and leaving a portion of the instrument in situ, or creating a perforation may not be negligent. However, with few exceptions, it is negligent not to recognize the complication, to omit to inform the patient, and not to make arrangements for remedial treatment/review. Patients are entitled to a prompt, honest explanation of any mishap or complication. Arrangements should be made to remedy the situation, in so far as is possible, and any referring dentist or other dentist involved in the patient's treatment, should be informed. Patients are entitled to receive, and should be offered referral for, a second opinion or specialist opinion/treatment where appropriate. All actions in relation to a mishap or complication should be recorded in the clinical notes.

PROTECTION OF THE PATIENT

If a dentist should fail to protect the oropharynx from ingestion of foreign bodies such as inhalation or swallowing of an endodontic instrument it is likely that any resultant claim will be indefensible. It is the dentist's duty to protect the patient from such harm/injury. The patient's professional advisors may well plead that the 'action speaks for itself' – 'res ipsa loquitur' and the burden of proof will shift from the patient to the dentist. Accordingly, the dentist will have to prove that he was not negligent and that he used all adequate precautions to prevent the damage. This may prove difficult because all responsible endodontic opinion advocates the use of a dental rubber dam as the only adequate and effective measure to prevent ingestion of endodontic instruments. Therefore, if small instruments are swallowed or inhaled the precautions taken were inadequate and the dentist may be successfully sued with all the attendant stress and publicity that this would entail.

Similarly, it is recommended that all patients undergoing treatment should wear protective spectacles, and that their clothing should be protected from spillages.

REFERRAL FOR TREATMENT

The responsibility for obtaining consent to endodontic treatment rests with all treating dentists. If the patient is being referred to an endodontic specialist some responsibility for the consent process remains with the referring dentist.

The requirements of the dentist depend on the reason for the referral. If the patient is referred for an opinion only, the referring dentist needs to ensure that the patient understands the reasons for the referral. If the patient is referred for treatment, the referring dentist should explore other treatment options with the patient and explain the endodontic treatment prior to referral.

It is the duty of the referring dentist to provide the endodontist with information concerning the history of the tooth, investigations and interventions carried out, as well as general information about the medical, dental and social histories of the patient. Relevant radiographs should be made available to the endodontist.

Likewise, the endodontist should communicate with the referring dentist, if appropriate following initial assessment, and always upon completion of treatment. Details of the root canal filling placed together with a final radiograph, type of temporization, recommendations for final restoration and any follow-up should be sent to the referring dentist.

References

Bolam v Friern Barnet Hospital Management Committee [1957] 1 WLR 582.

General Dental Council 1997 [and subsequent amendments] *Maintaining Standards – Guidance to Dentists on Professional and Personal Conduct.* GDC, London.

CASE STUDIES

Four cases are presented below which illustrate some of the problems that occur during endodontic treatment. All the cases were seen by an endodontist. A brief summary of the case is presented together with comments.

Case 1 (Figure 18.1)

Patient referred to an endodontist by his general dentist for root treatment of the mandibular right first molar. The patient had been informed during treatment that an instrument had separated in the root and they would be referred for specialized treatment.

Comments Unfortunately even with the most careful dentist endodontic instruments sometimes fracture. Provided the dentist was carrying out the canal preparation in line with what is expected by a responsible body of dental opinion (and this will no doubt be looked at if a claim ensues), the fracture of the instrument should be deemed an unfortunate mishap. The dentist was caring and honest, informing the patient of the mishap and with the patient's consent referred the patient for appropriate specialist care. While all dentists sympathize with patients faced with this occurrence no blame should be attached to this dentist.

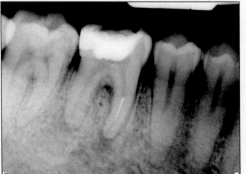

18.1

Case 2 (Figures 18.2 and 18.3)

Patient female, aged 44, attended dentist for emergency treatment with pain in mandibular right side. Dentist informed patient that he had removed an old crown and found and removed some decay and then informed the patient that more treatment would be required. No radiograph was taken during the appointment. The patient was told by the dentist that the tooth could be saved.

Radiograph shows furcation involvement and loss of all coronal hard tissue. The photograph shows a large perforation on the floor of the access cavity. The furcation lesion was probable from both lingual and buccal. When the patient was informed that the tooth required extraction she became upset and asked why the emergency dentist had not explained the hopeless prognosis and extracted the tooth himself.

Comments   Obviously the statement made to the patient by the emergency dentist that the tooth was saveable was inappropriate. Not surprisingly, misinformation does anger many patients particularly when they are faced with the surprise and disappointment of having to lose a tooth. Dentists should be careful to ensure that they have thoroughly assessed a situation before making bold statements. It is important to note, however, that while the dentist's ill-informed opinion could be readily criticized, it was felt that no actual damage had been caused to the patient by this careless comment and only for this reason litigation (alleging negligence) did not proceed.

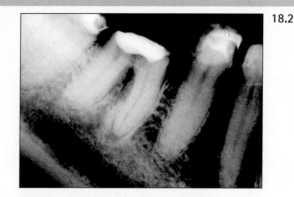

18.2

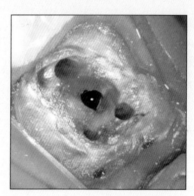

18.3

Case 3 (Figure 18.4)

Patient had the mandibular right first molar root treated. There was no previous root filling in that tooth. At no point was the patient informed of any problem relating to the treatment. Six months after treatment the patient experienced a dull ache in the right mandible. The first molar was slightly tender to percussion.

The radiograph shows that the first molar has been root treated with a metal point or instrument in the mesial root and paste or gutta percha in the distal root. There is extensive bone loss around both roots extending up into the furcation. A separated instrument is visible on the radiograph through the apex of the mesial root.

The second molar has distal caries with an impacted third molar apparently invading the carious cavity. The patient saw his/her dentist one month ago to complain of the discomfort and was referred for treatment of the first molar.

Comments   All dentists have a duty to be open and honest with patients. An endodontist examining this patient must inform the patient of the findings of the X-ray analysis of this region. It is essential that the patient is made aware of all the problems including the condition of the supporting tissues, the retained fractured instrument and the large cavity on the neighbouring tooth.

While such information should also be conveyed to the referring dentists, the endodontist's overriding duty is to the patient.

The dental problems for this patient must have been apparent at the time of the dentist taking his postoperative/endodontic radiograph if not during his efforts at endodontic treatment. It is not in line with any 'responsible dental opinion' to omit to point out to a patient these serious problems. Needless to say such a view might be very forcibly expressed by an independent dental expert when asked to prepare a report for the patient's solicitors!

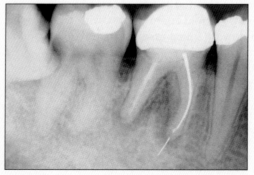

18.4

Case 4 (Figure 18.5)

A 45-year-old male complained of pain from a maxillary anterior tooth related to a bridge which had been fitted four months previously. A radiograph of the mesial abutment tooth showed a post in the left lateral incisor that has perforated the root. The post and bridge had been fitted at the same appointment according to the patient. No root filling is evident in the root canal. The patient stated that the dentist who had fitted the bridge told him that all was well and the treatment was completed.

Comments   Once more, any endodontist seeing this patient has a duty to inform the patient of what is apparent on X-ray analysis, including the post perforation of the root and the lack of any apparent root filling. Feasible treatment options (and costing) would also have to be discussed.

Naturally patients are aggrieved when difficulties and complications are not fully explained to them, particularly if they are misled into believing that 'all is well'.

Root perforations do occur but questions are bound to be raised as to whether this treatment (both the endodontics and the post preparation) would ever be felt to be reasonable care supported by a responsible body of dental opinion. Solicitors pursuing litigation in this matter (and assessing damages) will no doubt highlight the fact that, if this tooth is saveable, the patient will possibly have to endure further endodontic treatment, surgical repair of the perforation and replacement of the post.

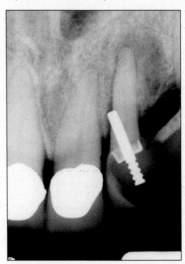

18.5

Index